Preterm Labour
Managing Risk in Clinical Practice

This volume summarises the most recent advances in the optimal clinical management of preterm labour, using the best available evidence. Preterm labour remains a challenge today, even with the latest developments discussed here. The contributors (mostly practising clinicians) are all actively involved in research into the mechanisms, aetiology, treatment and associated outcomes of preterm labour. The chapters are based on common clinical scenarios and each provides a comprehensive literature review followed by evidence-based recommendations on appropriate management. A summary of the pathophysiology of parturition is provided, and the obstetric scenarios cover management of threatened preterm labour, management of preterm premature ruptured membranes and management of preterm labour with specific complications (such as intrauterine growth restriction). Other chapters include the epidemiology, prediction and prevention of preterm labour. Anaesthetic and paediatric issues are explored in depth, and there are chapters on the legal and organisational issues surrounding preterm labour.

JANE NORMAN graduated in medicine from Edinburgh University in 1986. She did the early part of her postgraduate training in Edinburgh, and then moved to Glasgow where she is now Reader in Obstetrics and Gynaecology. For the last ten years, she has conducted research into parturition, at both the clinical and basic science level.

IAN GREER trained in internal medicine and obstetrics and gynaecology in Glasgow and Edinburgh. Prior to taking up his present post as Regius Professor of Obstetrics and Gynaecology, University of Glasgow, he was a clinical scientist at the MRC Reproductive Biology Unit in Edinburgh with a research programme on parturition. He has a continued interest in the mechanism of parturition and its pharmacological regulation.

Preterm Labour

Managing Risk in Clinical Practice

Edited by

Jane Norman
Reader (Honorary Consultant) in Obstetrics and Gynaecology
University of Glasgow

Ian Greer
Regius Professor of Obstetrics and Gynaecology
University of Glasgow

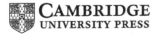

CAMBRIDGE
UNIVERSITY PRESS

CAMBRIDGE
UNIVERSITY PRESS

University Printing House, Cambridge CB2 8BS, United Kingdom

Cambridge University Press is part of the University of Cambridge.

It furthers the University's mission by disseminating knowledge in the pursuit of education, learning and research at the highest international levels of excellence.

www.cambridge.org
Information on this title: www.cambridge.org/9780521821865

First published 2005

A catalogue record for this publication is available from the British Library

ISBN 978-0-521-82186-5 Hardback

Contents

Contributors   vii

Preface   x
J. E. Norman and I. A. Greer

1   The epidemiology of preterm labour and delivery   1
Peter Danielian, Marion Hall

2   Biology of preterm labour   26
Andrew Thomson, Jane Norman

3   Transcriptional regulation of labour-associated genes   76
Tamsin Lindstrom, Jennifer Loudon, Phillip Bennett

4   Fetal outcome following preterm delivery   109
Malcom Levene, Lawrence Miall

5   The prediction of preterm labour   133
Philip Owen , Fiona Mackenzie

6   Prevention of preterm labour   153
John Morrison, Nandini Ravikumar

7   Management of preterm premature ruptured membranes   171
Donald Peebles

8   Management of threatened preterm labour   191
Manu Vatish, Katie Groom, Phillip Bennett, Steven Thornton

9   Management of preterm labour with specific complications   210
Mark Kilby, David Somerset

10   Anaesthetic issues in preterm labour, and intensive care management of the sick parturient   235
Anne May, Chris Elton

11   Management of the preterm neonate   260
      Richa Gupta, Michael Weindling

12   Organisation of high risk obstetric and neonatal services   307
      Karl Murphy and Sara Twaddle

13   The management of pregnancy and labour   329
      Sheila A. M. McLean, Sarah Elliston

14   Treating the preterm infant – the legal context   364
      Sarah Elliston

      Index   397

Contributors

Professor Phillip Bennett
Division of Paediatrics, Obstetrics and
Gynaecology
Institute of Reproductive and
Developmental Biology
Faculty of Medicine, Imperial College
Hammersmith Campus
Du Cane Road
London
W12 ONN

Dr Peter Danielian
Aberdeen Maternity Hospital
Cornhill Road
Aberdeen
AB25 2ZL

Dr Sarah Elliston
School of Law
Stair Building
5–9 The Square
University of Glasgow
G12 8QQ

Dr Chris Elton
Department of Anaesthesia
Leicester Royal Infirmary
Infirmary Square
Leicester
LE1 5WW

Dr Katie Groom
Division of Paediatrics, Obstetrics and
Gynaecology
Institute of Reproductive and
Developmental Biology
Faculty of Medicine, Imperial College
Hammersmith Campus
Du Cane Road
London
W12 ONN

Dr Richa Gupta
SpR in Neonatology
Neonatal Unit, Liverpool Women's Hospital
Crown Street
Liverpool
L8 7SS

Professor Marion Hall
Aberdeen Maternity Hospital
Cornhill Road
Aberdeen
AB25 2ZL

Dr Mark Kilby
Department of Fetal Medicine
Division of Reproduction and Child Health
Birmingham Women's Hospital
University of Birmingham
Edgebaston
Birmingham
B15 2TG

Professor M Levene
Department of Child Health and
Paediatrics
D floor, Clarendon Wing
The General Infirmary at Leeds
Leeds
LS2 9NS

Dr Tamsin Lindstrom
Division of Paediatrics, Obstetrics and
Gynaecology
Institute of Reproductive and
Developmental Biology
Faculty of Medicine, Imperial College
Hammersmith Campus
Du Cane Road
London
W12 ONN

Dr Jennifer Louden
Division of Paediatrics, Obstetrics and
Gynaecology
Institute of Reproductive and
Developmental Biology
Faculty of Medicine, Imperial College
Hammersmith Campus
Du Cane Road
London
W12 ONN

Dr Fiona Mackenzie
Princess Royal Maternity
Level 4
16 Alexandra Parade
Glasgow
G31 2ER

Prof SM McLean
School of Law
Stair Building
5–9 The Square
University of Glasgow
G12 8QQ

Dr Anne May
Ringwood
Forest Drive
Kirby Muxloe
Leicester LE9 2EA

Dr Lawrence Miall
Department of Child Health and Paediatrics
D floor, Clarendon Wing
The General Infirmary at Leeds
Leeds
LS2 9NS

Professor J Morrison
Department of Obstetrics and Gynaecology
National University of Ireland Galwav
Clinical Science Institute
University College Hospital
Newcastle Road
Galway
Ireland

Dr Karl Murphy
Department of Obstetrics and Gynaecology
St Mary's Hospital
Praed Street
London
W2 1NY

Dr Jane Norman
University of Glasgow Division of
Developmental Medicine
Glasgow Royal Infirmary
10 Alexandra Parade
Glasgow
G31 2ER

Dr Philip Owen
Princess Royal Maternity
Level 4
16 Alexandra Parade
Glasgow
G31 2ER

Dr Donald Peebles
Senior Lecturer/Honorary Consultant
Department of Obstetrics and Gynaecology
University College London
86–96 Chenies Mews
London
WC1E 6HX

Dr Nandi Ravikumar
Department of Obstetrics and
Gynaecology
National University of Ireland Galway
Clinical Science Institute
University College Hospital
Newcastle Road
Galway
Ireland

Dr David Somerset
Department of Fetal Medicine
Division of Reproduction and Child Health
Birmingham Women's Hospital
University of Birmingham
Edgebaston
Birmingham
B15 2TG

Dr Andrew Thomson
Deparment of Obstetrics and
Gynaecology
Royal Alexandra Hospital
Corsebar Road
Paisley
PA2 9PN

Professor Steve Thornton
The Sir Quinton Hazell Molecular
Medicine Research Centre
Department of Biological Sciences
University of Warwick
Gibbett Hill Road
Coventry
West Midlands
CV4 74L

Dr Sara Twaddle
9 Queen Street
Edinburgh
EH2 1JQ

Dr Manu Vatish
Lecturer in Obstetrics and Gynaecology
The Sir Quinton Hazell Molecular
Medicine Research Centre
Department of Biological Sciences
University Of Warwick
Gibbett Hill Road
Coventry
West Midlands
CV4 7AL

Professor Michael Weindling
Professor of Perinatal Medicine, University
of Liverpool
Consultant Neonatologist, Neonatal Unit,
Liverpool Women's Hospital
Crown Street
Liverpool
L8 7SS

Preface

J. E. Norman and I. A. Greer

Preterm labour and delivery remains the pre-eminent problem in modern obstetric practice. Around 6% of babies are delivered preterm in the UK and other developed countries. Prematurity has now overtaken congenital anomaly as the single biggest cause of perinatal mortality and morbidity. In view of the sequelae for the child and the mother and the high level of resource to manage this problem and its complications, preterm labour is a major healthcare problem in the developed world. Optimum management of the preterm parturient is informed by research into preterm labour, and significantly improves neonatal outcome. However, the rate of scientific advance in this area is enormous and it is difficult for the practising clinician to keep up to date, and translate this information into practice.

The purpose of this book is to provide an evidence-based approach for the prevention and treatment of preterm labour and its sequelae. We are fortunate to have been able to assemble a list of authors who are internationally acknowledged experts on the mechanisms, aetiology, treatment and associated outcomes of preterm labour. In additional, the majority are actively involved in the management of such problems in clinical practice, so bringing practical expertise to the underlying science. The authors have written an up-to-date clinically relevant text, based on evidence from both basic science and randomised clinical trials. It is not just the disease process and its management that is important. In modern practice the clinician is faced with the organisation of high-risk services, clinical risk management, and many legal and ethical issues surrounding preterm delivery and these issues are also addressed in this book providing a comprehensive text for contemporary practice.

This book is primarily aimed at practising obstetricians. The background science and detailed literature review make this book ideal for those with a special interest in the area. However, the structure of this book is such that information should be accessible to everyone involved in the case of the preterm-parturient from midwife to consultant.

We are indebted to the chapter authors who have each taken time to write a chapter that is both comprehensible and comprehensive, unstintingly sharing their knowledge and expertise. We are also grateful to Dr Alan Mathers for providing the ultrasound picture on the cover. We hope that those who buy this book will enjoy reading it and learning from it, as much as we have.

1

The epidemiology of preterm labour and delivery

Peter Danielian[1] and Marion Hall[2]

[1] Aberdeen Maternity Hospital
[2] Aberdeen Maternity Hospital

Defining the problem

The true incidence of preterm delivery and preterm labour can only be ascertained if a consistent definition is used, and if the data are population based. The reported incidence of preterm delivery is affected by the method of gestational age assessment, and by the differing definitions of viability used and therefore the registration of every preterm delivery. Further problems occur in the measurement of outcome because of the heterogeneity of preterm birth – delivery may occur near to the 37-week upper limit of gestation where there may be no pathological cause and the baby has relatively few if any problems, or it may occur at the extreme of prematurity at around 24 weeks' gestation, where survival rates are poor, and the risk of severe morbidity in those survivors is high. The birth may be spontaneous or elective (iatrogenic); the spontaneous delivery may be uncomplicated (and the outcome usually better (Chng 1981)) or complicated, for example by prelabour rupture of the membranes. The outcomes of such wide variations in aetiology and gestational age will obviously be dissimilar, and so comparisons are difficult and often of little clinical relevance.

Although there is widespread agreement that 'preterm' should refer to a gestational age below 37 completed weeks, there is poor agreement on the definition of the lower limit that defines fetal viability, and on the sub-division of the preterm period into intervals defined by outcome. There is often inaccuracy in the determination of gestational age, especially where there is no facility for routine checking of menstrual dates with early ultrasound scanning. Additionally, the group of women most likely to have inaccurate ascertainment of gestational age are often those women most likely to have the multiple socioeconomic risk factors associated with preterm delivery. These limitations must always be considered when comparisons are made between different countries, and when interpreting epidemiological data on the possible causes and outcomes of preterm delivery.

Preterm Labour Managing Risk in Clinical Practice, eds. Jane Norman and Ian Greer. Published by Cambridge University Press. © Cambridge University Press 2005.

Table 1.1. Conditions prompting elective preterm delivery

Maternal	Severe pre-eclampsia or eclampsia
	Major antepartum haemorrhage
	Chorioamnionitis
	Maternal disease: cardiac
	respiratory
	renal
Fetal	Rhesus (or other) isoimmunisation
	Severe intrauterine growth restriction
	Fetal compromise: anaemia
	hypoxia/acidosis
	cardiac/other organ
	failure
	Cord entanglement (monoamniotic twins)

Definition of preterm delivery

An agreed definition of 'preterm' is essential to enable the epidemiology of preterm delivery to be analysed, and comparisons between different populations to be made. Although the World Health Organization (WHO) has recommended that preterm be defined as a gestational age of less than 37 completed weeks (259 days) from the first day of the last menstrual period (WHO 1993), earlier WHO classifications were by birthweight (USPHS 1980) because this is more easily ascertained in countries where the routine ultrasound dating of pregnancy is not routinely or readily available. However gestational age is much more predictive of outcome than birthweight, especially in the developed world, and therefore the definition should be by gestational age if at all possible. There may also be some value in subdividing the definition of preterm to reflect prognostic significance: in the developed world, delivery at 36 weeks' gestation will usually have a vastly different outcome compared with delivery at 24 weeks. Although terms such as 'very preterm' and 'extremely preterm' have been suggested, at the present time, there is no widespread agreement on these subdivisions of the preterm period.

There is also no agreement on the defined lower limit of gestational age at which a delivery might be considered to be a birth – the WHO has suggested only including babies of birthweight more than 500 g, however this would exclude babies of relatively late gestations with severe in utero growth restriction (IUGR). Many countries have a legal definition of the lowest gestational age at which viability is deemed to be present, and will include all cases delivering above this limit in any statistics produced, but the definition varies greatly depending on the local provision of neonatal intensive care facilities, local definitions of viability and often other cultural factors. Countries with poorly developed neonatal facilities will thus often exclude any babies born below a certain birthweight on the grounds of non-viability, whatever the gestational age. Even within the United Kingdom, where the legal definition of viability is currently 24 weeks' gestational age and above throughout the country, there are local differences in the official data produced. For example Scotland considers all deliveries greater than 20 weeks in its official maternity statistics on the premise that the causes of pregnancy loss between 20 and 24 weeks will often be similar to those resulting in extreme preterm delivery at 24 to 26 weeks' gestation.

Determination of gestational age

Determination of gestational age is also of utmost importance in defining preterm delivery. Usually, unless the pregnancy has resulted from assisted conception, the exact date of conception is not known, and the first day of the last menstrual period is used to estimate gestational age. This assumes that the mother has a 28-day menstrual cycle, that she accurately recalls the date of her last period and that ovulation occurred mid-cycle. It is known that this method is inaccurate because of irregularity of the menstrual cycle, and because in many cases the first day of the last period is not known. This may be due to the taking of hormonal drugs for contraception which may affect the menstrual cycle, amenorrhoea because of breast feeding, or simply that the woman cannot recall the date accurately.

Because there is relatively little biological variation in size in early pregnancy, ultrasound examination at that time is a more accurate method of determining gestational age, and is used routinely in the developed world. The use of ultrasound can, however, lead to apparent higher rates of preterm birth (Yang *et al.* 2002). It has also been found that women with a known date of menstruation but with an early ultrasound scan that suggests that conception took place late in the menstrual cycle are more at risk of preterm delivery (Gardosi and Francis 2000). Whether this is a true risk factor is uncertain. There are, however, many developing countries that do not have the resources to offer this investigation to the majority of their pregnant population. In addition, in the developed world, women of poorer socioeconomic or educational backgrounds are more likely both to have uncertain menstrual dates and to attend so late in the antenatal period that ultrasound examination is no longer an accurate means of determining gestational age. The same group of women is also more likely to have poorer perinatal outcomes, including preterm delivery, and to be subject to many of the risk factors associated with preterm delivery (Hall and Carr-Hill 1985).

It is common practice in epidemiological studies of preterm delivery to describe the gestational age to the nearest completed week of pregnancy. Thus a pregnancy of 24 weeks and 6 days' gestation will usually be described as 24 weeks. This convention, especially if used in conjunction with ultrasound dating, can cause an apparent increase in the incidence of preterm delivery of up to 0.25% (Goldenberg *et al.* 1989).

Incidence and secular trends

The incidence of preterm delivery varies between 5% and 11% (Andrews *et al.* 2000). In the developed world the rate in general has been rising slowly or has been static over the past 10 to 20 years, but has fallen even in some developed countries. In New Zealand the singleton preterm birth rate rose from 4.3% in 1980 to 5.9% in 1999, a rise of 37% (Craig *et al.* 2002). Interestingly, the rate rose by 72% in high socioeconomic groups but only by 3.5% in the most deprived groups. This is due to the effects of delayed childbearing in affluent career-women, and to the increase in assisted reproduction in that group. In Canada the proportion of births to women aged over 35 years has increased from 8.4% in 1990 to 12.6% in 1996, an increase of more than 50%. Among these women the preterm delivery rate has increased by 14%. It is estimated that 36% of this increase is attributable to delayed childbearing, and there was also a 15% increase in twin rates and a 14% increase in triplet rates (Tough *et al.* 2002). This has lead to a reversal of the traditional socioeconomic risk in many western societies; in the USA the relative risk of preterm delivery in low socioeconomic-status and black ethnic groups, although still higher in absolute terms, diminished relative to the more affluent groups between 1981 and 1997 (Kogan *et al.* 2002); in another similar study, the preterm delivery rate in a black ethnic group hardly increased (15.5% to 16.0%) between 1975 and 1995, whereas the white ethnic group rate increased dramatically from 6.9% to 8.4%, a 22% increase (Ananth *et al.* 2001). In Finland, the rate of preterm birth fell from 9% in 1966 to 4.8% in 1986, however the proportion of the preterm deliveries that were spontaneous fell from 97% to 71%, and the iatrogenic cases rose from 3% to 29%. The iatrogenic births were commoner in the lower socio-economic groups in 1966, but this had been reversed by 1986 (Olsen *et al.* 1995). This increase in iatrogenic preterm delivery is due to improvements in neonatal care, and in the detection of IUGR and other fetal problems necessitating early delivery. In a Canadian (twin) study, the rate of preterm delivery had only increased from 42% to 48% over the period 1988–97, but the proportion of preterm induction of labour had risen from 3.5% to 8.6% (Joseph *et al.* 2001).

The other principal contributing factor to the preterm delivery rate is the increase in multiple births associated with the use of assisted reproduction techniques, and to the rise in iatrogenic preterm delivery of these women (Blondel *et al.* 2002). Although there had been a decline in twinning rates since the mid nineteenth century, there has been a rise more recently because of the increased use of assisted reproduction and ovulation induction techniques. The rate of triplet and higher-order births in the UK rose from 10 per 100 000 maternities before 1975 to 35 per 100 000 maternities in 1993, with a similar rise reported in France (Tuppin *et al.* 1993). It has been estimated that 15%–20% of twins and up to 69% of higher-order multiples are due to assisted reproduction.

The twin birth rate in the UK was approximately 1.25% up to 1960, then fell to a low of approximately 0.9% by 1980, then rose steadily to 1.24% in 1993 (Murphy 1995) and in some units is now nearly 2% of all deliveries.

An improvement in assisted reproduction techniques and reduction of the number of embryos replaced has been introduced over the past five years and can reduce the multiple pregnancy rate. Replacing two embryos rather than three has not had the desired effect on twin rates because of improvements in the effectiveness of assisted reproduction techniques (Martikainen *et al.* 2001; Ng *et al.* 2001) but replacing a single embryo (rather than two) can reduce the multiple pregnancy rate associated with in vitro fertilisation (IVF) from 27% to 15% (Dhont 2001), but there is usually a small reduction in the proportion of successful IVF cycles.

Causes of preterm delivery

Iatrogenic

A significant and increasing number of preterm deliveries are iatrogenic, especially in the developed world where they may account for as many as 30% of all preterm births (Olsen *et al.* 1995). Clinicians will elect to undertake preterm delivery if it is felt that continuation of the pregnancy is a greater risk to the life or health of the mother or fetus. Maternal conditions commonly causing such a decision to be considered would include severe pre-eclampsia or eclampsia; major obstetric haemorrhage; chorioamnionitis; and severe or deteriorating maternal cardiac, respiratory or renal disease.

Preterm delivery may also be necessary for any fetal condition that is deteriorating, and for which early delivery would confer benefit, either by removing the fetus from an adverse intrauterine environment (e.g. infection) or by allowing treatment of the condition only possible ex utero. Such complications that may necessitate preterm delivery include rhesus isoimmunisation, severe IUGR, and any other evidence of fetal compromise' e.g. abnormal fetal heart rate.

The contribution of operative delivery to the rate of preterm delivery arises in several ways. When term elective Caesarean section (CS) is decided upon antenatally, it is usually scheduled for 39 weeks (which may be up to three weeks before labour would have started spontaneously). Hence the whole distribution of gestational age at delivery is shifted to the left. This would not in itself increase the rate of preterm delivery, but occasionally elective CS may be inadvertently performed preterm.

Another problem arises when preterm labour seems to have started. It may be difficult to be sure whether labour is established or not. Evidence from trials of tocolytics show that many women recruited as being in active labour, but given placebo treatment, do not in fact deliver preterm. Hence if a woman scheduled for elective CS presents in apparent preterm labour, she may have a CS (and hence a preterm delivery) that might not have occurred if expectant management had been practised. In addition, even if elective CS were not the plan, when a woman presents preterm in possible labour, and has a breech presentation, early CS (for which there is no evidence of benefit in preterm delivery) may again cause delivery to be more preterm than necessary.

Whilst operative delivery may account for only a small proportion of preterm births, it is likely to be a bigger factor in units where there is a low threshold for delivery by CS than in units where the threshold is higher.

Idiopathic

Although in the past up to 50% of cases of preterm delivery were deemed to be idiopathic, this may represent an overestimate and, with improvements in the ability to detect probable causation, some authors have suggested that the term should be abandoned (Geary and Lamont 1993). However in clinical practice it is often impossible to determine a likely cause, and even in comparatively recent studies, idiopathic preterm delivery may account for up to 30% of cases (Hagan *et al.* 1996).

Infection

There is considerable evidence of an association between infection and preterm delivery, and a causative link is plausible and likely in some cases. Infection associated with or causing preterm labour may be lower genital tract, intrauterine or extra-uterine (generalised maternal infection).

Lower genital tract infections
Bacterial vaginosis

Bacterial vaginosis (BV) occurs when the normal vaginal microflora (principally lactobacilli) is replaced by other organisms, especially anaerobic bacteria, *Gardnerella vaginalis* and mycoplasmas. Women with BV detected antenatally are known to be at greater risk of preterm labour, although whether or not BV is a causal factor is more questionable. A systematic review of randomised trials of treatment of BV has concluded that antibiotic therapy is effective at eradicating BV

Table 1.2. Infections associated with preterm delivery

Genital	Bacterial vaginosis (BV)
	Group B streptococcus
	Chlamydia
	Mycoplasmas
Intrauterine	Ascending (from genital tract)
	Transplacental (blood-borne)
	Transfallopian (intraperitoneal)
	Iatrogenic (invasive procedures)
Extra-uterine	Pyelonephritis
	Malaria
	Typhoid fever
	Pneumonia
	Listeria
	Asymptomatic bacteriuria

during pregnancy (odds ratio (OR) 0.22, 95% confidence interval (CI) 0.17–0.27), and at reducing preterm delivery in the subgroup of women with a previous preterm birth (OR 0.37, 95% CI 0.23–0.60). There is also a trend towards reducing preterm delivery overall (McDonald *et al.* 2003). A recent randomised trial has found a significant reduction in preterm delivery and late miscarriage in women with BV who were treated with clindamycin (Ugwumadu *et al.* 2003), but there was no associated benefit in terms of neonatal intensive care admissions, proportions of low birthweight (LBW) or very low birthweight (VLBW) babies or in mean birthweight.

Group B streptococcus

Group B streptococcus (GBS) is a common vaginal pathogen, and many studies have found it to be more common in cases of preterm labour and preterm prelabour rupture of the membranes than in controls (Divers and Lilford 1993). Other studies, however, have not found any increased prevalence of GBS women delivering preterm (Kubota 1998). Whether GBS is a cause of preterm delivery rather than an association remains uncertain.

Chlamydia trachomatis

Genital chlamydial infection is now the commonest sexually transmitted disease in developed countries, especially in younger women, with infection rates in pregnancy of up to 20% in some groups (Goldenberg *et al.* 1996; Macmillan *et al.* 2000) and is associated with up to three times the risk of preterm delivery, even after controlling for confounding variables (Andrews *et al.* 2000a). There is little evidence of direct causation, but treatment has been shown to improve outcome in an observational study (Ryan *et al.* 1990).

Other genital organisms

Genital mycoplasmas (*Mycoplasma hominis, Ureaplasma urealyticum* and *Fusobacterium*) have been associated with preterm delivery (Divers and Lilford 1993; Hillier *et al.* 1995; Odendaal *et al.* 2002, but a causative role has not been established.

Other genital organisms that have been associated with an increased risk of preterm delivery include *Escherichia coli, Klebsiella, Haemophilus, Neisseia gonorrhoeae* and *Trichomonas vaginalis* (McDonald *et al.* 1991; Ekwo *et al.* 1993) but again the causative role is undetermined and some studies have either shown no effect of treatment on preterm delivery rate (Klebanoff *et al.* 2001; Gulmezoglu 2002) or have not even shown an association (McDonald *et al.* 1992).

Viral infections

Although there is little evidence that viruses are a common cause or association of preterm delivery, they may be implicated in some cases. One possible mechanism is that viral infection of the trophoblast could play a role in placental dysfunction, leading to complications including spontaneous miscarriage, pre-eclampsia, fetal growth restriction and preterm birth (Arechavaleta-Velasco *et al.* 2002), or preterm labour may occur secondary to host inflammatory responses to the viral infection (Salafia *et al.* 1991).

Intrauterine infection

Preterm delivery can result from intrauterine infection. Intrauterine infection may occur because of ascending infection from the vagina, blood-borne transmission via the placenta, transfallopian infection from the peritoneal cavity or by iatrogenic introduction following invasive procedures such as amniocentesis, chorion villus biopsy or fetal blood-sampling. The commonest cause of intrauterine infection is ascending infection from the lower genital tract. Ascending infection may follow rupture of the membranes, but can also occur with intact membranes. Pathogens ascend from the vagina through the cervix and cause infection of the decidua, the chorion, fetal blood vessels and can infect and cross the amnion to the amniotic fluid and the fetus. The fetus may inhale the infected amniotic fluid leading to pneumonia, or may become septicaemic from haematological infection secondary to decidual and villous infection.

There is a very strong association between intrauterine infection and preterm delivery. Up to 13% of women in preterm labour with intact membranes have positive amniotic fluid cultures, and these women are more likely to develop clinical chorioamnionitis, rupture the membranes and to go on to preterm delivery, than women with negative cultures. Similar results are found in women with preterm premature rupture of the membranes (pPROM) with 35% having positive amniotic fluid cultures. Positive cultures are more common in those women with pPROM who are in labour (75%) than those not in labour (Romero *et al.* 1988a). One study has also found that over 50% of women with suspected cervical incompetence (see p. 10) have positive amniotic fluid cultures (Romero *et al.* 1992). There is a greater concentration of bacterial endotoxin in women in preterm labour than in those not in preterm labour (Romero *et al.* 1988b).

There is also strong evidence that intrauterine infection causes preterm labour and delivery. There is a plausible mechanism in that bacterial products are known to include proteases and collagenases, which could weaken the membranes, and phospholipase A_2 and endotoxins known to be able to stimulate prostaglandin production in vitro and in vivo. Prostaglandins are known to be involved in the initiation of human labour and are of course widely used for the pharmacological induction of labour. In addition, the host inflammatory response to infection causes the release of inflammatory cytokines which are involved in cervical ripening and possibly membrane rupture.

Extra-uterine infection

Generalised maternal infections such as pyelonephritis (Lang *et al.* 1996), and malaria (Luxemburger *et al.* 2001) remain relatively common antecedents of preterm delivery, and timely antimicrobial treatment usually reduces the risk. Infections such as typhoid fever and maternal pneumonia although historically associated with preterm delivery are usually sensitive to antibiotics and are now less important in most regions.

Listeria monocytogenes

Listeriosis is an uncommon infection that can cause intrauterine and fetal infection and subsequent preterm delivery. Contaminated food is the usual source of infection and transmission appears to be blood-borne following gastrointestinal infection (Lennon *et al.* 1984; Romero *et al.* 1988c).

Asymptomatic bacteriuria

Asymptomatic urinary tract infection is common in pregnancy and is associated with preterm delivery. Two meta-analyses have shown that antimicrobial treatment reduces the risk of preterm delivery (Villar *et al.* 1998; Smaill 2001) and therefore causation appears likely. The exact mechanism is unknown, but there is evidence that there can be colonisation of the vagina with the same pathogen as found in the urine, and the bacteriuria may therefore be a surrogate marker for abnormal vaginal flora that could be the cause of preterm delivery (Thomsen *et al.* 1987).

Risk factors for preterm labour

There are many associated risk factors for spontaneous preterm delivery and often they are highly dependent on each other. This is particularly true for the socio-demographic variables, and therefore multivariate analysis is essential to account for possible confounding. In addition, there may be treatment paradox where an effective intervention reduces the incidence of preterm delivery and thus makes subsequent statistical proof of the effect more difficult to demonstrate. Although randomised controlled trials would be the most effective means of determining whether risk factors are causal or not, there are relatively few of these.

Maternal risk factors
Cervical incompetence

Cervical incompetence is a clinical diagnosis made when there appears to be dilation of the cervix in the absence of uterine contractions. The exact incidence of cervical incompetence is difficult to determine. It is possible that incompetence leads to preterm labour and delivery by allowing ascending infection or by causing rupture of the membranes and prostaglandin release, or that the delivery occurs simply because the fetus is too heavy to be retained in utero by the incompetent cervix. In a few cases incompetence of the cervix will be caused by previous surgery or by congenital abnormality of the genital tract. It is also possible that supposed cervical incompetence occurs as a result of vaginal and cervical infection causing ripening of the cervix as discussed above. In a randomised controlled trial of cervical cerclage in women thought to be at risk of preterm delivery, only 1 in 25 women benefited from the procedure (Macnaughton *et al.* 1993), which suggests that few patients have true incompetence.

Maternal reproductive risk factors
Previous preterm delivery

A previous preterm delivery is the most significant risk factor for subsequent preterm delivery and the relative risk increases with the number of prior preterm births, from 2.2 for one prior preterm birth to 4.9 for three or more (Hoffman and Bakketieg 1981). A study of only spontaneous onset preterm births from Aberdeen, Scotland found similar results, with a preterm delivery being three times more likely after a previous preterm delivery (Carr-Hill and Hall 1985).

Table 1.3. Risk factors for preterm delivery

Idiopathic	
Iatrogenic (elective)	severe maternal and/or fetal compromise
Infection	genital, intrauterine, extra-uterine/ systemic
Multiple pregnancy	assisted reproduction
Maternal factors	cervical incompetence
	psychiatric disease/stress
	other maternal disease, e.g. SLE,
Reproductive history	previous preterm delivery
	previous pPROM
	previous miscarriage/abortion
	short interpregnancy interval
	primiparity
	poor antenatal weight gain/low maternal weight
Sociodemographic	low or high maternal age
	lack of social support
	low socioeconomic status
	substance abuse
	environmental pollution/toxicity
	heavy physical work

The earlier the first preterm birth, the earlier the subsequent preterm birth: if the first is before 28 weeks, the relative risk of the subsequent birth also being before 28 weeks is 20.5, with an absolute risk of 8.2% (Hoffman and Bakketieg 1984). However most preterm births still occur in women without a prior event.

Previous preterm premature rupture of membranes

The risk of preterm delivery in women with previous pPROM has been estimated to range from 34% to more than 44%, and the risk of recurrent preterm rupture of the membranes to range from 16% to 32% (Naeye 1982; Lee *et al.* 2003).

Previous abortion

Although the Aberdeen study found that there was no increase in risk of preterm birth following spontaneous miscarriage or therapeutic termination of pregnancy (Carr-Hill and Hall 1985), and this finding has been more recently supported (Lao and Ho 1998), other studies have found that there is an increased risk, even after controlling for confounding variables, and that the risk increases with the number of prior miscarriages or induced abortions, from 1.3 after one previous abortion to 1.9 after 2 or more (Basso *et al.* 1998; Zhou *et al.* 1999; Henriet and Kaminski 2001).

Interpregnancy interval

Several studies have found an inverse relationship between the interval between pregnancies and the risk of preterm delivery. The risk of preterm delivery before 32 weeks is 30%–90% increased in women whose interpregnancy interval was less than 6 months compared with women with intervals of more than 12 months (Khoshnood *et al.* 1998; Klerman *et al.* 1998; Smith *et al.* 2003).

Parity

Preterm delivery is commoner in first pregnancies (Tough *et al.* 2001) and the risk decreases with successive pregnancies. Although early studies had found an increased risk of preterm delivery with higher parity, this was subsequently found to be an artefact, with in fact a lower risk with each successive pregnancy up to a parity of four (Hall 1985). Although there are few studies investigating the effects of parity greater than four, the earlier findings were confirmed in a recent study in Abu Dhabi which found no increase in preterm delivery rate (in fact there was a significant decrease) in a large study of women with a parity of ten and higher compared with those of parity less than five (Kumari and Badrinath 2002).

Multiple pregnancy

Multiple pregnancy is an important cause of preterm birth. Although multiple pregnancy accounts for only 1%–2% of births, it accounts for up to 12% of all preterm births (Gardner *et al.* 1995; Wright *et al.* 1998). Approximately 50% of twins will deliver preterm with modern obstetric practice in the developed world (Kogan *et al.* 2000), and for triplets and higher-order multiples, the likelihood of preterm delivery is often greater than 90% (Joseph *et al.* 2002). The mean gestational age at delivery is approximately 36 weeks for twin pregnancies and 33 weeks for triplet and higher-order pregnancies (Macfarlane *et al.* 1990; Levene *et al.* 1992).

Assisted reproduction

Ovulation induction and other forms of assisted conception such as IVF and other methods where ovulation induction drugs are utilised have been introduced in the industrialised nations over the past 20 to 30 years. Clomiphene was introduced in 1966 in the UK, and the number of prescriptions more than doubled between 1980 and 1993 to more than 60 000 per annum (Murphy 1995). The number of prescriptions for other ovulation induction agents has also increased. There has been a coincident increase in the prevalence of twin and higher-order multiple births over a similar time period, either because the ovulation induction drugs increase the likelihood of multiple ovulation, or multiple embryos are put into the uterus to increase the chances of a successful pregnancy. These assisted reproduction techniques have had a profound effect on preterm delivery rates mainly because of the increased associated risk of multiple pregnancy; however, the risk remains greater even when compared with naturally conceived multiple pregnancies (Pandian et al. 2001). In the USA, multiple births occur after 39% of IVF cycles, and in Europe, the figure is 26% (Katz et al. 2002). A review of all higher multiple pregnancies (triplets and higher) in 1989 in the UK showed that 69% of cases resulted from some form of assisted conception (ovarian stimulation in 34%, IVF in 24% and gamete intra fallopian transfer (GIFT) in 11%) whilst 31% of cases were spontaneous conceptions (Botting et al. 1987). It has been estimated that 15%–20% of twins are due to assisted conception techniques (Murphy 1995); use of clomiphene can lead to multiple pregnancy rates of up to 7.9% and use of gonadotrophins to rates of 25%–30% (Navot et al. 1991). There is some evidence that assisted conception leads to an increased incidence of monozygotic twins relative to dizygotic, with rates of 13% of twin pregnancies following ovulation induction, and 22% of triplets containing monozygotic twins (Derom et al. 1987). Monochorionic twins have been found to occur eight times more often following assisted reproduction than after natural conception (Wenstrom et al. 1993). Monochorionic twins are more likely to deliver preterm than dichorionic twins, with consequent implications for perinatal mortality and morbidity, and for long-term outcome.

In a recent Canadian study it was estimated that IVF accounted for 21% of all twins, and all triplet pregnancies; IVF accounted for 66% of the increase in preterm delivery below 30 weeks' gestation (Tough et al. 2000).

The prevalence of multiple pregnancy, especially that of higher-order multiples, has increased markedly over the past 10 to 20 years, largely because of the effects of assisted conception techniques. The twinning rate has been increased by between 4% and 10%, and the triplet rate by over 300% by such treatment. Approximately 70% of triplet pregnancies are likely to be a result of assisted reproduction. In addition, assisted conception leads to a relative increase in monochorionicity, with further impact on preterm delivery rates.

Sociodemographic risk factors
Maternal age

Both extremes of maternal age have been associated with an increased risk of preterm birth. Teenagers have an increased risk of preterm birth even when other socioeconomic variables are taken into account (Gortzak-Uzan et al. 2001;

Kogan *et al.* 2002). A large study in Sweden has found that the risk (compared with controls aged 20–24) is greatest (odds ratio 4.8) for maternal age 13–15 years delivering at fewer than 33 weeks' gestation (Olausson *et al.* 2001). The risk at age 16–17 years is still double that of the controls. The risks for moderately preterm delivery are also increased in the younger age groups, but to a lesser extent. Similar results have been found in multiparous teenagers in the USA with odds ratios of 4.22 at 10–14 years of age, 2.19 at 15–17 years of age and 1.69 at 18–19 years (Akinbami *et al.* 2000).

Women aged over 35 to 40 years of age have been found to have twice the rate of preterm delivery compared with controls aged between 20 and 30 years (16% vs. 8%) (Seoud *et al.* 2002); an increase in risk still remains even when only nulliparous women were considered (Ezra *et al.* 1995), and when other potential confounders were taken into account (Martius *et al.* 1998). The higher rate of elective Caesarean section as the method of delivery in older women may also be a contributing factor.

Marital status

Single mothers are known to be at increased risk of preterm delivery, but often it is difficult to separate this from other linked social factors. A recent European study has found that the impact of marital status on the risk of preterm birth varies in relation to marital practices in the population, defined by the proportion of out-of-marriage births. They found a significantly elevated risk of preterm birth associated with both cohabitation and single motherhood (OR 1.61) for women living in countries where fewer than 20% of births occur outside marriage. In contrast, there was no excess risk in countries where out-of-marriage births are more common (Zeitlin *et al.* 2002). It seems likely therefore that in most societies, marital status is a poor indicator of preterm delivery risk; lack of social support for the mother is probably a more relevant measure of social deprivation and thus a better indicator of risk.

Race

Preterm delivery is much more common in black and hispanic populations in the USA and in ethnic minority groups in most developed countries, but again it is often difficult to exclude the confounding effects of associated poor socio-economic status and often lack of access to health care. In a study of black and white US army personnel with identical healthcare access, although only small differences in preterm delivery were found, there was still an excess in the black population, especially for very preterm delivery (Adams *et al.* 1993). A recent UK study (controlling for other confounding factors) found similar results, with an increased risk of preterm delivery in Afro-Caribbeans with the greatest difference for delivery below 28 weeks; this difference remained significant even when social deprivation was accounted for. Although there was an excess of preterm delivery in Africans, this became non-significant once social deprivation was controlled for. There was no increased risk in Asian women, and Asians were the only group in which social deprivation was not associated with an increase in preterm delivery (Aveyard *et al.* 2002). It seems therefore that although social deprivation accounts for a significant proportion of the excess risk of preterm delivery in ethnic minority groups, other factors may be involved; it is possible that there could be a difference in the length of gestation in different racial groups, thereby giving an apparent change in the preterm delivery rate.

Socioeconomic status

As socioeconomic status increases the rate of preterm delivery decreases, but it is always difficult to control for the often multiple and closely-associated factors. Women in poor socioeconomic groups are more likely to be younger, unmarried, to drink and smoke more, abuse illegal drugs and utilise antenatal care less than more affluent groups (Johnson *et al.* 2002). However, low socioeconomic status has been found to be an independent risk factor. In an intergenerational study in the USA, although the preterm birth rate was higher for African-Americans compared with white women, the rate improved in both ethnic groups over three generations as socioeconomic status improved (Foster *et al.* 2000). Preterm labour is also more common in women who have suffered physical violence during the year prior to delivery (Cokkinides *et al.* 1999).

Psychiatric disease and stress

Although there is a plausible mechanism for stress initiating preterm labour via raised corticotrophin-releasing hormone (CRH) levels, a definitive link has yet to be established. Conflicting results have been obtained (Whitehead *et al.* 2002). Differences in CRH levels have been found to be associated with preterm labour in preliminary studies (Ruiz *et al.* 2002). Anxiety (but not depression) has been found to be related to preterm labour, but the association was weaker in those women who had no pregnancy-related morbidity to worry about (Dole *et al.* 2003). Women with high levels of stress are likely to smoke more and to drink more alcohol than non-stressed controls.

Preterm delivery is linked with a wide range of psychiatric disorders (Kelly *et al.* 2002), and a large Swedish study found that schizophrenia carried a 2.4-fold risk of preterm delivery, even when all known factors were controlled for, including smoking (Nilsson *et al.* 2002). There is no evidence that increasing social support during the pregnancy reduces the risk of preterm delivery (Hodnett 2003).

Maternal work

A meta-analysis of 29 studies has found that heavy physical work (OR 1.22), prolonged standing (OR up to 2.72) and shift and night work (OR 1.24) are all associated with preterm birth. (Teitelman *et al.* 1990; Mozurkewich *et al.* 2000). Although employed women may be healthier than the unemployed and have less socioeconomic deprivation, the effects of standing and heavy physical work appear to be significant risk factors for preterm delivery.

Nutrition and maternal weight

Low maternal weight, low maternal body mass index (BMI) and poor nutrition have all been associated with preterm birth. Improved analysis of these factors taking into account confounding variables has more recently found no independent effect of nutrition, and nutritional intervention in pregnancy has not been found to have any effect on preterm delivery rates. There is conflicting evidence on maternal weight and BMI, but there does seem to be an association between low maternal weight or poor weight gain during pregnancy and preterm delivery (Kramer *et al.* 1992; Siega-Riz *et al.* 1996; Carmichael *et al.* 1997; Cohen *et al.* 2001).

Substance abuse
Alcohol

Alcohol intake in the third trimester has been found to be associated with a *reduced* risk of preterm delivery (Wright *et al.* 1998) but this effect may be reversed in heavier drinkers. The relative risk was lower (0.69–0.89) in women who drank up to nine drinks per week, but the relative risk for those who were still drinking ten or more drinks per week at 30 weeks' gestation was 3.56 (Kesmodel *et al.* 2000).

Tobacco

Many studies have found an association between cigarette-smoking and preterm birth, and there appears to be a dose-related effect: the more cigarettes smoked the higher the risk. Women who smoke more than 10 cigarettes per day have a 1.7 times risk of delivery before 32 weeks (Peacock *et al.* 1995; Kyrklund-Blomberg and Cnattingius 1998). A more recent study has shown a stronger relation between smoking and preterm birth resulting from prelabour rupture of the membranes (Savitz *et al.* 2001). Antismoking interventions do not have a significant effect on the rate of preterm delivery.

Other drugs

Opiate drug dependency is associated with an increase in preterm delivery, but the mechanism is unclear. There are often several associated social factors, including multiple drug abuse such as cigarettes and alcohol. Mothers who take cocaine have up to a 37% absolute risk of preterm delivery (Calhoun and Watson 1991); this may be due to an increase in circulating catecholamines and also to the increased risk of antepartum haemorrhage. Caffeine intake has also been dose-related to preterm rupture of the membranes (Williams *et al.* 1992) and preterm delivery (Eskenazi *et al.* 1999), but more recent studies suggest that caffeine intake has no effect on preterm delivery rate, although it may be associated with IUGR (Fortier *et al.* 1993; Peacock *et al.* 1995; Santos *et al.* 1998).

Environmental pollution

Preterm delivery is more common in areas of high industrial air pollution even when other demographic variables are taken into account (Lin *et al.* 2001). Other environmental toxins are also implicated: agricultural nitrate contamination (Bukowski *et al.* 2001) and maternal serum dichlorodiphenyltrichloroethane (DDT) metabolite levels (Longnecker *et al.* 2001) both have a dose-related effect on preterm delivery risk; arsenic contamination of drinking water (Ahmad *et al.* 2001) has also been implicated.

Other maternal factors

Preterm delivery may also be caused by, or be associated with, other factors' e.g. chronic disease such as antiphospholipid syndrome or systemic lupus erythematosus (SLE) (Rai and Regan 1997; Yasmeen *et al.* 2001), or by physical abnormalities of the uterus, either congenital (Cooney *et al.* 1998) or secondary to tumours such as fibroids.

Fetal sex

There is a small but significant effect of fetal sex on the rate of preterm delivery, with an excess of male infants (Hall and Carr-Hill 1982; Astolfi and Zonta 1999). National figures for Sweden have shown that males account for 55%–60% of births between 23 and 32 weeks' gestation.

Antenatal care

Lack of access to good-quality antenatal care is associated with IUGR and preterm delivery, but whether this is a causal relationship is uncertain. A recent US review of over 14 million pregnancies found that for both black and white ethnic groups, absence of antenatal care was associated with a 2.8 relative risk for preterm delivery. Although there could be many other associated risk factors, there was an inverse dose-response relationship between the number of perinatal visits and gestational age at delivery suggesting possible causation (Vintzileos *et al.* 2002).

The strength of these sociodemographic associations of preterm delivery is small compared with the effect of previous obstetric history, and with the medical and obstetric complications of the index pregnancy, which lead to iatrogenic or spontaneous preterm delivery. Some studies have found that sociodemographic factors do not have any substantial impact on the rates of preterm delivery, with low maternal age the only factor that retained a significant association after accounting for other factors (Wildschut *et al.*1997)

Summary

Preterm delivery is the most important single cause of perinatal mortality and morbidity, and represents a considerable cost both in terms of direct perinatal health care and the resulting long-term health, educational and care requirements necessary for the survivors of very preterm delivery. There are also important, but largely unascertained financial and emotional costs to the families of such children. The magnitude of the problems presented by preterm delivery is difficult to quantify because of the diversity of methods used to determine gestation and the differing definitions of fetal viability, but it is certain that worldwide it represents an enormous clinical, financial and human burden.

The causation of preterm delivery is multifactorial and comprises a complex interaction of previous obstetric history, sociodemographic risk factors and obstetric complications in the index pregnancy.

Although the main risk factor for preterm delivery is a previous preterm delivery, there is no evidence that this knowledge can be successfully used to prevent a further preterm delivery in the next pregnancy in the majority of cases. The second most important cause of preterm delivery is intrauterine infection. There is some evidence that treating certain infections such as bacterial vaginosis and asymptomatic bacteriuria may prevent preterm delivery, but only in a relatively small subset of cases.

The many risk factors associated with low socioeconomic status are not readily amenable to correction in many societies, and even when equal access to health services has been achieved, significant differences still remain between ethnic and other groups, often for generations, and often despite improvement in financial and social circumstances.

In the past 20 to 30 years, there has been an increase in preterm delivery rates in most but not all developed countries, largely as a result of iatrogenic delivery. The stimulus for this increase has primarily been the great improvement in neonatal care in the developed world that has enabled increasingly premature babies to survive. Added to this has been the impact of assisted reproduction techniques which has led to an increase in preterm delivery rates, not only because of the increase in multiple pregnancy rates, but also because of the increase in preterm delivery in singleton pregnancies conceived in this manner. Because these technologies are often restricted to the relatively affluent in many countries, the expected inverse relationship between socioeconomic status and preterm delivery rates has been reversed in recent years.

REFERENCES

Adams, M. M., Read, J. A., Rawlings, J. S. *et al.* (1993) Preterm delivery among black and white enlisted women in the United States Army. *Obstet. Gynecol.* **81**, 65–71.

Ahmad, S. A., Sayed, M. H., Barua, S. *et al.* (2001) Arsenic in drinking water and pregnancy outcomes. *Environ. Health Perspect.* **109**, 629–31.

Akinbami, L. J., Schoendorf, K. C. and Kiely, J. L. (2000) Risk of preterm birth in multiparous teenagers. *Arch. Pediatr. Adolesc. Med.* **154**, 1101–7.

Ananth, C. V., Misra, D. P., Demissie, K. and Smulian, J. C. (2001) Rates of preterm delivery among Black women and White women in the United States over two decades: an age-period-cohort analysis. *Am. J. Epidemiol.* **154**, 657–65.

Andrews, W. W., Goldenberg, R. L., Mercer, B. *et al.* (2000a) The Preterm Prediction Study: association of second-trimester genitourinary chlamydia infection with subsequent spontaneous preterm birth. *Am. J. Obstet. Gynecol.* **183**, 662–8.

Andrews, W. W., Hauth, J. C. and Goldenberg, R. L. (2000b) Infection and preterm birth *Am. J. Perinatol.* **17**: 357–65.

Arechavaleta-Velasco, F., Koi, H., Strauss, J. F. III and Parry, S. (2002) Viral infection of the trophoblast: time to take a serious look at its role in abnormal implantation and placentation? *J. Reprod. Immunol.* **55**, 113–21.

Astolfi, P. and Zonta, L. A. (1999) Risks of preterm delivery and association with maternal age, birth order and fetal gender. *Hum. Reprod.* **14**, 2891–4.

Aveyard, P., Cheng, K. K., Manaseki, S. and Gardosi, J. (2002) The risk of preterm delivery in women from different ethnic groups. *BJOG* **109**, 894–9.

Basso, O., Olsen, J. and Christensen, K. (1998) Risk of preterm delivery, low birthweight and growth retardation following spontaneous abortion: a registry-based study in Denmark *Int. J. Epidemiol.* **27**, 642–6.

Blondel, B., Kogan, M. D., Alexander, G. R. *et al.* (2002) The impact of the increasing number of multiple births on the rates of preterm birth and low birthweight: an international study. *Am. J. Public Health* **92**, 1323–30.

Botting, B. J., Davies, I. M. and Macfarlane, A. J. (1987) Recent trends in the incidence of multiple births and associated mortality. *Arch. Dis. Child.* **62**, 941–50.

Bukowski, J., Somers, G. and Bryanton, J. (2001) Agricultural contamination of groundwater as a possible risk factor for growth restriction or prematurity. *J. Occup. Environ. Med.* **43**, 377–83.

Calhoun, B. C. and Watson, P. T. (1991) The cost of maternal cocaine abuse: I. Perinatal cost. *Obstet. Gynecol.* **78**, 731–4.

Carmichael, S. Abrams, B. and Selvin, S. (1997) The association of pattern of maternal weight gain with length of gestation and risk of spontaneous preterm delivery. *Pediat. Perinatal Epidemiol.* **11**, 392–406.

Carr-Hill, R. A. and Hall, M. H. (1985) The repetition of spontaneous preterm labour. *BJOG* **92**, 921–8.

Chng, P. K. (1981) An analysis of preterm singleton deliveries and associated perinatal deaths in a total population. *BJOG* **88**, 814–18.

Cohen, G. R., Curet, L. B., Levine, R. J. *et al.* (2001) Ethnicity, nutrition, and birth outcomes in nulliparous women. *Am. J. Obstet. Gynecol.* **185**, 660–7.

Cokkinides, V. E., Coker, A. L., Sanderson, M., Addy, C. and Bethea, L. (1999) Physical violence during pregnancy: maternal complications and birth outcomes. *Obstet. Gynecol.* **93**, 661–6.

Cooney, M. J., Benson, C. B. and Doubilet, P. M. (1998) Outcome of pregnancies in women with uterine duplication anomalies. *J. Clin. Ultrasound* **26**, 3–6.

Craig, E. D., Thompson, J. M. and Mitchell, E. A. (2002) Socioeconomic status and preterm birth: New Zealand trends, 1980 to 1999. *Arch. Dis. Child. Fetal Neonatal Ed.* **86**, F142–6.

Derom, C., Vlietinck, R., Derom, R., Van den Berghe, H. and Thiery, M. (1987) Increased monozygotic twinning rates after ovulation induction. *Lancet* **i**, 1236–8.

Dhont, M. (2001). Single-embryo transfer. *Semin. Reprod. Med.* **19**, 251–8.

Divers, M. J. and Lilford, R. J. (1993) Infection and preterm labor: a meta-analysis. *Contemp. Rev. Obstet. Gynaecol.* **5**, 71–4.

Dole, N., Savitz, D. A., Hertz-Picciotto, I., Siega-Riz, A. M., McMahon, M. J., and Buekens, P. (2003) Maternal stress and preterm birth. *Am. J. Epidemiol.* **157**, 14–24.

Ekwo, E. E., Gosselink, C. A., Woolson, R. and Moawad, A. (1993) Risks for premature rupture of amniotic membranes. *Intl. J. Epidemiol.* **22**, 495–503.

Eskenazi, B., Stapleton, A. L., Kharrazi, M. and Chee, W. Y. (1999) Associations between maternal decaffeinated and caffeinated coffee consumption and fetal growth and gestational duration. *Epidemiol.* **10**, 242–9.

Ezra, Y., McParland, P. and Farine, D. (1995) High delivery intervention rates in nulliparous women over age 35. *Eur. J. Obstet. Gynecol. Reprod. Biol.* **62**, 203–7.

Fortier, I., Marcoux, S. and Beaulac-Baillargeon, L. (1993) Relation of caffeine intake during pregnancy to intrauterine growth retardation and preterm birth. *Am. J. Epidemiol.* **137**, 931–40.

Foster, H. W., Wu, L., Bracken, M. B. *et al.* (2000) Intergenerational effects of high socio-economic status on low birthweight and preterm birth in African Americans. *J. Natl Med. Assoc.* **92**, 213–21.

Gardner, M. O., Goldenberg, R. L., Cliver, S. P. *et al.* (1995) The origin and outcome of preterm twin pregnancies. *Obstet. Gynecol.* **85**, 553–7.

Gardosi, J. and Francis, A. (2000) Early pregnancy predictors of preterm birth: the role of a prolonged menstruation–conception interval. *BJOG* **107**, 228–37.

Geary, M. and Lamont, R. (1993) Prediction of preterm birth. In M. G. Elder, R. F. Lamont and R. Romero, eds., *Preterm Labor*. New York NY: Churchill Livingstone, pp. 51–63.

Goldenberg, R. L., Davis, R. O., Cutter, G. R. *et al.* (1989) Prematurity, postdates, and growth retardation: the influence of use of ultrasonography on reported gestational age. *Am. J. Obstet. Gynecol.* **160**, 462–70.

Goldenberg, R. L., Klebanoff, M. A., Nugent, R. *et al.* (1996) Bacterial colonization of the vagina during pregnancy in four ethnic groups. Vaginal Infections and Prematurity Study Group. *Am. J. Obstet. Gynecol.* **174**, 1618–21.

Gortzak-Uzan, L., Hallak, M., Press, F., Katz, M. and Shoham-Vardi, I. (2001) Teenage pregnancy: risk factors for adverse perinatal outcome. *J. Matern. Fetal Med.* **10**, 393–7.

Gulmezoglu, A. M. (2002) Interventions for trichomoniasis in pregnancy. *Cochrane Database Syst. Rev.* **3**, CD000220.

Hagan, R., Benninger, H., Chiffings, D., Evans, S. and French, N. (1996) Very preterm birth – a regional study. Part 1: Maternal and obstetric factors. *BJOG* **103**, 230–8.

Hall, M. H. (1985) Incidence and distribution of preterm labour. In R. W. Beard and F. Sharp eds., *Preterm Labour and Its Consequences*. London: RCOG, pp. 5–13.

Hall, M. and Carr-Hill, R (1982) Impact of sex-ratio on onset and management of labour. *BMJ* **285**, 401–3.

Hall, M. H. and Carr-Hill, R. A. (1985) The significance of uncertain gestation for obstetric outcome. *BJOG.* **92**, 452–60.

Henriet, L. and Kaminski, M. (2001) Impact of induced abortions on subsequent pregnancy outcome: the 1995 French national perinatal survey. *BJOG* **108**, 1036–42.

Hillier, S. L., Nugent, R. P., Eschenbach, D. A. *et al.* (1995) Association between bacterial vaginosis and preterm delivery of a low-birth-weight infant. The Vaginal Infections and Prematurity Study Group *N. Engl. J. Med.* **333**, 1737–42.

Hodnett ED (2003) Support during pregnancy for women at increased risk of low birthweight babies. (Cochrane Review). Cochrane Database Syst. Rev. **2**, CD000198

Hoffman, H. J. and Bakketeig, L. S. (1981) Epidemiology of preterm birth: results from a longitudinal study of births in Norway. In M. G. Elder and C. H. Hendricks, eds., *Preterm Labour*. London: Butterworths, pp. 93–115.

Hoffman, H. J. and Bakketeig, L. S. (1984) Risk factors associated with the occurrence of preterm birth. *Clin. Obstet. Gynecol.* **27**, 539–52.

Johnson, D., Jin, Y. and Truman, C. (2002) Influence of aboriginal and socioeconomic status on birth outcome and maternal morbidity. *J. Obstet. Gynaecol. Can.* **24**, 633–40.

Joseph, K. S., Allen, A. C., Dodds, L., Vincer, M. J. and Armson, B. A. (2001) Causes and consequences of recent increases in preterm birth among twins. *Obstet. Gynecol.* **98**, 57–64.

Joseph, K. S., Marcoux, S., Ohlsson, A. *et al.* (2002) Preterm birth, stillbirth and infant mortality among triplet births in Canada, 1985–96. *Paediatr. Perinatal Epidemiol.* **16**, 141–8.

Katz, P., Nachtigall, R. and Showstack, J. (2002) The economic impact of the assisted reproductive technologies. *Nat. Cell. Biol.* **4**, S29–32.

Kelly, R. H., Russo, J., Holt, V. L. *et al.* (2002) Psychiatric and substance use disorders as risk factors for low birth weight and preterm delivery. *Obstet. Gynecol.* **100**, 297–304.

Kesmodel, U., Olsen, S. F. and Secher, N. J. (2000) Does alcohol increase the risk of preterm delivery? *Epidemiology.* **11**, 512–18.

Khoshnood, B., Lee, K. S., Wall, S., Hsieh, H. L. and Mittendorf, R. (1998) Short interpregnancy intervals and the risk of adverse birth outcomes among five racial/ethnic groups in the United States. *Am. J. Epidemiol.* **148**, 798–805.

Klebanoff, M. A., Carey, J. C., Hauth, J. C. *et al.*; National Institute of Child Health and Human Development Network of Maternal-Fetal Medicine Units. (2001) Failure of metronidazole to prevent preterm delivery among pregnant women with asymptomatic *Trichomonas vaginalis* infection. *N. Engl. J. Med.* **345**, 487–93.

Klerman, L. V., Cliver, S. P. and Goldenberg, R. L. (1998) The impact of short interpregnancy intervals on pregnancy outcomes in a low-income population. *Am. J. Public Health* **88**, 1182–5.

Kogan, M. D., Alexander, G. R., Kotelchuck, M. *et al.* (2000) Trends in twin birth outcomes and prenatal care utilization in the United States, 1981–1997. *JAMA* **284**, 335–41.

Kogan, M. D., Alexander, G. R., Kotelchuck, M., MacDorman, M. F., Buekens, P. and Papiernik, E. (2002) A comparison of risk factors for twin preterm birth in the United States between 1981–82 and 1996–97. *Matern. Child Health J.* **6**, 29–35.

Kramer, M. S., McLean, F. H., Eason, E. L. and Usher, R. H. (1992) Maternal nutrition and spontaneous preterm birth. *Am. J. Epidemiol.* **136**, 574–83.

Kubota, T. (1998) Relationship between maternal group B streptococcal colonization and pregnancy outcome. *Obstet. Gynecol.* **92**, 926–30.

Kumari, A. S. and Badrinath, P. (2002) Extreme grandmultiparity: is it an obstetric risk factor? *Eur. J. Obstet. Gynecol. Reprod. Biol.* **101**, 22–5.

Kyrklund-Blomberg, N. B. and Cnattingius, S. (1998) Preterm birth and maternal smoking: risks related to gestational age and onset of delivery. *Am. J. Obstet. Gynecol.* **179**, 1051–5.

Lang, J. M., Lieberman, E. and Cohen, A. (1996) A comparison of risk factors for preterm labor and term small-for-gestational-age birth. *Epidemiology* **7**, 369–76.

Lao, T. T. and Ho, L. F. (1998) Induced abortion is not a cause of subsequent preterm delivery in teenage pregnancies. *Hum. Reprod.* **13**, 758–61.

Lee, T., Carpenter, M. W., Heber, W. W. and Silver H. M. (2003) Preterm premature rupture of the membranes: risks of recurrent complications in the next pregnancy among a population-based sample of gravid women. *Am. J. Obstet. Gynecol.* **188**, 209–213.

Lennon, D., Lewis, B., Mantell, C. *et al.* (1984) Epidemic perinatal listeriosis. *Pediatr. Infect. Dis.* **3**, 30–4.

Levene, M. I., Wild, J. and Steer, P. J. (1992) Higher multiple births and the modern management of infertility in Britain. *BJOG* **99**, 607–13.

Lin, M. C., Chiu, H. F., Yu, H. S. *et al.* (2001) Increased risk of preterm delivery in areas with air pollution from a petroleum refinery plant in Taiwan. *J. Toxicol. Environ. Health A.* **64**, 637–44.

Longnecker, M. P., Klebanoff, M. A., Zhou, H. and Brock, J. W. (2001) Association between maternal serum concentration of the DDT metabolite DDE and preterm and small-for-gestational-age babies at birth. *Lancet* **358**, 110–4.

Luxemburger, C., McGready, R., Kham, A. *et al.* (2001) Effects of malaria during pregnancy on infant mortality in an area of low malaria transmission. *Am. J. Epidemiol.* **154**, 459–65.

McDonald, H. M., O'Loughlin, J. A., Jolley, P., Vigneswaran, R. and McDonald, P. J. (1991) Vaginal infection and preterm labour. *BJOG* **98**, 427–35.

(1992) Prenatal microbiological risk factors associated with preterm birth. *BJOG.* **99**, 190–6.

McDonald, H., Brocklehurst, P., Parsons, J. and Vigneswaran, R. (2003) Antibiotics for treating bacterial vaginosis in pregnancy. *Cochrane Database Syst. Rev.* **2**, CD000262.

Macmillan, S., McKenzie, H., Flett, G. and Templeton, A. (2000) Which women should be tested for *Chlamydia trachomatis*? *BJOG* **107**, 1088–93.

Macnaughton, M. C., Chalmers, I. G., Dubowitz, V. *et al.* (1993) Final report of the Medical Research Council/Royal College of Obstetricians and Gynaecologists Multicentre Randomised Trial of Cervical Cerclage *BJOG.* **100**, 516–23.

Martikainen, H., Tiitinen, A., Tomas, C. *et al.* Finnish ET study group. (2001) One versus two embryo transfer after IVF and ICSI: a randomized study. *Hum. Reprod.* **16**, 1900–3.

Martius, J. A., Steck, T., Oehler, M. K. and Wulf K. H. (1998) Risk factors associated with preterm (<37+0 weeks) and early preterm birth (<32+0 weeks): univariate and multivariate analysis of 106 345 singleton births from the 1994 statewide perinatal survey of Bavaria. *Eur. J. Obstet. Gynecol. Reprod. Biol.* **80**, 183–9.

Mozurkewich, E. L., Luke, B., Avni, M. and Wolf, F. M. (2000) Working conditions and adverse pregnancy outcome: a meta-analysis. *Obstet. Gynecol.* **95**, 623–35.

Murphy, M. F. G. (1995) The association of twinning with long-term disease. In R. H. Ward and M. Whittle, eds., *Multiple pregnancy* London: RCOG, pp. 14–29.

Navot, D., Goldstein, N., Mor-Josef, S., Simon, A., Relou, A. and Birkenfeld, A. (1991) Multiple pregnancies: risk factors on prognostic variables during induction of ovulation with human menopausal gonadotrophin. *Hum. Reprod.* **6**: 1152–5.

Naeye, R. L. (1982) Factors that predispose to premature rupture of the fetal membranes. *Obstet. Gynecol.* **60**, 93–98.

Ng, E. H., Lau, E. Y., Yeung, W. S. and Ho, P. C. (2001) Transfer of two embryos instead of three will not compromise pregnancy rate but will reduce multiple pregnancy rate in an assisted reproduction unit. *J. Obstet. Gynaecol. Res.* **27**: 329–35.

Nilsson, E., Lichtenstein, P., Cnattingius, S., Murray, R. M. and Hultman, C. M. (2002) Women with schizophrenia: pregnancy outcome and infant death among their offspring. *Schizophr. Res.* **58**, 221–9.

Odendaal, H. J., Popov, I., Schoeman, J. and Grove, D. (2002) Preterm labour: is *Mycoplasma hominis* involved? *S. Afr. Med. J.* **92**, 235–7.

Olausson, P. O., Cnattingius, S. and Haglund, B. (2001) Does the increased risk of preterm delivery in teenagers persist in pregnancies after the teenage period? *BJOG* **108**, 721–5.

Olsen, P., Laara, E., Rantakallio, P. *et al.* (1995) Epidemiology of preterm delivery in two birth cohorts with an interval of 20 years. *Am. J. Epidemiol.* **142**, 1184–93.

Pandian, Z., Bhattacharya, S. and Templeton, A. (2001) Review of unexplained infertility and obstetric outcome: a 10 year review. *Hum. Reprod.* **12**, 2593–7.

Peacock, J. L., Bland, J. M. and Anderson, H. R. (1995) Preterm delivery: effects of socioeconomic factors, psychological stress, smoking, alcohol, and caffeine. *BMJ* **311**, 531–5.

Rai, R. and Regan, L. (1997) Obstetric complications of antiphospholipid antibodies. *Curr. Opin. Obstet. Gynecol.* **9**, 387–90.

Romero, R., Quintero, R., Oyarzun, E. *et al.* (1988a) Intraamniotic infection and the onset of labor in preterm premature rupture of the membranes. *Am. J. Obstet. Gynecol.* **159**, 661–6.

Romero, R., Roslansky, P., Oyarzun, E. *et al.* (1988b) Labor and infection. II. Bacterial endo-toxin in amniotic fluid and its relationship to the onset of preterm labor. *Am. J. Obstet. Gynecol.* **158**, 1044–9.

Romero, R., Winn, H.N., Wan, M. and Hobbins, J.C. (1988c) *Listeria monocytogenes chorioamnionitis* and preterm labor. *Am. J. Perinatol.* **5**, 286–8.

Romero, R., Gonzalez, R., Sepulveda, W. *et al.* (1992) Infection and labor. VIII. Microbial invasion of the amniotic cavity in patients with suspected cervical incompetence: prevalence and clinical significance. *Am. J. Obstet. Gynecol.* **167**, 1086–91.

Ruiz, R.J., Fullerton, J., Brown, C.E. and Dudley, D.J. (2002) Predicting risk of preterm birth: the roles of stress, clinical risk factors and corticotropin-releasing hormone. *Biol. Res. Nurs.* **4**, 54–64.

Ryan, G.M.Jr., Abdella, T.N., McNeeley, S.G., Baselski, V.S. and Drummond, D.E. (1990) *Chlamydia trachomatis* infection in pregnancy and effect of treatment on outcome. *Am. J. Obstet. Gynecol.* **162**, 34–9.

Salafia, C.M., Vogel, C.A., Vintzileos, A.M. *et al.* (1991) Placental pathologic findings in preterm birth. *Am. J. Obstet. Gynecol.* **165**, 934–8.

Santos, I.S., Victora, C.G., Huttly, S. and Carvalhal, J.B. (1998) Caffeine intake and low birth weight: a population-based case-control study. *Am. J. Epidemiol.* **147**, 620–7.

Savitz, D.A., Dole, N., Terry, J.W.Jr, Zhou, H. and Thorp, J.M.Jr. (2001) Smoking and pregnancy outcome among African-American and white women in central North Carolina. *Epidemiology* **12**, 636–42.

Seoud, M.A., Nassar, A.H., Usta, I.M. *et al.* (2002) Impact of advanced maternal age on pregnancy outcome. *Am. J. Perinatol.* **19**, 1–8.

Siega-Riz, A.M., Adair, L.S. and Hobel, C.J. (1996) Maternal underweight status and inadequate rate of weight gain during the third trimester of pregnancy increases the risk of preterm delivery. *J. Nutrit.* **126**, 146–53.

Smaill, F. (2001) Antibiotics for asymptomatic bacteriuria in pregnancy. *Cochrane Database Syst Rev* **2**, CD000490.

Smith, G.C.S., Pell, J.P. and Dobbie, R. (2003) Interpregnancy interval and risk of preterm birth and neonatal death: retrospective cohort study. *BMJ* **327**, 313–19.

Teitelman, A.M., Welch, L.S., Hellenbrand, K.G. and Bracken, M.B. (1990) Effect of maternal work activity on preterm birth and low birth weight. *Am. J. Epidemiol.* **131**, 104–13.

Thomsen, A.C., Morup, L. and Hansen, K.B. (1987) Antibiotic elimination of group-B streptococci in urine in prevention of preterm labour. *Lancet* **i**, 591–3.

Tough, S.C., Greene, C.A., Svenson, L.W. and Belik, J. (2000) Effects of in vitro fertilization on low birth weight, preterm delivery, and multiple birth. *J. Pediatr.* **136**, 618–22.

Tough, S.C., Svenson, L.W., Johnston, D.W. and Schopflocher, D. (2001) Characteristics of preterm delivery and low birthweight among 113 994 infants in Alberta: 1994–1996. *Can. J. Public Health* **92**, 276–80.

Tough, S.C., Newburn-Cook, C., Johnston, D.W. *et al.* (2002) Delayed childbearing and its impact on population rate changes in lower birth weight, multiple birth, and preterm delivery. *Pediatrics* **109**, 399–403.

Tuppin, P., Blondell, B. and Kaminski, M. (1993) Trends in multiple deliveries and infertility treatments in France. *BJOG* **100**, 383–5.

Ugwumadu, A., Manyonda, I., Reid. F. and Hay, P. (2003) Effect of early oral clindamycin on late miscarriage and preterm delivery in asymptomatic women with abnormal vaginal flora and bacterial vaginosis: a randomised controlled trial. *Lancet* **361**, 983–8.

US public Health Services (USPHS). (1980) *Internaltional Classification of Disedses*. Ninth Revision: Clinicial Modification, 2nd edn. Washington DC: US Department of Health and Human Resources Publication PH801260.

Villar, J., Gulmezoglu, A. M. and de Onis, M. (1998) Nutritional and antimicrobial interventions to prevent preterm birth: an overview of randomized controlled trials. *Obstet. Gynecol. Surv.* **53**, 575–85.

Vintzileos, A. M., Ananth, C. V., Smulian, J. C., Scorza, W. E. and Knuppel, R. A. (2002) The impact of prenatal care in the United States on preterm births in the presence and absence of antenatal high-risk conditions. *Am. J. Obstet. Gynecol.* **187**, 1254–7.

Wenstrom, K. D., Syrop, C. H., Hammett, E. G. and Van Voorhis, B. J. (1993) Increased risk of monochorionic twinning associated with assisted reproduction. *Fertil. Steril.* **60**, 510–514.

Whitehead, N., Hill, H. A., Brogan, D. J. and Blackmore-Prince, C. (2002) Exploration of threshold analysis in the relation between stressful life events and preterm delivery. *Am. J. Epidemiol.* **155**, 117–24.

World Health Organization (WHO). (1993) *International Statistical Classification of Diseases and Related Health Problems*. 10th revision, vol. II. Geneva, Switzerland: WHO.

Wildschut, H. I., Nas, T. and Golding, J. (1997) Are sociodemographic factors predictive of preterm birth? A reappraisal of the 1958 British Perinatal Mortality Survey. *BJOG* **104**, 57–63.

Williams, M. A., Mittendorf, R., Stubblefield, P. G. *et al.* (1992) Cigarettes, coffee, and preterm premature rupture of the membranes. *Am. J. Epidemiol.* **135**, 895–903.

Wright, S. P., Mitchell, E. A., Thompson, J. M. *et al.* (1998) Risk factors for preterm birth: a New Zealand study. *N. Z. Med. J.* **111**, 14–16.

Yang, H., Kramer, M. S., Platt, R. W., *et al.* (2002) How does early ultrasound scan estimation of gestational age lead to higher rates of preterm birth? *Am. J. Obstet. Gynecol.* **186**, 433–7.

Yasmeen, S., Wilkins, E. E., Field, N. T., Sheikh, R. A. and Gilbert, W. M. (2001) Pregnancy outcomes in women with systemic lupus erythematosus. *J. Matern. Fetal. Med.* **10**, 91–6.

Zeitlin, J. A., Saurel-Cubizolles, M. J. and Ancel, P. Y. (2002) EUROPOP Group. Marital status, cohabitation, and risk of preterm birth in Europe: where births outside marriage are common and uncommon. *Pediat. Perinatal Epidemiol*, **16**, 124–30.

Zhou, W., Sorensen, H. T. and Olsen, J. (1999) Induced abortion and subsequent pregnancy duration. *Obstet. Gynecol.* **4**, 948–53.

Biology of preterm labour

Andrew Thomson[1] and Jane Norman[2]

[1] Royal Alexandra Hospital, Paisley
[2] Glasgow Royal Infirmary

Introduction

The prevention of preterm labour remains one of the primary goals of obstetric research. To achieve this effectively, we need to understand the mechanisms regulating uterine contractility, cervical ripening and activation of the fetal membranes. Whether preterm labour represents an acceleration of the mechanisms involved in term labour remains controversial. Romero *et al.* (1997) propose that the fundamental difference between term and preterm labour is that the former results from physiological activation of the components of a common terminal pathway, while preterm labour results from disease processes activating one or more of the components of this pathway. In contrast, Challis *et al.* (2000) suggest that the causes of preterm labour may vary at different times during pregnancy and will not necessarily reflect acceleration of the processes occurring during labour at term. At present, the factors maintaining myometrial quiescence during pregnancy, and those that stimulate the onset of uterine contractions and cervical ripening at term remain obscure. Until these factors are elucidated, it seems unlikely that effective strategies for the treatment of preterm labour will be found (Goldenberg and Rouse 1998).

Myometrial contractions

The uterus is spontaneously active and, using electromyographic measurements, contractile activity can be detected in both pregnant and non-pregnant women (Morrison 1996). Two different types of electromyographic activity have been described in the myometrium of the pregnant rhesus monkey, referred to as contractures and contractions, and are believed to be present in most species (Nathanielsz *et al.* 1992). Contractures represent low-amplitude, long-acting uterine activity, which commences early in pregnancy; in women these were first observed by Braxton Hicks in 1873. Contractions are high-amplitude and of short

Preterm Labour Managing Risk in Clinical Practice, eds. Jane Norman and Ian Greer. Published by Cambridge University Press. © Cambridge University Press 2005.

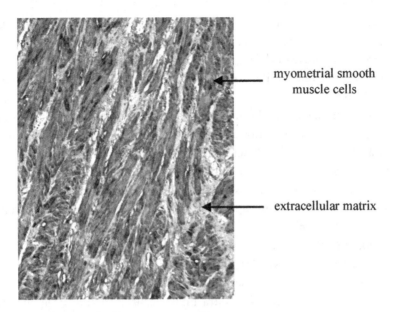

myometrial smooth
muscle cells

extracellular matrix

Figure 2.1   Photomicrograph of human myometrium.

duration, and are characterised by nocturnal or labour uterine activity (Nathanielsz *et al.* 1992). The level of activity in the uterus throughout pregnancy is regarded as relatively low, compared with that measured both during labour and the immediate puerperium, when strong contractions occur to expel the fetus and placenta, and then maintain haemostasis.

Organisation of myometrial smooth muscle

The myometrium is composed of interlacing bundles of long, spindle-shaped smooth muscle fibres arranged in ill-defined layers (Figure 2.1). The myometrial smooth muscle cells are surrounded by extracellular material composed of collagen fibres, fibroblasts and bone-marrow-derived cells (Garfield and Yallampalli 1994). During pregnancy, the myometrium grows dramatically owing to hypertrophy and an increase in the number of smooth muscle cells by division (Carsten 1968). The myometrial cells communicate with one another through intercellular channels called gap junctions, which were first observed in myometrial cells in rats just prior to and during parturition (Garfield *et al.* 1977). Gap junctions consist of channels that connect the interiors of two cells. The channels are composed of proteins, termed connexins, which span the plasma membranes to form a pore. They provide a low-resistance pathway between individual myometrial smooth muscle cells and allow the passage of inorganic ions and small molecules (Cole *et al.* 1988). Within the pregnant myometrium, two connexin proteins, connexin-43 (Cx-43) and Cx-26, are particularly abundant, but exhibit temporally distinct patterns of expression. The expression of Cx-43 is low throughout most of pregnancy, but increases dramatically immediately before the onset of labour (Lye *et al.* 1993). In contrast, the expression of Cx-26 is highest during late pregnancy, but falls to low levels during labour (Orsino *et al.* 1996). Although Cx-43 is generally thought to mediate the increased electrical coupling within the myometrium during labour, the contribution of Cx-26 to the regulation of myometrial contractility remains to be determined. The number of gap junctions increases in the myometrium at the time of labour in most if not all species. They are under hormonal control, with progesterone inhibiting, and oestradiol stimulating their formation. In addition prostaglandins regulate gap junction formation and function (Garfield 1994).

Unlike striated muscle, the actin and myosin filaments of myometrial smooth muscle are not organised into fibres and fibrils, but instead occur in random bundles throughout the myocyte (Somlyo 1980; Garfield 1984). However, like skeletal muscle, myometrial contractions occur from a sliding of actin and myosin filaments, without any change in the length of either filament (Huxley 1971). A rise in intracellular calcium (Ca^{2+}) promotes the binding of calcium to calmodulin. Calcium-calmodulin activates myosin light chain kinase (MLCK) which itself phosphorylates myosin. The phosphorylated myosin filaments bind to actin, and contraction occurs with the hydrolysis of adenosine triphospate (ATP).

Electrical activity

The myometrial smooth muscle cells are spontaneously active, such that isolated strips of pregnant or non-pregnant uterus will produce regular spontaneous contractions. These spontaneous contractions are preceded by action potentials. Myometrial cells have a negative resting membrane potential of approximately $-50\,mV$ (Inoue *et al.* 1990). Changes in the myometrial membrane potential, occurring from ion flow across the membrane, are fundamental to the control of uterine activity (Wray 1993). When the magnitude of this potential is reduced beyond a certain threshold, an action potential may be stimulated. The basis of this myogenic mechanism is the spontaneous depolarisation of pacemaker cells within the myometrium. Unlike cardiac muscle, the pacemaker cells in the myometrium are not anatomically fixed or defined and it is unclear why some cells or groups of cells should become pacemakers.

Calcium and uterine contractions

An increase in intracellular calcium is essential for uterine contractility. In the resting state, intracellular calcium is maintained at a concentration of about 10^{-7} M which increases to 10^{-6} M during contraction (Thornton and Gillespie 1992). The extracellular calcium concentration is 10^{-3} M. Intracellular calcium can be increased by several mechanisms, and different agents are thought to operate via different routes. Voltage-dependent and receptor-operated calcium channels are two important mechanisms (Hurwitz 1986). When the membrane is depolarised to an appropriate level, voltage-dependent calcium channels convert to an activated or open state, thus allowing a substantial calcium influx into the cell down its concentration gradient. In contrast, receptor-operated calcium channels are opened in response to activating ligands, such as hormones or neurotransmitters, which bind to specific receptors associated with the channel.

Calcium may be released into the cytoplasm from stores within the cell. The sarcoplasmic reticulum represents the major intracellular store for calcium and in the myometrium it is well developed, though less well so than in skeletal and cardiac muscles (Garfield and Somlyo 1985; Somlyo *et al.* 1985). Calcium release from the sarcoplasmic reticulum store can occur through inositol 1,4,5-trisphosphate-gated channels (Carsten and Miller 1985) or ryanodine-gated channels. Ryanodine channels are physiologically activated by calcium itself, resulting in calcium-induced calcium release. The contribution of sarcoplasmic reticulum calcium in smooth muscle contraction has been questioned following data obtained in non-pregnant rat myometrium (Taggart and Wray 1998). These data demonstrated no effect of sarcoplasmic reticulum inhibition on either spontaneous force or calcium transients. Indeed, further studies in pregnant human myometrium indicated that the sarcoplasmic reticulum may act to limit contractions and act as a calcium sink rather than to amplify contractions (Kupittayanant *et al.* 2002).

Relaxation occurs with the dephosphorylation of myosin light chains by a phosphatase. Further, cell repolarisation results in a lowering of intracellular calcium by extrusion across the sarcolemma and uptake into the internal stores, thus inactivating the calcium-calmodulin MLCK complex.

In summary, contraction of the myometrium at term or preterm, depends upon conformational changes in the actin and myosin molecules that allow actin and myosin filaments to slide over each other, ultimately leading to a shortening of the myocyte. An increase in intracellular calcium is crucial to this process. Agents that stimulate myometrial activity generally increase intracellular levels via an influx of calcium through receptor-activated channels, or perhaps also through the release of calcium from intracellular stores, including the sarcoplasmic reticulum. Agents that inhibit uterine activity do so by increasing intracellular levels of cyclic nucleotides cAMP or cGMP, which in turn inhibit release of calcium from intracellular stores or reduce MLCK activity.

Control of myometrial function

Neuronal modulation

It has been recognised for more than a century that the uterus receives an extensive autonomic innervation (Krantz 1959), yet the contribution of neuronal modulation of uterine activity has been less well characterised than the hormonal factors involved. Myometrial smooth muscle cells possess all four main types of adrenergic receptors (α_1, α_2, β_1 and β_2) (Bottari et al. 1985). It has been postulated that α_1-receptors mediate contraction and β_2-receptors are predominantly responsible for relaxation (Bulbring and Tomito 1987). Activation of the α_2-receptors seem to have no effect on contractile activity (Hoffman et al. 1981). Both β_1- and β_2-receptors are coupled to adenylate cyclase via an intermediate G-protein (G_s). Activation of adenylate cyclase results in an increase in cAMP that activates cAMP-dependent kinase. This in turn leads to a reduction in phosphorylation of myosin light chains and hence relaxation (Price and Bernal 2001). Other mechanisms whereby cAMP may result in relaxation include calcium sequestration and efflux of calcium through the cell membrane (Diamond 1990; Thornton and Gillespie 1992). The α-adrenoceptor is coupled to adenylate cyclase by an inhibitory G-protein (G_i). This G_i may directly reduce adenylate cyclase activity or may prevent stimulation of the enzyme by G_s.

Cholinergic stimulation (acetylcholine acting on muscarinic M_1 and M_3 receptors) causes uterine contractions by increasing inositol 1,4,5-trisphosphate and hence elevating intracellular calcium (Marc et al. 1986). Other neurotransmitters that are known to be present within the uterus include vasoactive intestinal polypeptide (Alm et al. 1977; Huang et al. 1984), neuropeptide Y (Owman et al. 1986), substance P (Alm et al. 1978), calcitonin gene-related peptide (Gibbins et al. 1985; Samuelson et al. 1985), galanin and gastrin-releasing peptide (Stjernquist et al. 1986).

However, it is well established that contractions and expulsion of the fetus can proceed in the absence of neuronal activity (Reynolds 1965) suggesting that the role of these nerves in the contractile activity of the uterus is of minor importance (Wray 1993).

Hormonal modulation

Oestrogen and progesterone

Changes in hormonal conditions have profound effects on uterine activity; the steroid hormones oestrogen and progesterone have long been known to influence myometrial contractility (Bozler 1941; Fuchs 1978). Human pregnancy is characterised by a state of markedly increased oestrogen levels, predominantly 17β-oestradiol and oestriol. Although oestrogens are known to stimulate prostaglandin production in the decidua, promote the formation of gap junctions and

Table 2.1. Control of myometrial function

		Stimulatory	Inhibitory
Neuronal	Adrenaline/ noradrenaline	α_1-receptors	β_1- and β_2-receptors
	Acetylcholine	✔	
	Vasoactive intestinal polypeptide		✔
	Neuropeptide Y		Inhibits neurally induced contraction
	Substance P	✔	
	Calcitonin gene-related peptide		✔
	Galanin	✔	
	Gastrin-releasing peptide	✔	
Hormonal	Oestrogen	✔	
	Progesterone		✔
	Oxytocin	✔	
	Prostaglandins	PGE_2 & $PGF_{2\alpha}$ ✔	
	Endothelins	✔	
	Nitric oxide		✔
	Inflammatory mediators (e.g. interleukins)	✔	
Metabolic modulation	Myometrial blood flow		Decreased blood flow
	Hypoxia		✔
	pH		Acidosis ✔
	Stretch	✔	

increase the synthesis of oxytocin receptors, their role in the initiation of parturition in the human remains uncertain (Batra 1994).

Progesterone is essential in the maintenance of pregnancy (Csapo 1956), and has traditionally been perceived as having a 'relaxing' effect on human myometrium. The proposed mechanisms for this have included diminished myometrial cell membrane permeability for calcium, increased adenosine monophosphate synthesis and an inhibition of decidual prostaglandin formation (Egarter and Husslein 1992). Progesterone and synthetic progestational agents have been employed as tocolytic agents in the management of suspected preterm labour (Fuchs and Stakeman 1960; Keirse 1990). A recent double-blind, placebo-controlled trial has found that weekly injections of 17 α-hydroxyprogesterone caproate resulted in a substantial reduction in the rate of recurrent preterm delivery among women who were at particularly high risk for preterm delivery and reduced the likelihood of several complications in their infants (Meis *et al.* 2003). Furthermore, treatment with an antiprogesterone, such as mifepristone, increases both uterine activity and myometrial sensitivity to prostaglandins (Swahn and Bygdeman 1988).

In human parturition, progesterone withdrawal and oestrogen activation are not mediated by changes in progesterone and oestrogen levels. Instead, Mesiano *et al.* (2002) have shown that these events could be mediated by changes in the responsiveness of the myometrium to progesterones and oestrogens via changes in progesterone and oestrogen receptor expression. In term human myometrium, responsiveness to progesterone is controlled by the expression of progesterone receptor type A relative to progesterone receptor type B. A significant increase in the type A to type B progesterone receptor ratio underlies functional progesterone withdrawal. Functional oestrogen activation occurs by increased expression of oestrogen receptor type α and is linked to functional progesterone withdrawal.

Oxytocin

Oxytocin is a powerful stimulator of uterine activity and can enhance the force, the frequency and the duration of uterine contractions. Oxytocin is a 9 amino acid peptide, which is synthesised within the supraoptic and paraventricular nuclei of the hypothalamus as a large precursor molecule (Dawood and Khan-Dawood 1985). This molecule is subsequently broken down to the active hormone and its neurophysin, which are transported along neurones to the posterior pituitary gland. In 1909, Blair-Bell demonstrated the uterotonic action of posterior pituitary extracts at a Caesarean section. Since then, the pituitary extracts, and later purified oxytocin, have been used to arrest postpartum haemorrhage and to induce or augment labour. Whilst oxytocin has classically been described as being released from the posterior lobe of the pituitary gland, it is also expressed in amnion, chorion and decidua (Chibbar *et al.* 1993).

Oxytocin stimulates uterine contraction by a variety of mechanisms that may include a small contribution from calcium released by inositol 1,4,5-trisphosphate from the sarcoplasmic reticulum, but which is predominantly on activation of receptor-operated calcium channels. Calcium-independent oxytocin contraction has also been described (Matsuo *et al.* 1989) and is probably due to a protein phosphorylating either a contractile or cytosolic protein (Oishi *et al.* 1991). Although the involvement of oxytocin in the initiation of human parturition remains controversial (see Zeeman *et al.* 1997 for review), three lines of evidence provide support for a role for oxytocin and its receptor in the regulation of human labour. Firstly, concentrations of circulating oxytocin hormone and decidual and myometrial oxytocin receptors increase before parturition. Secondly, infusions of oxytocin stimulate myometrial contractions that are indistinguishable from normal labour (Mitchell and Schmid 2001). Thirdly, antagonists to oxytocin can inhibit both myometrial contractions in vitro (Kinsler *et al.* 1996; Nilsson *et al.* 2003) and uterine contractions in preterm labour (Worldwide Atosiban versus Beta-Agonists Study Group 2001).

There is a marked gestational difference in the pharmacological ability of oxytocin to cause uterine contractions, oxytocin being most effective in the third trimester. This is due to the presence of a higher concentration of oxytocin receptors at this time and is the basis of human uterine sensitivity to oxytocin throughout pregnancy (Theobald *et al.* 1969; Fuchs *et al.* 1984). Fetal oxytocin and local uterine and decidual sources of oxytocin can act on the myometrium in an endocrine and paracrine manner to initiate and maintain effective uterine contractions (Chard *et al.* 1971).

Prostaglandins

It is well established that an increase in prostaglandin synthesis, particularly PGE_2 and $PGF_{2\alpha}$, occurs in uterine and fetal tissues during labour (Slater *et al.* 1998, 1999; Erkinheimo *et al.* 2000). Prostaglandins are formed from arachadonic acid by the enzyme cyclo-oxygenase (COX), of which there are three isoforms. Cyclo-oxygenase-1 is a constitutive and ubiquitous isoform, whilst COX-2 is an inducible isoform (Slater *et al.* 1998; Wallace 1999). Both of these isoforms are expressed in human fetal membranes and myometrium. Studies have suggested that COX-2 expression increases in myometrium during labour, along with prostaglandin production, while COX-1 expression is not altered (Slater *et al.* 1999; Erkinheimo *et al.* 2000). Sadovsky *et al.* (2000), found that PGE_2 synthesis increases in myometrium during term and preterm labour, and that this is inhibited by selective COX-2 inhibitors, but not significantly altered by a selective COX-1 inhibitor. This suggests the prominent role of COX-2 in forming PGE_2 in the myometrium during labour. Cyclo-oxygenase-2 expression is greater in amnion and chorio-decidua during labour, and prostaglandins produced in fetal membranes act on myometrium as paracrine agents (Slater *et al.* 1994, 1998; Sawdy *et al.* 2000). Recent evidence suggests that the labour-associated increase in fetal membrane COX-2 mRNA concentration is due to the accumulation of stable mRNA, rather than increased activity (Johnson *et al.* 2002). The effects of COX-2 in fetal membranes are likely to be balanced by those of prostaglandin dehydrogenase, which metabolises prostaglandins and which is itself stimulated by endogenously produced corticotrophin-releasing hormone in fetal membranes

(McKeown and Challis 2003). At present, it is unclear whether COX-3 is involved in the synthesis of prostaglandins during term or preterm labour (for review, see Mitchell and Olson 2004).

Cytokines are thought to play an important role in the regulation of prosta-glandin biosynthesis in gestational tissues (Hansen *et al.* 1999). The production of prostaglandin biosynthesis from amnion, chorion, decidua and myometrium is increased by the inflammatory cytokines interleukin(IL)-1 and tumour necrosis factor-α (TNFα)(Bowen *et al.* 2002). This effect is likely to occur through increased expression of COX-2 (Rauk and Chiao 2000). Prostaglandin concentrations can be increased through inhibition of metabolic inactivation. The enzyme that catabolises prostaglandins to inactive metabolites, 15-hydroxyprostaglandin dehy-drogenase (PGDH), is abundant in chorion, placental trophoblast and, to a lesser extent, decidua (Germain *et al.* 1994). Its activity may prevent prostaglandins in the amniotic fluid from acting upon the myometrium. Activity and PGDH protein in chorionic trophoblast of the lower uterine segment decrease with term labour, possibly contributing to the activation of the myometrium (Van Meir *et al.* 1997).

Prostaglandin E_2 and $PGF_{2\alpha}$ increase uterine contractile activity in association with a rise in intracellular free calcium, which seems to be due primarily to an influx of extracellular calcium (Morrison and Smith 1994). In contrast to oxyto-cin, prostaglandins do not increase inositol 1,4,5-trisphosphate production in human myometrium or release intracellular calcium stores in cultured myometrial cells (Thornton and Gillespie 1992).

Endothelins

Endothelin-1 (ET-1), a potent vasoconstrictor, is capable of contracting several non-vascular smooth muscles including non-pregnant and pregnant rat myometrium (Calixto and Rae 1991) and human myometrium in vitro (Word *et al.* 1990). The concentration of ET-1 in maternal blood is increased during pregnancy and reaches a peak at term (Carbonne *et al.* 1998). Human myometrium is sensitive to ET-1, and ET-1-induced uterine contraction is markedly increased at the end of pregnancy (Osada *et al.* 1997). In addition, rat uterine contractile responsiveness to ET-1 is elevated during labour and diminished postpartum. The increased responsiveness is associated with an increase in the density of ET-1 receptors in myometrium (Yallampalli and Garfield 1994). Taken together, these data suggest a role for ET-1 in the initiation and maintenance of labour.

Endothelin$_A$ (ET$_A$) receptors and a smaller proportion of ET$_B$ receptors have been identified in human myometrium (Bacon *et al.* 1995), but only the propor-tion of the ET$_A$ receptor is increased in pregnant myometrium (Honore *et al.* 2000). Activation of the myometrial ET$_A$ receptor generates two intracellular messengers: inositol 1,4,5-trisphosphate, which releases calcium from the

Table 2.2. Clinical scenarios employing the myometrial relaxant effects of nitric oxide donors

Correction of uterine inversion	(Altabef *et al.* 1992; Bayhi *et al.* 1992; Dayan and Schwalbe 1996)
To facilitate external cephalic version	(Belfort 1993)
To aid manual removal of placenta	(Barnes 1882)
To allow internal podalic version of the second twin	(Wessen *et al.* 1995)
To relieve intrapartum fetal distress related to uterine hypertonicity	(Mercier *et al.* 1997)
To facilitate delivery at Caesarean section	(Mayer and Weeks 1992; David *et al.* 1998)
Tocolysis in preterm labour	(Lees *et al.* 1994; Rowlands *et al.* 1996; Duckitt and Thornton 2002)

sarcoplasmic reticulum, and diacylglycerol, which acts in concert with free calcium to stimulate protein kinase C(PKC) (Eude *et al.* 2000). Di Liberto *et al.* (2003) have demonstrated that PKC zeta and not PKC delta is necessary for ET-1-induced human myometrial contraction at the end of pregnancy.

Nitric oxide

Nitric oxide is a reactive gas with a very short physiological half-life. It is synthesised from L-arginine by the enzyme nitric oxide synthase (NOS), of which three isoforms have been identified. Nitric oxide is a crucial biological mediator, involved in diverse activities such as smooth muscle relaxation, neurotransmission, inflammation and regulation of the immune response (Nathan 1992). Nitric oxide is also known to play an important role in several aspects of reproductive physiology including menstruation and conception by means of its effects on the release luteinising hormone-releasing hormone, sperm motility, ovarian function and implantation (Chwalisz *et al.* 1996; Rosselli 1997).

There is now considerable evidence that nitric oxide is involved in the regulation of myometrial contractility during pregnancy (Ledingham *et al.* 2000a for review). The L-arginine-nitric oxide system has been identified within human myometrium, placenta and fetal membranes and several studies have attempted to determine whether a downregulation in NOS activity occurs at the onset of human labour at term (Di Iulio *et al.* 1995; Ramsay *et al.* 1996; Thomson *et al.* 1997b; Bao *et al.* 2002). These studies concluded that there was no significant fall in NOS activity during human parturition; indeed, Ramsay *et al.* (1996) found a slight increase in myometrial NOS activity in tissue collected during labour compared with that collected before labour. Further studies indicated that NOS activity in myometrium is downregulated in the third trimester suggesting a role for the L-arginine-nitric oxide system in the maintenance of uterine quiescence during pregnancy (Bansal *et al.* 1997; Norman *et al.* 1999); these data have not consistently been reproduced by others (Dennes *et al.* 1999).

In vitro and in vivo studies have demonstrated that drugs that act by liberating nitric oxide (nitric oxide donors) can induce myometrial relaxation. In human studies, when nitric oxide donors have been applied to myometrium in vitro, an inhibition of spontaneous and oxytocin-induced activity was found when amplitude or force of contractions were measured (Buhimschi *et al.* 1995; Lee and Chang 1995; Norman *et al.* 1997). It has long been recognised that nitric oxide donors relax the human uterus in vivo. As early as 1882, Barnes reported the use of amyl nitrite to facilitate manual removal of a retained placenta. More recently, intravenous glyceryl trinitrate (GTN) has been reported in uncontrolled case reports to allow correction of uterine inversion (Altabef *et al.* 1992; Bayhi *et al.* 1992; Dayan and Schwalbe 1996), to facilitate intrapartum external cephalic version (Belfort 1993), and to allow internal podalic version of a second twin (Wessen *et al.* 1995). In a prospective observational study, intravenous GTN produced relief of intrapartum fetal distress related to uterine hyperactivity (Mercier *et al.* 1997). This agent has also been used to facilitate fetal delivery during Caesarean section (Mayer and Weeks 1992), although a randomised trial found that administration of GTN leads to no clinically relevant effect on fetal extraction (David *et al.* 1998).

Two uncontrolled, observational studies investigating the effects of GTN patches in women with a diagnosis of preterm labour, concluded that GTN can arrest such labour (Lees *et al.* 1994; Rowlands *et al.* 1996). Randomised controlled trials were then undertaken to investigate the tocolytic effects of nitric oxide donors in preterm labour; a review of these trials has concluded that there is currently insufficient evidence to support the routine administration of nitric oxide donors in the management of threatened preterm labour (Duckitt and Thornton 2002).

Inflammatory mediators

Leukocytes, predominantly neutrophils and macrophages, infiltrate myometrium during spontaneous labour at term (Thomson *et al.* 1999), and it seems likely that this process is regulated by an increased expression of cell adhesion molecules (Winkler *et al.* 1998; Thomson *et al.* 1999; Ledingham *et al.* 2001).

The infiltrating leukocytes are a rich source of inflammatory mediators. These include plasminogen activators, eicosanoids, collagenase and elastase, and pro-inflammatory cytokines, including IL-1β, IL-6, IL-8 and TNF-α (Nathan 1987; Osmers *et al.* 1992; Casatella 1995; Young *et al.* 2002). Since these mediators have many diverse functions, the inflammatory infiltrate could have different roles in different regions of the uterus. Within the lower segment, it could be involved in tissue remodelling and thereby facilitate cervical dilatation and passage of the fetus. In the upper segment, leukocyte products, including eicosanoids, interleukins and TNF-α, may stimulate uterine contractions directly or indirectly by facilitating the production of uterotonic prostaglandins (Casey *et al.* 1990). Furthermore, inflammatory mediators may also initiate tissue remodelling in the uterine body. Granstrom *et al.* (1989) demonstrated that the connective tissue of the uterine isthmus (lower segment) and the uterine body undergo a biochemical ripening process similar to that found in the cervix, with an increase in collagenolytic activity following the onset of labour. A breakdown of the connective tissue within the myometrium may facilitate the coordination of uterine contractions by allowing the formation of gap junctions (Garfield and Hayashi 1981).

Metabolic modulation

A variety of metabolic factors are thought to play a crucial role in the control of myometrial contractility. These include myometrial blood flow, uterine phosphorus metabolites, hypoxia and pH, and have been reviewed by Wray (1993) and Morrison (1996). Metabolic inhibition/hypoxia exerts a profound and rapid inhibitory action on human myometrium, even in the presence of oxytocin (Monir-Bishty *et al.* 2003). It is likely that the inhibitory effects of hypoxia feed back and limit the contractions occurring in human labour. Stretch of the myometrial smooth muscle cells is also thought to be involved in the control of myometrial contractility. Multiple pregnancies are at increased risk of preterm labour; one reason for this may be that the increased intrauterine volume in multiple pregnancy imposes an increase in tension within the uterine wall and hence, a stretch or distension of the uterine myocytes. Within smooth muscle tissues including myometrium, stretch has been shown to induce depolarisation of the cell membrane, increase action potential frequency and subsequent contraction (Johansson and Mellander 1975; Manabe *et al.* 1985; Coburn 1987; Harder *et al.* 1987). Studies in rat myometrium have shown that stretch or distension of the uterus is required for full expression of Cx-43, the major protein forming myometrial gap junctions (Ou *et al.* 1997).

Cervical ripening

During pregnancy, the cervix must remain firm and closed to retain the conceptus within the uterine cavity. With the onset of cervical ripening, it is converted into a soft and easily dilating structure that allows the uterine contractions to deliver the fetus through the birth canal. Our understanding of the physiological mechanisms involved in cervical ripening is far from complete. Interest in this process has mainly been concerned with the development of pharmacological agents to ripen the cervix in order to facilitate induction of labour. In contrast, research on preterm labour and therapeutic strategies aimed at preventing it have concentrated on abolishing the associated uterine contractions whilst largely ignoring the cervix (Olah and Gee 1992). This interest in tocolytic agents has arisen since the presence of uterine contractions is the most obvious manifestation of preterm labour. Yet it is clear that the process of cervical ripening is likely to begin prior to the onset of myometrial activity, as in normal labour at term, or at least concurrently. Hence a better understanding of the processes involved in cervical ripening may lead to new therapeutic strategies in the prevention of preterm delivery.

Structure of the cervix

The main formed element of the cervical stroma is extracellular connective tissue matrix. The extracellular matrix is made up of type I (66%) and type III (33%) collagen, (Kleissl *et al.* 1978) with a small amount of type IV collagen in the basement membranes. The fibrils of collagen are bound together into dense bundles that confer on the cervix the rigidity that characterises its non-pregnant and early pregnant condition. A small amount of elastin is also present within the cervix. While the collagen confers rigidity, elastin may be responsible for providing elasticity; this assists in closing the cervix after delivery and thereafter returning it to its non-pregnant shape.

The collagen is embedded in a ground substance consisting of large molecular weight proteoglycan complexes containing a variety of glycosaminoglycans (GAGs). Glycosaminoglycans are long chains of highly negatively charged repeating disaccharides containing one hexosamine (glucosamine or galactosamine) and one uronic acid (glucuronic or iduronic). There are several different GAGs, such as heparin and heparan sulphate and dermatan and chondroitin sulphate. These vary in their composition with regard to the exact combination of hexosamine and uronic acid residues, and each varies intrinsically with regard to chain length. In cervical tissue the most abundant GAGs are chondroitin and its epimer, dermatan sulphate (von Maillot *et al.* 1979; Uldbjerg *et al.* 1983c). As well as forming the ground substance of the tissue, proteoglycans invest collagen fibrils (Scott and Orford 1981), with their protein cores attaching to the collagen. The relationship between the GAG side-chains and the collagen fibrils is important in orientating the collagen and conferring on the cervix its mechanical strength (Lindahl and Hook 1978). The binding affinity of GAGs to collagen increases with increasing chain length and charge density. Hyaluronic acid binds least strongly of the GAG molecules and will act to destabilise the collagen fibrils. Glycosaminoglycans such as dermatan sulphate, containing iduronic as opposed to glucuronic acid, bind strongly and promote tissue stability (Obrink 1973). Changes in the

Table 2.3. Changes in the cervix during pregnancy

Increase in hydration
Disruption of collagen bundles
Decrease in collagen concentration
Decrease in the size of collagen fibrils
Mature collagen is replaced with new collagen with fewer cross links
Alteration in the ground substance proteoglycan/glycosaminoglycan composition
An influx of inflammatory cells to the cervical stroma with cervical ripening

proteoglycans/GAG composition can therefore alter collagen binding and facilitate collagen breakdown.

The major cellular component of cervical connective tissue is the fibroblast. These cells appear to be responsible for the synthesis of both collagen and ground substance. Whilst the bulk of the cervix consists of fibrous tissue, there is a varying amount of smooth muscle – usually about 10%, but it can vary between 2% and 40%. The functional role of this smooth muscle is controversial, although it is capable of both spontaneous and drug-induced contractions (Nixon 1951; Hillier and Karim 1970). It seems that the connective tissue in the cervix is more important than the muscle component. The muscle is unlikely to act as a sphincter mechanism, both on the basis of its low concentration and also its spatial arrangement within the cervix. It is proposed that it protects important blood vessels during labour and brings about prompt closure of the cervix following delivery (Calder 1994).

The cervix during pregnancy

During pregnancy the cervix becomes metabolically more active. In the non-pregnant state, the cervix consists of around 80% water (Liggins 1978) and this increases to around 86% in late pregnancy (Uldbjerg *et al.* 1983d). This water interacts with the matrix proteins and facilitates the function of elastin. Since GAGs are hydrophilic, these molecules may be important in controlling tissue hydration, with increased hydration destabilising the collagen fibrils and promoting ripening. There does not seem to be a change in cervical water content immediately before or after delivery in humans (Leppert 1992). Whilst messenger RNA for tropoelastin, the precursor for elastin, is increased in pregnancy, the cervical elastin content does not appear to change throughout gestation (Leppert 1992). The smooth muscle cells of the cervix become enlarged and prominent during pregnancy. Smooth muscle enlargement may play a role in cervical tissue rearrangement as collagen bundles are aligned in close approximation to the smooth muscle bundles.

The collagen content of the cervix, both type I and type III, undergoes marked changes in pregnancy. The spaces between the collagen bundles become dilated as early as 8–14 weeks' gestation. Although there is an increase in the total collagen content of the cervix at term, the collagen concentration is reduced by 30%–50% compared to the non-pregnant cervix (Fosang *et al.* 1984; Kokenyesi and Woessner 1990; Jeffrey 1991). The cervical collagen concentration measured biochemically also decreases (Danforth *et al.* 1974; Uldbjerg *et al.* 1983a; Granstrom *et al.* 1989). This arises because other components of the cervix, the water and non-collagen proteins, are increasing in relatively greater amounts. In addition, the collagen fibrils are reduced in size (Danforth *et al.* 1960). This decline in cervical collagen appears to be even more marked when studied histologically using stains specifically intended for polymerised collagen. A much lower proportion of the collagen exists as intact fibres in the dilated cervix at term (Obrink 1973). Several mechanisms have been proposed to explain these changes in collagen composition; essentially, these are increased enzymatic collagen degradation and/or alteration in the proteoglycan/GAG composition of the ground substance.

Collagen is amenable to breakdown by the action of lytic enzymes. These include collagenases (matrix metalloproteinase(MMP)-1, MMP-8 and MMP-13), which are produced by fibroblasts and leukocytes; and leukocyte elastase, produced by macrophages, neutrophils and eosinophils. Collagenase is secreted in a latent form, procollagenase, which is activated by cleavage of the proenzyme by plasmin or stromelysin (MMP-3) to the active form. The activated collagenase specifically breaks down the triple helix of the collagen fibril by hydrolysing peptide bonds (Wooley 1984; Stricklin and Hibbs 1988). Radiolabel studies suggest that the cells critically involved in collagen degradation during cervical dilatation are not the cervical fibroblasts, but rather neutrophils migrating from blood vessels. The neutrophils secrete both elastase and collagenase (MMP-8) (Osmers *et al.* 1992). Elastase breaks down collagen by acting on the telopeptide non-helical domains. Elastase can degrade not only elastin and collagen, but also proteoglycans, and it may act synergistically with collagenase on collagen. As the cervical collagen content decreases through pregnancy, the leukocyte elastase and collagenase activities increase (Uldbjerg *et al.* 1983a). In addition, the amount of soluble collagen (reflecting partly degraded collagen) in the tissue increases in parallel with the increased enzyme activities (Ito *et al.* 1979; Uldbjerg *et al.* 1983a). Mature collagen with many cross links may be broken down during pregnancy and replaced with new collagen that has fewer cross links and is more amenable to rapid breakdown at the time of parturition. As the pregnancy advances, collagen is more easily extracted from cervical tissues, with the immature cross links in newly synthesised collagen contributing to this phenomenon.

In addition to increased collagen breakdown, there are changes in the cervical proteoglycan and GAG content as pregnancy advances. The total GAG content of the cervix increases substantially by term, indicating active synthesis although the concentrations of GAGs may remain relatively constant (Golichowski 1980). Whilst some studies have shown an increase in the hyaluronic acid concentration in pregnancy (von Maillot *et al.* 1979; Golichowski 1980), other studies have found no increase (Uldbjerg *et al.* 1983d; Fosang *et al.* 1984; Uldbjerg and Malmstrom 1991). Although this could reflect variation between species, these discrepancies could also be attributed to variations in the site of the cervical biopsies used in each study (Leppert 1995). Studies employing more recently developed biochemical techniques have demonstrated that the concentration of hyaluronic acid increases almost 12-fold at 2–3 cm dilatation (Leppert 1992). This GAG may help to 'loosen' the collagenous network of the cervix whilst an increase in the hyaluronic acid available to bind water may be associated with an increase in tissue hydration and tissue deformability. There may be a relative decrease in chondroitin and dermatan sulphate, compared to the non-pregnant cervix. It has been proposed that tissues become more rigid with increasing chondroitin sulphate concentration. Thus, a reduction in the chondroitin sulphate concentration might result in increased compliance and is likely to reduce the mechanical strength of collagen fibrils, and make them more amenable to breakdown by proteolytic enzymes.

The predominant proteoglycan in the non-pregnant, human cervix is dermatan sulphate proteoglycan II (decorin or DSPG II), a small proteoglycan with one dermatan sulphate side-chain (Uldbjerg *et al.* 1983c). In addition, there are small amounts of two other proteoglycans, one with two dermatan sulphate side-chains, biglycan (DSPG I) and a larger one with chondroitin/dermatan sulphate side-chains called large proteoglycan(PGL) (Norman *et al.* 1991). It is proposed that the amount of decorin increases in the pregnant cervix (Leppert 1995), until late pregnancy when the proteoglycan concentration decreases to about 50% of that in the non-pregnant cervix. After the onset of cervical ripening, the amount of decorin still dominates in the cervix, but there is an increase in the other proteoglycans (Norman *et al.* 1993). Such an alteration in the proteoglycan and collagen composition of the ground substance might explain the altered biomechanical properties of the cervix (Greer 1992). In the rat, a strong correlation exists between the cervical linear circumference and the decorin–collagen ratio (Kokenyesi and Woessner 1990) supporting this contention.

The increase in total GAGs probably reflects an increased production by fibroblasts that become increasingly active as pregnancy advances (Junqueira *et al.* 1980; Parry and Ellwood 1981). Additionally, the increase could reflect breakdown of the proteoglycan complexes to provide free hyaluronic acid and proteoglycans.

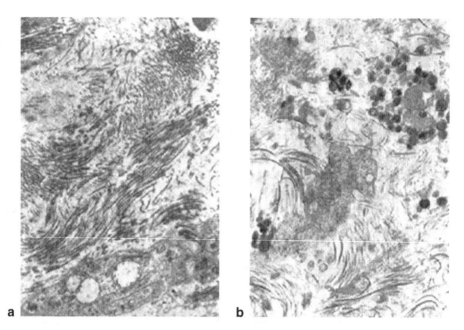

Figure 2.2   Electron micrographs of cervical stroma (a) before and (b) after the onset of spontaneous labour at term. The cervical connective tissue at term shows widely scattered fibrils of collagen and a marked increase in ground substance when compared to the non-pregnant or early pregnant cervix. Following the onset of labour (b), there is further disruption and dissociation of the cervical collagen fibrils, compared with cervix before labour(a).

The proteases required for this could come from the activated fibroblasts, or the leukocytes that infiltrate the cervical connective tissue .

Cervical ripening

The phenomenon of cervical ripening is a prelude to the onset of labour and is most obvious during the last five or six weeks of pregnancy although it may have its origins even earlier. Clinically, ripening refers to the increased softening, distensibility, effacement and early dilatation that can be detected by pelvic examination. These changes are the result of profound alterations in the biomechanical properties of cervical tissue and include a reduction in collagen concentration, an increase in water content and a change in proteoglycan/GAG composition (Calder and Greer 1992). One important change involved in cervical ripening is a rearrangement and realignment of collagen (Leppert 1995) (Figure 2.2). The cervical connective tissue at term shows widely scattered and dissociated fibrils of collagen and a marked increase in the ground substance when compared to the non-pregnant or early pregnant cervix. The process of cervical ripening has been compared to an inflammatory reaction (Liggins 1981) and infiltration of cervical

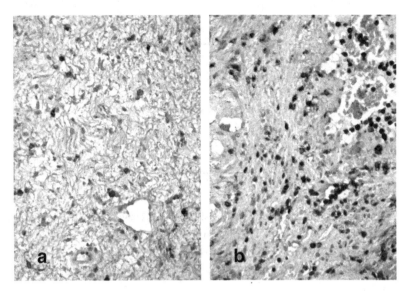

Figure 2.3   Micrograph of human cervical biopsy obtained (a) before the onset of labour and (b) after the
onset of labour. An antibody against the common leukocyte antigen CD45 was used to stain
leukocytes (staining brown).

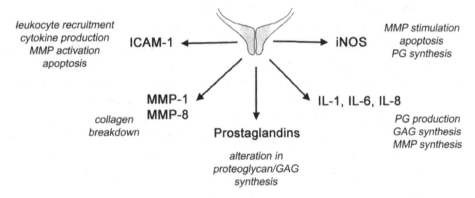

Figure 2.4   Mechanisms of cervical ripening. ICAM-1, intercellular adhesion molecule-1; iNOS,
inducible NOS.

tissue with inflammatory cells has been shown in experimental circumstances
(Junqueira *et al.* 1980; Chwalisz 1988; Rath *et al.* 1988; Bokstrom *et al.* 1997)
and during human parturition at term (Osman *et al.* 2003) (Figure 2.3).

The control of cervical ripening

Cervical ripening appears to be an active process in view of the changes that occur
within the cervical connective tissue and cellular components (Figure 2.4).

Table 2.4. The control of cervical ripening

Prostaglandins
Oestrogens
Progesterone withdrawal
Inflammatory mediators (e.g. interleukin-8)
Nitric oxide
Relaxin
Apoptosis

Furthermore, animal studies have shown that cervical ripening occurs even when the cervix is physically isolated from the uterus (Stys *et al.* 1980; Ledger *et al.* 1985). Those factors controlling cervical ripening, and which may be implicated in the pathophysiology of preterm labour, are incompletely understood.

Prostaglandins

Prostaglandins undoubtedly play a role in the control of cervical ripening in the human. The main prostaglandins produced by the cervix are PGE_2, PGI_2, and to a lesser extent $PGF_{2\alpha}$, and their production increases in association with cervical ripening (Ellwood *et al.* 1980). Physiologically, PGE_2 is probably much more important than $PGF_{2\alpha}$, while the role of PGI_2 in cervical ripening is rather uncertain. Amniotic fluid concentrations of PGE_2 and $PGF_{2\alpha}$ correlate directly with the cervical score in women at term who are not in labour (Calder 1980). In addition, receptors for PGE_2 and $PGF_{2\alpha}$ can be demonstrated in the cervix (Crankshaw *et al.* 1979). These data suggest that prostaglandins have a physiological role in cervical ripening; there is no doubt that natural and synthetic prostaglandins are effective pharmacological agents for ripening the cervix at any stage in pregnancy (Calder 1980; Calder and Greer 1991). Prostaglandins might effect cervical ripening by inducing the breakdown of collagen. Alternatively, they could modify the binding of collagen and the hydration of tissue by altering the GAG/proteoglycan composition. Prostaglandin E_2 treatment will reduce collagen concentration similar to the changes seen in physiological ripening (Uldbjerg *et al.* 1981; Ekman *et al.* 1986), but it is uncertain whether this is the result of collagenolysis. While some studies have shown an increase in collagenase activity following the administration of PGE_2 (Ding *et al.* 1990), others have shown no such change (Ellwood *et al.* 1981; Uldbjerg *et al.* 1983b; Rath *et al.* 1987). While these conflicting results may, to some extent, reflect difficulties in assessing collagenase activity, Rath *et al.* (1987) supported their findings by demonstrating an absence of collagen breakdown fragments on electrophoresis following prostaglandin therapy. In this study significant cervical ripening occurred in the treated group.

There is evidence that prostaglandins act by altering the ground substance in cervical tissue (Uldbjerg *et al.* 1981, 1983b). An increase in hydration and hyaluronic acid concentration has been demonstrated in animal studies, after PGE_2 administration (Cabrol *et al.* 1987). Prostaglandin E_2 can influence cervical fibroblast production of collagen and GAG. The production of these two substances is inversely related such that an increase in GAG production occurs when collagen synthesis is reduced (Norstrom 1984; Norstrom *et al.* 1985); Johnston *et al.* (1993) have shown that PGE_2 administration in late pregnancy results in an increase in circulating levels of chondroitin sulphate, similar to those seen in spontaneous labour. Thus, PGE_2-mediated cervical ripening may be explained by alterations in GAG/proteoglycan content that will disperse and destabilise the collagen fibrils thereby increasing tissue compliance.

Oestrogens

Other naturally occurring agents also act to control cervical structural changes. Oestrogens such as oestradiol have been used to bring about cervical ripening in the clinical situation (Gordon and Calder 1977; Allen *et al.* 1989; Magann *et al.* 1995). The mechanism underlying the effects of oestradiol may be due in part to the induction of prostaglandin synthesis within the tissues (Horton and Poyser 1976). Oestradiol might also be responsible for the influx of protease-producing leukocytes which could induce ripening (Calder and Greer 1992). A systematic review examining the effectiveness and safety of oestrogens for third trimester cervical ripening and induction of labour concluded that there were insufficient data to draw any conclusions regarding the efficacy of oestrogen as an induction agent (Thomas *et al.* 2001)

Progesterone and antiprogesterones

Progesterone inhibits the effects of collagenase within the uterine corpus (Jeffrey *et al.* 1971) and may have a similar role within the cervix. It has an inhibitory effect on cervical ripening and parturition in those animals where a decrease in progesterone at term results in ripening and labour. Such a decrease does not occur in the human but progesterone is a potent anti-inflammatory agent (Sitteri *et al.* 1977), and could still be an important physiological inhibitor of the ripening process in vivo by inhibiting neutrophil influx and activation (Jeffrey and Koob 1980). This is supported by the observation of the cervical softening effect of the antiprogesterones prior to termination of pregnancy (Gupta and Johnson 1990; Radestad *et al.* 1990), and which is associated with a neutrophil influx in animal models (Chwalisz 1988). In addition, antiprogesterones might exert their effects through prostaglandins as they appear to stimulate prostaglandin synthesis and reduce catabolism in vitro (Kelly *et al.* 1986; Kelly and Bukman 1990). Morphological and biochemical studies in humans and animals, have shown evidence of collagenolysis in the cervix after treatment with antiprogesterones (Hegele-Hartung *et al.* 1989; Radestad *et al.* 1993). Other workers, however, have failed to show any change in cervical collagen content (Norman 1992; Bokstrom and Norstrom 1995).

Relaxin

There is good theoretical evidence that relaxin, a 6-kD dimeric peptide hormone, plays a role in the process of cervical ripening in the human. Relaxin increases collagenase activity (von Maillot *et al.* 1977) perhaps via a mitogenic effect on fibroblasts, which are known to exhibit relaxin receptors (McMurty *et al.* 1980). While the specific role of relaxin during human pregnancy is unknown, increased relaxin concentrations in the maternal circulation are associated with preterm labour, perhaps by altering cervical connective tissue (Petersen *et al.* 1992; Weiss *et al.* 1993). Pharmacologically, porcine relaxin has been shown to cause cervical ripening in women (MacLennan *et al.* 1980; Evans *et al.* 1983). More recently, the efficacy of recombinant human relaxin, administered vaginally, has been investigated; while no adverse effects could be attributed to the preparation, recombinant human relaxin had no appreciable effects on cervical ripening (Bell *et al.* 1993; Brennand *et al.* 1997). Further trials are required to determine the role of relaxin, either purified porcine or recombinant human, as an induction or cervical ripening agent in clinical practice (Kelly *et al.* 2001).

Inflammatory mediators

Cervical ripening is considered to be a physiological inflammatory process, characterised by an accumulation of neutrophils and macrophages in the cervical stroma (Junqueira *et al.* 1980; Liggins 1981; Bokstrom *et al.* 1997; Osman *et al.* 2003). The putative effects of these leukocytes include breakdown and remodelling of cervical tissue via release of MMPs, prostaglandins, cell adhesion molecules and nitric oxide (Thomson *et al.* 1999; Ledingham *et al.* 2000b, 2001). The leukocytes and other cell types within the cervix release pro-inflammatory cytokines including IL-1β, IL-6 and IL-8, which may also contribute to this process, not least by promoting further leukocyte invasion (Young *et al.* 2002). Interleukin-8 is an inflammatory cytokine that is capable of producing a selective neutrophil chemotaxis and activation (Baggiolini *et al.* 1989). This cytokine can be produced by fibroblasts in the human cervix (Barclay *et al.* 1993), and can induce cervical ripening in non-pregnant and pregnant rabbits (El Maradny *et al.* 1994). Interleukin-8 may have a synergistic interaction with prostaglandin E$_2$ in promoting cervical ripening (Colditz 1990). The increase in IL-8 during cervical ripening correlates with increases in leukocyte infiltration and concentrations of MMPs in the tissue (Osmers *et al.* 1995; Winkler *et al.* 1999). Other cytokines, including IL-1β (El Maradny *et al.* 1995) and TNF α (Chwalisz *et al.* 1994a) have been shown to produce cervical ripening in animal studies. These cytokines have been shown to affect production of MMPs and tissue inhibitors of matrix metalloproteinases (TIMPs) by human cervical fibroblasts and smooth muscle cells (Ito *et al.* 1990; Sato *et al.* 1990; Ogawa *et al.* 1998; Watari *et al.* 1999). Increases in granulocyte-colony stimulating factor and monocyte chemotactic protein1(MCP-1), cyto-kines, which stimulate proliferation and activation of immune cells, also occur with cervical ripening (Denison *et al.* 2000; Sennstrom *et al.* 2000).

Nitric oxide

The results of both animal and human studies on nitric oxide production and NOS expression in the cervix indicate that nitric oxide may play a role in cervical ripening. The nitric oxide generating system is present in the rat cervix and, in contrast to the body of the uterus, it is downregulated during pregnancy, but upregulated during term and preterm labour (Buhimschi *et al.* 1996). Treatment of pregnant guinea-pigs with the NOS inhibitor N(4)-nitro-L-arginine methyl ester(L-NAME) induced preterm labour but delayed physiological cervical ripening, resulting in prolonged deliveries (Chwalisz *et al.* 1994b). Furthermore, L-NAME treatment of pregnant rats significantly prolonged the duration of labour, suggestive of cervical dystocia, whilst a decrease in cervical extensibility was observed after in vitro incubation with L-NAME (Buhimschi *et al.* 1996). Chwalisz *et al.* (1997) demonstrating that the local application of the nitric oxide donor, sodium nitroprusside, produced effective ripening of the guinea-pig cervix, assessed by both force-resistance measurements and morphological evaluation. It seems that, at least in animal pregnancy, nitric oxide represents a final metabolic pathway of cervical ripening. Acting in concert with prostaglandins, particularly PGE$_2$, nitric oxide might induce local vasodilatation and increase vascular permeability and leukocyte infiltration, and perhaps also activate MMPs and other mechanisms responsible for the extracellular matrix remodelling (Chwalisz *et al.* 1997).

The L-arginine-nitric oxide system is present in the human cervix and is upregulated during labour at term (Tschugguel *et al.* 1999; Ledingham *et al.* 2000b; Bao *et al.* 2001). The level of nitric oxide metabolites increases in cervical fluid after cervical ripening or cervical manipulation, supporting a role for nitric oxide in cervical ripening (Vaisanen-Tommiska *et al.* 2003). Furthermore, nitric oxide donors have been shown to produce effective ripening of the human cervix in the first trimester of pregnancy (Thomson *et al.* 1997a, 1998; Facchinetti *et al.* 2000), and at term (Chanrachakul *et al.* 2000). The mechanisms of nitric oxide-induced cervical ripening remain uncertain, but may involve the production of PGE$_2$ (Ekerhovd *et al.* 2002) and PGF$_{2\alpha}$ (Ledingham *et al.* 1999; Ekerhovd *et al.* 2002), and the production of MMP-1 from cervical fibroblasts (Yoshida *et al.* 2001).

Apoptosis

Cervical ripening occurs spontaneously in a timely, species-specific manner suggesting that apoptosis, or programmed cell death, may be involved (Leppert 1995). Apoptosis is a phenomenon characterised by the shrinkage of cells, compaction of chromatin into uniformly dense bundles and clear halo nuclei. One study in pregnant rats showed that, as gestation advanced, the numbers of dying smooth muscle cells in the cervix increased along with DNA degradation fragments and cervical softening (Leppert and Yu 1994). In a subsequent study, Leppert (1998) found that the incidence of apoptotic cells in the rat cervix increased throughout gestation. Apoptosis in cervical stromal cells has also been described in human pregnancy with an increase in the number of cells undergoing apoptosis during labour (Allaire *et al.* 2001).

Biology of membrane rupture

Rupture of the fetal membranes is a vital part of normal parturition. During spontaneous labour at term, the membranes remain intact until after the onset of labour in 90% of women. In only 10% do they rupture prematurely, prior to the onset of labour (premature rupture of membranes(PROM)). In contrast, in only 60%–70% of women in preterm labour do the membranes remain intact until after the onset of labour, leaving 30%–40% who have preterm premature rupture of the fetal membranes prior to the onset of labour (pPROM). These data suggest that specific pathophysiological events lead to pPROM, and that pPROM and preterm labour may have different aetiologies. The biochemical and molecular evidence emerging about these conditions support this assertion and is reviewed below.

Structure of fetal membranes

The histological structure of the fetal membranes is shown in Figure 2.5. There are three main components, the amnion and the chorion, which are fetally derived tissues, and maternal decidua, which adheres to the amnion and chorion. The amnion is composed of a single layer of cuboidal epithelium lying on a basement membrane, under which lies a compact and a fibroblast layer of connective tissue. These layers are mirrored in the chorion, with a connective tissue layer made of

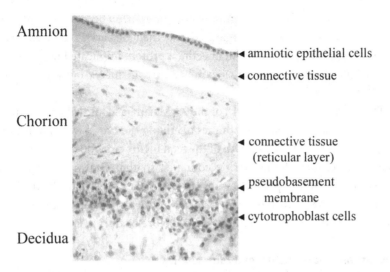

Amnion — amniotic epithelial cells

— connective tissue

Chorion

— connective tissue (reticular layer)

— pseudobasement membrane

— cytotrophoblast cells

Decidua

Figure 2.5   Haematoxylin and eosin stain of human fetal membranes.

reticular cells, an intervening pseudobasement membrane and then a multilayered epithelium of cytotrophoblast cells. Immediately below this is the decidual layer.

There is a considerable reserve in the tensile strength of the fetal membranes during normal pregnancy. The main tensile strength in the fetal membranes is generated by the extracellular matrix of the connective tissue, principally collagens type I and III (Malak *et al.* 1993). These collagens are denser and more organised in the compact layer of the amnion than in the fibroblast layer of the amnion or the reticular layer of the chorion. Collagen type VI stabilises the network of collagens I and III by attachment to basement membranes and to stromal collagen type IV and to laminin. Another important structural component of the extracellular matrix is fibronectin, and indeed identification of fetal fibronectin in the maternal cervix and vagina is a marker for preterm birth (Goldenberg *et al.* 1996). Within this extracellular matrix lies a cellular population of fibroblasts, myofibroblasts and macrophages.

Morphological changes associated with membrane rupture at term

The morphological events associated with membrane rupture at term have been well characterised. Membrane rupture arises in a morphologically distinct area called the zone of altered morphology (ZAM) (Malak and Bell 1994). This zone is characterised by marked thinning of the cytotrophoblast layer (with associated loss of cells) and decidua, and swelling of the connective tissue components with an increase in the total number of cells in the reticular layer, particularly the myofibroblasts. A reduction in elements neccessary for structural integrity of individual cells and a decrease in cell–cell contacts is also observed, which will further weaken this area. The amnion and the chorion become separated. Collagen fibres are disrupted and disorganised and their density is reduced (particularly collagen types I, III and V). Osteonectin, a protein implicated in the regulation of extracellular matrix turnover is expressed by an increasing proportion of cells (McParland *et al.* 2001).

The morphological hallmarks of the ZAM can be identified prior to the onset of labour in an area of fetal membranes overlying the cervix (McLaren *et al.* 1999).

It has been shown that growth of the fetal membranes does not keep up with the increased volume of the uterine contents, so that fetal membranes are under increasing tension as pregnancy advances (Millar *et al.* 2000). With the development of the ZAM, which produces a local weakness in fetal membranes, membrane rupture eventually occurs, either shortly before or during labour.

Biochemical events associated with membrane rupture at term

The MMPs are a family of proteins that break down collagens (Woessner 1994). Their natural inhibitors, with which the MMPs form 1:1 complexes are the tissue inhibitors of matrix metalloproteinase (TIMPs). Since collagens provide the main tensile strength to the fetal membranes it is no surprise that fetal membrane rupture is associated with an increase in MMP expression and activity and a decrease in TIMP expression and activity. Using Northern analysis, examination of chorio-decidua at various time points throughout labour at term showed high MMP-1 expression prior to the onset of labour, increased expression of MMP-3 and MMP-9 during labour but prior to delivery and increased TIMP-1 post delivery (Bryant-Greenwood and Yamamoto 1995). Amniotic fluid MMP-3 levels increase in association with each of term and preterm labour but not spontaneous membrane rupture (Park *et al.* 2003). In contrast a rise in amniotic fluid MMP-9 activity (Maymon *et al.* 2000c) and expression (determined by enzyme-linked immunosorbert assay(ELISA)) (Locksmith *et al.* 2001) occurs in association with membrane rupture at term. Immunohistochemical and cell culture data suggest that MMP-9 is produced in the amnion epithelial cells and chorion trophoblast cells (Xu *et al.* 2002). The hypothesis that MMPs have a causative effect on membrane rupture is further strengthened by a study showing a local increase in MMP-9 activity and protein concentration in the cervical area of the fetal membranes prior to labour – i.e. the area of the ZAM where membrane rupture occurs (McLaren *et al.* 2000a).

The signals that stimulate MMP activity remain incompletely understood. However, PGE_2 stimulates MMP-9 in fetal membranes ex vivo (McLaren *et al.* 2000b), and $PGF_{2\alpha}$ stimulates MMP-2 and MMP-9, and inhibits TIMP-1 production in decidua ex vivo (Ulug *et al.* 2001). Additionally, IL-1 increases biosynthesis of collagenase (MMP-1, -8 and -13) in cultured human chorionic cells ex vivo

(Katsura *et al.* 1989). Since COX-2, which produces prostaglandins, and IL-1 both increase in fetal membranes co-incident with the onset of labour (Slater *et al.* 1999; Osman, *et al.* 2003), the increase in MMP activity at term is probably stimulated (at least in part) by increased endogenous prostaglandin and IL-1 expression.

Preterm premature rupture of the membranes (pPROM)

Morphometric alterations similar to those occurring in the ZAM also occur in pPROM, but not in preterm labour in the absence of ruptured membranes (Malak *et al.* 1994). An increase in MMP activity has also been demonstrated in association with pPROM, and a greater number of MMP types appear to be involved, as would be expected with the multiple aetiology of this condition. An increase in amniotic fluid MMP-1, MMP-8 and MMP-9 activity (Maymon *et al.* 2000a, 2000d) and fetal membrane MMP-2 expression (Fortunato *et al.* 2000) has been demonstrated in association with pPROM. Additionally, in pPROM in association with intrauterine infection MMP-7 is elevated (Maymon *et al.* 2000b). Distinct biochemical events seem to occur in each of pPROM and preterm labour. Specifically, pPROM membranes have greater MMP-2, -9 and membrane type 1(MT-1) MMP and decreased TIMP-2 mRNA expression compared with fetal membranes from women in preterm labour without pPROM (Fortunato and Menon 2001). These molecular events are paralleled by protein concentrations in amniotic fluid by ELISA.

There are several possible pathophysiologic pathways that might lead to MMP elevation and subsequently pPROM. Macrophage and neutrophil derived MMP-7 and MMP-8 respectively might be stimulated by lipopolysaccharides and pro-inflammatory cytokines present in the uterine cavity in association with infection. Similarly, TNFα, which is elevated in intra-amniotic infection, can stimulate chorionic production of MMP-1 (So *et al.* 1992).

Apoptosis may also play a part. Activation of the apoptosis pathway (DNA fragmentation, elevated bax and p53 transcription and decreased bcl-2 transcription) are present in fetal membranes during pPROM, but not term or preterm labour (Fortunato *et al.* 2000). Matrix Metalloproteinase-2 production is stimulated by p53, providing a pathway through which apoptosis might stimulate membrane rupture in pPROM (Bian and Sun 1997). However, the mechanism by which apoptosis is stimulated in pPROM is unclear.

Where pPROM occurs in association with placental abruption, thrombin may play a causative role by stimulating decidual protease production (Lockwood *et al.* 1996). Support for this hypothesis is given by data showing that second trimester levels of thrombin-antithrombin complex (a marker of thrombin production) are very much higher in those destined to develop pPROM, compared with controls (Rosen *et al.* 2001).

Summary

The tensile strength of the fetal membranes derives largely from the collagen fibres that contribute to its composition. Prior to the onset of labour at term, the membranes become weakened in an area overlying the cervix known as the ZAM. Coincident with this MMP expression increases. Together these weaken the fetal membranes leading to rupture.

The histological events associated with pPROM have been less extensively identified. However, MMP activation again plays a role, with a wider variety of MMPs implicated with pPROM than membrane rupture at term. Matrix metalloproteinase activation might be the final common pathway through which infection and placental abruption provoke pPROM. Since the molecular and biochemical events associated with pPROM differ from those of preterm labour alone, different pharmacotherapeutic strategies might be required to prevent or treat each of these conditions.

Biology of labour at term

Despite major advances in molecular biology and the science of reproduction, the signals controlling the onset of human parturition remain elusive. The search for the triggering mechanism initiating human labour, which focused on oxytocin in the early twentieth century, has since included prostaglandin production, growth factors, cytokines, endothelins, gap junction formation and, more recently, placental corticotrophin-releasing hormone(CRH) (Karalis *et al.* 1996) and nitric oxide withdrawal (Izumi *et al.* 1993). In non-primate mammals, the end of pregnancy is associated with a fall in maternal progesterone concentrations (Csapo 1977), which, together with increasing oestradiol concentrations, activates multiple pathways, including stimulation of oxytocin release, oxytocin receptors and prostaglandin synthesis, which contribute to the initiation of labour (Casey and MacDonald 1988; Liggins 1994).

It would seem reasonable that the fetus should trigger the onset of labour when maturity is adequate for extra-uterine survival, and this is certainly the case in sheep. In sheep, fetal cortisol triggers parturition by increasing the activity of placental enzymes, including 17α-hydroxylase and P450 C-17,20 lyase, which enable progesterone conversion to oestradiol (Flint *et al.* 1975). The resultant increase in the ratio of oestradiol to progesterone stimulates myometrial oxytocin receptors, gap junction formation, prostaglandin production and maternal pituitary oxytocin release, events leading directly to labour and delivery (Schwartz 1997). These same pathways are activated at term in human pregnancy when circulating levels of fetal plasma cortisol are also raised. However, the target for cortisol action in the ovine placenta, 17α-hydroxylase, is absent in human placenta, and there is no consistent rise in maternal plasma concentrations of oestrogens or any consistent decline in progesterone concentrations before the onset of labour in woman (Tulchinsky *et al.* 1972; Flint 1979). Hence, if fetal cortisol is a factor controlling the onset of human parturition, its mode of action must be different from that in sheep.

The onset of human parturition is associated with an increase in the production of prostaglandins within the uterus. As discussed earlier, prostaglandins are synthesised from arachidonic acid via the enzyme cyclo-oxygenase, of which there are three isoforms. With the onset of labour at term, there is an increase in COX-2 expression in the amnion and chorio-decidua (Slater *et al.* 1995, 1998) and an increase in the production of prostaglandins E_2 and $F_{2\alpha}$ by these tissues (Keirse 1979; Mitchell 1984; Casey and MacDonald 1988). Prostaglandin production is stimulated by platelet-activating factor and by various cytokines, including IL-1, IL-6 and TNF (Challis and Mitchell 1994). Loss of chorionic prostaglandin dehydrogenase activity may be significant in initiating labour, particularly in preterm labour (Keirse 1995), although in vitro studies have not found any change in prostaglandin metabolism with labour at term (Brennand *et al.* 1998).

The myometrium is stimulated directly by both prostaglandins and oxytocin derived from the chorion-decidua (Fuchs *et al.* 1984). Other myometrial stimulants, such as platelet-activating factor and endothelin, may also be involved in the initiation of myometrial contractions (Wolff *et al.* 1996). Simultaneously, the connective tissue of the cervix undergoes complex biochemical changes that lead to softening and distensibility. Cervical ripening has been compared to an inflammatory reaction and is characterised by an accumulation of leukocytes in the cervical stroma (Junqueira *et al.* 1980; Liggins 1981; Bokstrom *et al.* 1997).

The signal to this chain of events is unknown although the progesterone-withdrawal theory remains the leading hypothesis. Progesterone inhibits human myometrial contractions and decreases gap junction formation (Beck *et al.* 1978; Ambrus and Rao 1994). Labour is an inflammatory process (Kelly 1996) and progesterone is recognised to be an anti-inflammatory agent (Sitteri *et al.* 1977). Whilst exogenous progesterone does not postpone the onset of parturition at term in humans as it does in sheep, antiprogesterones activate many of the pathways involved in the onset of labour and induce uterine contractility and cervical ripening (Chwalisz 1994; Lelaidier *et al.* 1994). These observations propose a role for progesterone in the maintenance of pregnancy and suggest that a decline in progesterone sensitivity, or an uncoupling of progesterone action in late pregnancy, without an actual fall in the hormone's concentration, could be an important factor in the initiation of human labour. Possible uncoupling mechanisms include local metabolism of progesterone and progesterone inactivation by a specific binding protein (Westphal *et al.* 1977), by an endogenous antiprogesterone (Casey and MacDonald 1993; Wilson and Parsons 1996) or by a change in the number or affinity of progesterone receptors (Khan-Dawood and Dawood 1984; Mesiano *et al.* 2002).

A role for CRH in the initiation of human labour has been proposed (Reis *et al.* 1999 for review). Corticotrophin-releasing hormone is a peptide hormone that was originally recognised as a hypothalamic releasing factor, and is now known to be secreted by placental trophoblast into the maternal circulation (Keelan *et al.* 1997). Maternal plasma CRH levels rise exponentially during pregnancy and elevated plasma CRH levels have been associated with preterm labour (Kurki *et al.* 1991). The bioavailability of circulating CRH is known to be influenced by the CRH-binding protein (CRH-BP) that binds to the hormone in an equimolar ratio and prevents its recognition at the CRH receptor. Corticotrophin-releasing hormone-binding protein is present in the maternal circulation in concentrations that will block the bioactivity of CRH until the final three weeks before the onset of spontaneous labour (McLean *et al.* 1995). At this time the continuing rise in plasma CRH concentrations is accompanied by an abrupt fall in CRH-BP concentrations in the maternal circulation and amniotic fluid (Florio *et al.* 1997). Corticotrophin-releasing hormone receptors are present in the myometrium (Hillhouse *et al.* 1993) and fetal membranes (Petraglia *et al.* 1990), and CRH stimulates the release of prostaglandins from human amnion and decidua in vitro (Jones and Challis 1989) and has been reported to potentiate the action of oxytocin and $PGF_{2\alpha}$ in stimulating myometrial contraction in vitro (Benedetto *et al.* 1994) and in vivo (McLean *et al.* 1994). Corticotrophin releasing hormone is present in the amniotic fluid and fetal circulation where it is capable of stimulating the fetal pituitary–adrenal axis to increase fetal adrenal glucocorticoid secretion, promoting fetal organ maturation. Further, CRH induces the synthesis of prostaglandins and glucocorticoids, which in turn stimulate further placental CRH secretion, creating positive feedback loops in the maternal, fetal and amniotic compartments, which may drive the onset of labour (Challis and Hooper 1989).

Role of infection

Accumulating evidence indicates that subclinical infection is implicated in the pathogenesis of spontaneous preterm labour, with approximately 30%–40% of preterm labours being associated with an underlying infective process. This evidence is derived from systemic, intrauterine and intracervical inoculation studies in pregnant animals (Dombroski *et al.* 1990; Heddleston *et al.* 1993), from case-control and cohort studies of cervico-vaginal microbial colonisation in women with preterm labour, and from the higher rate of histological chorioamnionitis found after spontaneous preterm labour and birth (Russell 1979; Naeye and Peters

Table 2.5. Organisms/infections implicated in spontaneous preterm labour

Gardnerella vaginalis
Ureaplasma urealyticum
Chlamydia trachomatis
Neisseria gonorrhoeae
group B streptococci
Escherichia coli
Klebsiella spp.
Haemophilus influenzae
Mycoplasma hominis
Trichomonas vaginalis
Peridontal infection
Asymptomatic bacteriuria

1980; Guzick and Winn 1985). Furthermore, in bacteriological cultures of amniotic fluid taken from women presenting with spontaneous preterm labour, microbial organisms have been found in 10%–15% of cases (Gomez *et al.* 1997).

It is likely that infection contributes to preterm labour and to preterm rupture of the fetal membranes through inflammation and the triggering of the cytokine cascade. Bacterial organisms secrete phospholipases resulting in an increase in arachadonic acid release from intrauterine tissues and prostaglandin production. In addition, bacterial endotoxin, such as lipopolysaccharide, acts on macrophages within the fetal membranes, causing either prostaglandin release or further cytokine production (Bennett *et al.* 1987; Romero *et al.* 1988). The organisms that have the strongest associations with spontaneous preterm labour are *Gardnerella vaginalis* and *Ureaplasma urealyticum*, and the sexually transmitted organisms *Chlamydia trachomatis* and *Neisseria gonorrhoeae*. Other organisms such as group B streptococci, *Escherichia coli*, *Klebsiella* spp., *Haemophilus influenzae* and *Mycoplasma hominis* have also been implicated in the pathogenesis of spontaneous preterm delivery. The Vaginal Infections and Prematurity Study showed that pregnant women colonised with *Trichomonas vaginalis* had a 30% higher risk of delivering an infant with low birthweight or delivering before term, a 40% higher risk of giving birth to an infant who was both preterm and of low birth weight, and nearly twice the risk of stillbirth or neonatal death, as compared with women without *Trichomonas vaginalis* colonisation (Cotch *et al.* 1997). Prospective studies have shown a significant association between periodontal infection and preterm birth (Jeffcoat *et al.* 2001). One pilot study has suggested that performing scaling and root planning in pregnant women with periodontitis may reduce preterm birth (Jeffcoat *et al.* 2003). Asymptomatic bacteriuria has been associated with preterm labour and antibiotic treatment of this is associated with a reduction in the incidence of preterm delivery (Smaill 2002).

There have been many randomised trials of antibiotics for the prevention of preterm labour in asymptomatic women, with disappointing results. Klebanoff *et al.* (2001) found that treatment of pregnant women with asymptomatic trichomoniasis, using oral metronidazole, does not prevent preterm delivery. Similarly, Carey *et al.* (2000) found that the treatment of asymptomatic bacterial vaginosis in pregnant women using oral metronidazole did not reduce the occurrence of preterm delivery or other adverse perinatal outcomes, whilst Kekki *et al.* (2001) found that vaginal clindamycin did not decrease the rate of preterm deliveries in women with asymptomatic bacterial vaginosis. The current evidence does not support screening and treating all pregnant women for bacterial vaginosis to prevent preterm labour. For women with a history of a previous preterm birth there is some suggestion that detection and treatment of bacterial vaginosis early in pregnancy may prevent a proportion of these women having a further preterm birth (Brocklehurst *et al.* 2002). The ORACLE trial, which was reported in 2001 (Kenyon *et al.* 2001), and which investigated the role of antibiotics in pregnant women in spontaneous preterm labour, concluded that antibiotics should not be routinely prescribed to women in spontaneous preterm labour without clinical evidence of infection or preterm, prelabour rupture of the fetal membranes.

Summary

Parturition requires the myometrium, which has been maintained in a state of relative quiescence during pregnancy, to develop coordinated contractions, and the cervix to dilate and allow passage of the fetus through the birth canal. Challis *et al.* (2000) have proposed that it is useful to divide the uterine phenotype during parturition into different stages, to facilitate understanding of the mechanisms controlling labour. During most of pregnancy, the myometrium is in a state of relative quiescence, and this corresponds to phase 0 of parturition. During this phase a variety of different inhibitors may act upon the myometrium; these include progesterone, relaxin, prostacyclin, nitric oxide and endogenous β-adrenergic agonists. The switch from myometrial quiescence to myometrial activation is described as phase 1 of parturition, and is essential to enable the muscle to respond to the stimulation provided by increasing levels of uterotonic agents. Further, the changes occurring during phase 1 allow the generation of synchronous, high-amplitude, high-frequency contractions of labour. Challis and Lye (1994) have proposed that myometrial activation results from coordinated expression of a variety of proteins, termed contraction-association proteins. These proteins include ion channels (Boyle *et al.* 1987), agonist receptors (e.g. for oxytocin and prostaglandins) (Negishi *et al.* 1995) and gap junctions (Garfield 1994). Stimulation corresponds to phase 2, when endogenous uterotonins, including oxytocin, prostaglandins and CRH, act on the activated myometrium. Postpartum involution of the uterus corresponds to phase 3 of parturition.

At present, most agents used in the management of preterm labour (inhibitors of prostaglandin synthesis, calcium channel blockers, oxytocin antagonists and β-adrenoceptor agonists), are directed at myometrial stimulation (phase 2), in which myometrial activation has already taken place. It seems likely that future strategies aimed at the diagnosis and management of preterm labour should address uterine activation (Challis *et al.* 2000).

REFERENCES

Allaire, A. D.. D'Andrea, N., Truong McMahon, M. J. and Lessey, B. A. (2001) Cervical stroma apoptosis in pregnancy. *Obstet. Gynecol.* **97**(3), 399–403.

Allen, J., Uldbjerg, N., Petersen, L. K. and Secher, N. J. (1989) Intracervical 17-β oestradiol before induction of second trimester abortion with a prostaglandin E_1 analogue. *Eur. J. Obstet. Gynecol. Reprod. Biol.* **32**, 123–7.

Alm, P., Alumets, J., Hakanson, R. and Sundler, F. (1977) Peptidergic (vasoactive intestinal peptide) nerves in the genito-urinary tract. *Neurosci.* **2**, 751–4.

Alm, P., Alumets, J., Brodin, G. *et al.* (1978) Peptidergic (substance P) nerves in the genito-urinary tract. *Neurosci.* **3**, 419–25.

Altabef, K. M., Spencer, J. T. and Zinberg, S. (1992) Intravenous nitroglycerin for uterine relaxation for an inverted uterus. *Am. J. Obstet. Gynecol.* **166**, 1237–8.

Ambrus, G. and Rao, Ch. V. (1994) Novel regulation of pregnant human myometrial smooth muscle cell gap junctions by human chorionic gonadotrophin. *Endocrinology* **135**, 2772–9.

Bacon, C. R., Morrison, J. J., O'Reilly, G., Cameron, I. T. and Davenport, A. P. (1995) ET_A and ET_B endothelin receptors in human myometrium characterised by the subtype selective ligands BQ123, BQ3020, FR139317 and PD151242. *J. Endocrinol.* **144**, 127–34.

Baggiolini, M., Wakz, A. and Kunkel, S. L. (1989) Neutrophil activating peptide-1/interleukin-8 a novel cytokine that activate neutrophils [review]. *J. Clin. Invest.* **246**, 1045–9.

Bansal, R. K., Goldsmith, P. C., He, Y. *et al.* (1997) A decline in myometrial nitric oxide synthase expression is associated with labor and delivery. *J. Clin. Invest.* **99**, 2502–8.

Bao, S., Rai, J. and Schreiber, J. (2001) Brain nitric oxide synthase expression is enhanced in the human cervix in labor. *J. Soc. Gynecol. Investig.* **8**(3), 158–64

(2002) Expression of nitric oxide synthase isoforms in human pregnant myometrium at term. *J. Soc. Gynecol. Investig.* **9**(6), 351–6.

Barclay, C. G., Brennand, J. E., Kelly, R. W. and Calder, A. A. (1993) Interleukin-8 production by the human cervix. *Am. J. Obstet. Gynecol.* **169**, 625–32.

Barnes, F. (1881) Hourglass contraction of the uterus treated with nitrate of amyl. *BMJ* **1**, 377.

Batra, S. (1994) Hormonal control of myometrial function. In T. Chard and J. G. Grudzinskas, eds., *The Uterus*. Cambridge: Cambridge University Press. 173–92.

Bayhi, D. A., Sherwood, C. D. and Campbell, C. E. (1992) Intravenous nitroglycerin for uterine inversion. *J. Clin. Anaesth.* **4**, 487–8.

Beck, P., Adler, P., Szlachter, N., Steinetz, B. G. and Weiss, G. (1978) Synergistic effect of human relaxin and progesterone concentration preceding normal labor. *Obstet. Gynecol.* **51**, 686–90.

Belfort, M. A. (1993) Intravenous nitroglycerin as a tocolytic agent for intrapartum external cephalic version. *S. Afr. Med. J.* **83**, 656.

Bell, R. J., Permezel, M., MacLennan, A. *et al.* (1993) A randomized, double-blind, placebo-controlled trial of the safety of vaginal recombinant human relaxin for cervical ripening. *Obstet. Gynecol.* **82**, 328–33.

Benedetto, C., Petraglia, F., Marozio, L. *et al.* (1994) Corticotropin-releasing hormone increases prostglandin $F_{2\alpha}$ activity on human myometrium. *Am. J. Obstet. Gynecol.* **171**, 126–31.

Bennett, P. R., Rose, M. P., Myatt, L. and Elder, M. G. (1987) Preterm labor: stimulation of arachidonic acid metabolism in human amnion cells by bacterial products. *Am. J. Obstet. Gynecol.* **156**(3), 649–55.

Bian, J. and Sun, Y. (1997) Transcriptional activation by p53 of the human type IV collagenase (gelatinase A or matrix metalloproteinase 2) promoter. *Mol. Cell. Biol.* **17**(11), 6330–8.

Bokstrom, H. and Norstrom, A. (1995) Effects of mifepristone and progesterone on collagen synthesis in the human uterine cervix. *Contraception* **51**, 249–54.

Bokstrom, H., Brannstrom, M., Alexandersson, M. and Norstrom, A. (1997) Leukocyte sub-populations in human uterine cervical stroma at early and term pregnancy. *Hum. Reprod.* **12**, 586–90.

Bottari, S. P., Vokaer, A., Kaivez, E., Lescrainier, J. P. and Vauquelin, G. (1985) Regulation of α- and β-adrenergic receptor subclasses by gonadal steroids in human myometrium. *Acta Physiol. Hung.* **65**, 335–46.

Bowen, J. M., Chamley, L., Keelan, J. A. and Mitchell, M. D. (2002) Cytokines of the placenta and extra-placental membranes: roles and regulation during human pregnancy and parturition. *Placenta* **23**(4), 257–73.

Boyle, M. B., MacLusky, N. J., Naftolin, F. and Kaczmarek, L. K. (1987) Hormonal regulation of K+-channel messenger RNA in rat myometrium during oestrus cycle and in pregnancy. *Nature* **330**(6146), 373–5.

Bozler, E. (1941) Influence of estrone on the electrical characteristics and the mobility of uterine muscle. *Endocrinology* **29**, 225–7.

Brennand, J. E., Calder, A. A., Leitch, C. R. *et al.* (1997) Recombinant human relaxin as a cervical ripening agent. *BJOG*, **104**, 775–80.

Brennand, J., Leask, R., Kelly, R., Greer, I. and Calder, A. (1998) The influence of amniotic fluid on prostaglandin synthesis and metabolism in human fetal membranes. *Acta Obstet. Gynecol. Scand.* **77**, 142–50.

Brocklehurst, P., Hannah, M. and McDonald, H. (2002) Interventions for treating bacterial vaginosis in pregnancy (Cochrane Review). In *The Cochrane Library*, Issue 3, Oxford: Update Software.

Bryant-Greenwood, G. D. and S. Y. Yamamoto (1995) Control of peripartal collagenolysis in the human chorion-decidua. *Am. J. Obstet. Gynecol.* **172**(1 Pt 1), 63–70.

Buhimschi, I., Yallampalli, C., Dong, Y-L. and Garfield, R. E. (1995) Involvement of a nitric oxide-cyclic guanosine monophosphate pathway in control of human uterine contractility during pregnancy. *Am. J. Obstet. Gynecol.* **172**, 1577–84.

Buhimschi, I., Ali, M., Jain, V., Chwalisz, K. and Garfield, R. E. (1996) Differential regulation of nitric oxide in the rat uterus and cervix during pregnancy in labour. *Hum. Reprod.* **11**, 1755–66.

Bulbring, E. and Tomito, T. (1987) Catecholamine action on smooth muscle. *Pharmacol. Rev.* **39**, 49–96.

Cabrol, D., Dubois, P., Sedbon, E. *et al.* (1987) Prostaglandin E_2-induced changes in the distribution of glycosaminoglycans in the isolated rat cervix. *Eur. J. Obstet. Gynecol.* **26**, 359–65.

Calder, A. A. (1980) Pharmacological management of the unripe cervix in the human. In F. Naftolin and P. G. Stubblefield, eds., *Dilatation of the Uterine Cervix*. New York: Raven Press, pp. 147–56.

(1994) The cervix during pregnancy. In T. Chard and J. G. Grudzinskas, eds., *The Uterus*. Cambridge: Cambridge University Press, pp. 288–307.

Calder, A. A. and Greer, I. A. (1991) Pharmacological modulation of cervical compliance in the first and second trimesters of pregnancy. *Semin. Perinatol.* **15**, 162–72.

(1992) Cervical physiology and induction of labour. In J. Bonnar, ed., *Recent Advances in Obstetrics and Gynaecology*. Edinburgh: Churchill Livingstone, **17**, 33–56.

Calixto, J. B. and Rae, G. A. (1991) Effects of endothelin, Bay K8644 and other oxytocics in non-pregnant and late pregnant rat isolated uterus. *Eur. J. Pharmacol.* **192**, 109–16.

Carbonne, B., Mignot, T. M., Tsatsaris, V. and Ferre, F. (1998) Changes in plasma and amniotic fluid endothelin levels during pregnancy: facts or artefacts? *Eur. J. Obstet. Gynecol. Reprod. Biol.* **76**(1), 15–19.

Carey, J. C., Klebanoff, M. A., Hauth, J. C. *et al.* (2000) Metronidazole to prevent preterm delivery in pregnant women with asymptomatic bacterial vaginosis. National Institute of Child Health and Human Development Network of Maternal-Fetal Medicine Units. *N. Engl. J. Med.* **342** 534–40.

Carsten, M. E. (1968) Regulation of myometrial composition, growth and activity. In N. S. Assali, ed., *The Maternal Organism, Vol 1 of the Biology of Gestation Series*. New York: Academic Press, pp. 355–425.

Carsten, M. E. and Miller, J. D. (1985) Calcium release by inositol trisphosphate from calcium-transporting microsomes derived from uterine sarcoplasmic reticulum. *Biochem. Biophys. Res. Commun.* **130**, 1027–31.

Casatella, M. N. (1995) The production of cytokines by polymorphonuclear neutrophils. *Immunol. Today* **16**, 21–6.

Casey, M. L. and MacDonald, P. C. (1988) Biomolecular processes in the onset of parturition: decidual activation. *Clin. Obstet. Gynecol.* **31**, 533–52.

(1993) Human parturition: distinction between the initiation of parturition and the onset of labor. *Semin. Reprod. Endocrinol.* **11**, 272–84.

Casey, M. L., Cox, S. M., Word, A. and MacDonald, P. C. (1990) Cytokines and infection-induced preterm labour. *Reprod. Fertil. Dev.* **2**, 499–510.

Challis, J. R. G. and Hooper, S. (1989) Birth: Outcome of a positive cascade. *Bailliere's Clin. Endocrinol. Metab.* **3**, 781–93.

Challis, J. R. G. and Lye, S. J. (1994) Parturition. In E. Knobil and J. D. Neil eds., *The Physiology of Reproduction.* New York: Raven Press, pp. 985–1031.

Challis, J. R. and Mitchell, M. D. (1994) Basic mechanisms of preterm labour. *Res. Clin. Forums* **16**, 39–58.

Challis, J. R. G., Matthews, S. G., Gibb, W. and Lye, S. J. (2000) Endocrine and paracrine regulation of birth at term and preterm. *Endocr. Rev.* **21**, 514–50.

Chanrachakul, B., Herabutya, Y. and Punyavachira, P. (2000) Randomized comparison of glyceryl trinitrate and prostaglandin E_2 for cervical ripening at term. *Obstet. Gynecol.* **96**, 549–53.

Chard, T., Boyd, N. R. H., Edwards, C. R. W. and Boyd, N. (1971) Release of oxytocin and vasopressin by human fetus during labour. *Nature (Lond.)* **234**, 352–4.

Chibbar, R., Miller, F. D. and Mitchell, B. F. (1993) Synthesis of oxytocin in amnion, chorion and decidua may influence the timing of human parturition. *J. Clin. Invest.* **91**, 185–92.

Chwalisz, K. (1988) Cervical ripening and induction of labour with progesterone antagonists. *Proceedings of the XI European Congress of Perinatal Medicine.* Rome: CIC Edizioni Internaziolini, p. 60.

(1994) The use of progesterone antagonists for cervical ripening as an adjunct to labour and delivery. *Hum. Reprod.* **9**, 131–63.

Chwalisz, K., Benson, M., Scholz, P. *et al.* (1994a) Cervical ripening with the cytokines interleukin 8, interleukin 1β and tumour necrosis factor α in guinea pigs. *Hum. Reprod.* **9**, 2173–81.

Chwalisz, K., Ciesla, I. and Garfield, R. E. (1994b) Inhibition of nitric oxide (NO) synthesis induces preterm parturition and pre-eclampsia-like conditions in guinea pigs. *Soc. Gynecol. Investig., 41st Annual Meeting.* A36.

Chwalisz, K., Buhimschi, I. and Garfield R. E. (1996) Role of nitric oxide in obstetrics. *Prenat. Neonat. Med.* **1**, 292–329.

Chwalisz, K., Shao-Qing, S., Garfield, R. E. and Bier, H. M. (1997) Cervical ripening in guinea-pigs after a local application of nitric oxide. *Hum. Reprod.* **12**, 2093–101.

Coburn RF. (1987) Stretch-induced membrane depolarization in ferret trachealis smooth muscle cells. *J. Appl. Physiol.* **62**, 2320–5.

Colditz, I. G. (1990) Effects of exogenous prostaglandin E_2 and actinomycin-D on plasma leakage induced by neutrophil activating peptide-1/interleukin-8. *Immunol. Cell. Biol.* **68**, 397–403.

Cole, W. C., Garfield, R. E. and Kirkaldy, J. S. (1988) Gap junctions and direct intercellular communication between rat uterine smooth muscle cells. *Am. J. Physiol.* **249**, C20–31.

Cotch, M. F., Pastorek, J. G. 2nd, Nugent, R. P., *et al.* (1997) Trichomonas vaginalis associated with low birth weight and preterm delivery. The Vaginal Infections and Prematurity Study Group. *Sex. Transm. Dis.* **24**, 353–60.

Crankshaw, D. J., Crankshaw, J., Brenda, L. A. and Daniel, E. E. (1979) Receptors for E type prostaglandins in the plasma membrane of non-pregnant myometrium. *Arch. Biochem. Biophys.* **198**, 459–65.

Csapo, A. L. (1956) Progesterone 'block'. *Am. J. Anat.* **98**, 273–91.

(1977) The "see-saw" theory of parturition. *Ciba Found. Symp.* **47**, 159–210.

Danforth, D. N., Buckingham, J. C. and Roddick, J. W. (1960) Connective tissue changes incident to cervical effacement. *Am. J. Obstet. Gynecol.* **86**, 939–45.

Danforth, D. N., Veis, A., Breen, M. *et al.* (1974) The effect of pregnancy and labor on the human cervix: changes in collagen, glycoproteins and glycosaminoglycans. *Am. J. Obstet. Gynecol.* **120**, 641–9.

David, M., Halle, H., Lichtenegger, W., Sinha, P. and Zimmermann, T. (1998) Nitroglycerin to facilitate fetal extraction during cesarean delivery. *Obstet. Gynecol.* **91**, 119–24.

Dawood, M. Y. and Khan-Dawood, F. S. (1985) Oxytocin. In R. F. Shearman, ed., *Clinical Reproductive Endocrinology.* New York: Churchill Livingstone. 233–49.

Dayan, S. S. and Schwalbe, S. S. (1996) The use of small dose intravenous nitroglycerin in a case of uterine inversion. *Anesth. Analg.* **82**, 1091–3.

Denison, F. C., Riley, S. C., Elliott, C. L. *et al.* (2000) The effect of mifepristone administration on leukocyte populations, matrix metalloproteinases and inflammatory mediators in the first trimester cervix. *Mol. Hum. Reprod.* **6**(6), 541–8.

Dennes, W. J., Slater, D. M., Poston, L. and Bennett, P. R. (1999) Myometrial nitric oxide synthase messenger ribonucleic acid expression does not change throughout gestation or with the onset of labor. *Am. J. Obstet. Gynecol.* **180**(2 Pt 1), 387–92.

Di Iulio, J. L., Gude, N. M., King, R. G. and Brennecke, S. P. (1995) Human placental and fetal membrane nitric oxide synthase activity before, during, and after labor at term. *Reprod. Fertil. Dev.* **7**, 1505–8.

Di Liberto, G., Dallot, E., Eude-Le Parco, I. *et al.* (2003) A critical role for PKC zeta in endothelin-1-induced uterine contractions at the end of pregnancy. *Am. J. Physiol. Cell. Physiol.* **285**, C599–607.

Diamond, J. (1990) Beta-adrenoreceptors, cyclic AMP and cyclic GMP in control of uterine motility. In M. E. Carsten and J. D. Miller, eds., *Uterine Function: Molecular and Cellular Aspects.* New York: Plenum Press, pp. 249–75.

Ding, J. Q., Granberg, S. and Norstrom, A. (1990) Clinical effects and cervical tissue changes after treatment with 16, 16 dimethyl-trans delta 2 PGE_1 methylester. *Prostaglandins* **39**, 281–5.

Dombroski, R. A., Woodard, D. S., Harper, M. J. and Gibbs, R. S. (1990) A rabbit model for bacteria-induced preterm pregnancy loss. *Am. J. Obstet. Gynecol.* **163**(6 Pt 1), 1938–43.

Duckitt, K. and Thornton, S. (2002) Nitric oxide donors for the treatment of preterm labour. *Cochrane Database Syst. Rev.* 3, CD002860.

Egarter, C. H. and Husslein, P. (1992) Biochemistry of myometrial contractility. *Clin. Obstet. Gynecol.* **6**, 755–69.

Ekerhovd, E., Weijdegard, B., Brannstrom, M., Mattsby-Baltzer, I. and Norstrom, A. (2002) Nitric oxide induced cervical ripening in the human: Involvement of cyclic guanosine monophosphate, prostaglandin F(2 alpha), and prostaglandin E(2). *Am. J. Obstet. Gynecol.* **186**(4), 745–50.

Ekman, G., Malmstrom, A. and Uldbjerg, N. (1986) Cervical collagen: an important regulator of cervical function in term labour. *Obstet. Gynecol.* **67**, 633–6.

El Maradny, E., Kanayama, N., Halim, A. *et al.* (1994) Interleukin-8 induces cervical ripening in rabbits. *Am. J. Obstet. Gynecol.* **171**, 77–83.

(1995) The effect of interleukin-1 in rabbit cervical ripening. *Eur. J. Obstet. Gynecol. Reprod. Biol.* **60**, 75–80.

Ellwood, D. A., Mitchell, M. D. and Anderson, A. B. M. (1980) The in vitro production of prostanoids by the human cervix during pregnancy: preliminary observations. *BJOG*, **87**, 210–14.

Ellwood, D. A., Anderson, A. B. M., Mitchell, M. D. *et al.* (1981) Prostanoids, collagenase and cervical softening in sheep. In D. A. Ellwood and A. B. M. Anderson, eds., *The Cervix in Pregnancy and Labour: Clinical and Biochemical Investigations.* Edinburgh: Churchill Livingstone, pp. 57–73.

Erkinheimo, T. L., Saukkonen, K., Narko, K. *et al.* (2000) Expression of cyclo-oxygenase-2 and prostanoid receptors by human myometrium. *J. Clin. Endocrinol. Metab.* **85**(9), 3468–75.

Eude, I., Paris, B., Cabrol, D., Ferre, F. and Breuiller-Fouche, M. (2000) Selective protein kinase C isoforms are involved in endothelin-1-induced human uterine contraction at the end of pregnancy. *Biol. Reprod.* **63**(5), 1567–73.

Evans, M. I., Dougan, M. B., Moawad, A. H. *et al.* (1983) Ripening of the human cervix with porcine ovarian relaxin. *Am. J. Obstet. Gynecol.* **147**, 410–14.

Facchinetti, F., Piccinini, F. and Volpe, A. (2000) Chemical ripening of the cervix with intra-cervical application of sodium nitroprusside: a randomized controlled trial. *Hum. Reprod.* **15**(10), 2224–7.

Flint, A. P. F. (1979) Role of progesterone and estrogen in the control of the onset of labor in man: a continuing controversy. In M. J. N. C. Keirse, A. B. M. Anderson and J. Bennebroek-Gravenhorst, eds., *Human Parturition. New Concepts and Developments.* The Netherlands: Leiden University Press, pp. 85–100.

Flint, A. P. F., Anderson, A. B. M., Steele, P. A. and Turnbull, A. C. (1975) The mechanism by which fetal cortisol controls the onset of parturition in the sheep. *Biochem. Soc. Trans.* **3**, 1189–94.

Florio, P., Woods, R. J., Genazzani, A. R., Lowry, P. J. and Petraglia, F. (1997) Changes in amniotic immunoreactive corticotrophin-releasing factor (CFR) and CRF-binding protein levels in pregnant women at term and during labor. *J. Clin. Endocrinol. Metab.* **82**, 835–8.

Fortunato, S. J. and Menon, R. (2001). Distinct molecular events suggest different pathways for preterm labor and premature rupture of membranes. *Am. J. Obstet. Gynecol.* **184**, 1399–405; discussion 1405–6.

Fortunato, S. J., Menon, R., Bryant, C. *et al.* (2000). Programmed cell death (apoptosis) as a possible pathway to metalloproteinase activation and fetal membrane degradation in premature rupture of membranes. *Am. J. Obstet. Gynecol.* **182**(6), 1468–76.

Fosang, A. J., Handley, C. J., Santer, V., Lowther, D. A. and Thorburn, G. D. (1984) Pregnancy-related changes in the connective tissue of the ovine cervix. *Biol. Reprod.* **30** 1223–35.

Fuchs, A. R. (1978) Hormonal control of myometrial function during pregnancy and parturition. *Acta Endocrinol.* **221**, 3–71.

Fuchs, F. and Stakeman, G. (1960) Treatment of threatened premature labour with large doses of progesterone. *Am. J. Obstet. Gynecol.* **79**, 172–6.

Fuchs, A. R., Fuchs, F., Husslein, P. and Soloff, M. S. (1984) Oxytocin receptors in the human uterus during pregnancy and parturition. *Am. J. Obstet. Gynecol.* **150**, 734–41.

Garfield, R. E. (1984) Myometrial ultrastructure and uterine contractility. In S. Bottari, J. P. Thomas and A. Vokaer, eds., *Uterine Contractility*. New York: Mason, pp. 81–109.

(1994) Role of cell-to-cell coupling in control of myometrial contractility and labor. In R. E. Garfield and T. N. Tabb, eds., *Control of Uterine Contractility*. Boca Raton: CRC Press, pp. 39–81.

Garfield, R. E., and Hayashi, R. H. (1981) Appearance of gap junctions in the myometrium of women during labor. *Am. J. Obstet. Gynecol.* **140**, 254–60.

Garfield, R. E. and Somlyo, A. P. (1985) Structure of smooth muscle. In A. K. Groves and E. E. Daniel, eds., Calcium and Contractility. Clifton, NJ: Humana Press, pp.1–36.

Garfield, R. E. and Yallampalli, C. (1994) Structure and function of uterine muscle. In T. Chard and J. G. Grudzinskas, eds., *The Uterus*. Cambridge: Cambridge University Press, pp .54–93.

Garfield, R. E., Sims, S. M., Daniel, E. E. (1977) Gap junctions: their presence and necessity in myometrium during parturition. *Science*, **198**, 958–960.

Germain, A. M., Smith, J., Casey, M. L. and MacDonald, P. C. (1994) Human fetal membrane contribution to the prevention of parturition: uterotonin degradation. *J. Clin. Endocrinol. Metab.* **78**, 463–70.

Gibbins, I. L., Furness, J. B., Costa, M. *et al.* (1985) Co-localization of calcitonin gene-related peptide-like immunoreactivity with substance P in cutaneous, vascular and visceral sensory neurons of guinea pigs. *Neurosci. Lett.* **57**, 125–30.

Goldenberg, R., Mercer, B., Meis, P. J. *et al.* (1996). "The preterm preduction study: fetal fibronectin testing and spontanous preterm birth." *Obstet. Gynecol.* **87**, 643–8.

Goldenberg, R. L. and Rouse, D. J. (1998) Prevention of premature birth. *N. Engl. J. Med.* **339**, 313–320.

Golichowski, A. (1980) Cervical stromal interstitial polysaccharide metabolism in pregnancy. In F. Naftolin and P. G. Stubblefield, eds., *Dilatation of the Uterine Cervix: Connective Tissue Biology and Clinical Management*. New York: Raven Press, pp. 99–112.

Gomez, R., Romero, R., Mazor, M. *et al.* (1997) The role of infection in preterm labour and delivery. In M. G. Elder, R. Romero and R. F. Lamont, eds., *Preterm Labor*. New York: Churchill Livingstone, pp. 85–126.

Gordon, A. J. and Calder, A. A. (1977) Oestradiol applied locally to ripen the unfavourable cervix. *Lancet* **ii**, 1319–21.

Granstrom, L., Ekman, G., Ulmsten, U. and Malmstrom, A. (1989) Changes in connective tissue of corpus and cervix uteri during ripening and labour in term pregnancy. *BJOG* **96**, 1198–202.

Greer, I. A. (1992) Cervical ripening. In J. O. Drife and A. A. Calder, eds., *Prostaglandins and the Uterus*. London: Springer-Verlag, pp. 191–209.

Gupta, J. K. and Johnson, N. (1990) Effect of mifepristone on dilatation of the pregnant and non-pregnant cervix. *Lancet* **i**, 1238–40.

Guzick, D. S. and Winn, K. (1985) The association of chorioamnionitis with preterm delivery. *Obstet. Gynecol.* **65**, 11–16.

Hansen, W. R., Keelan, J. A., Skinner, S. J. and Mitchell, M. D. (1999). Key enzymes of prostaglandin biosynthesis and metabolism. Coordinate regulation of expression by cytokines in gestational tissues: a review. *Prostaglandins Other Lipid Mediat.* **57**, 243–57.

Harder, D. R., Gilbert, R. and Lombard, J. H. (1987) Vascular muscle cell depolarization and activation in renal arteries on elevation of transmural pressure. *Am. J. Physiol.* **253**(4 Pt 2), F778–81.

Heddleston, L., McDuffie, R. S. Jr. and Gibbs, R. S. (1993) A rabbit model for ascending infection in pregnancy: intervention with indomethacin and delayed ampicillin-sulbactam therapy. *Am. J. Obstet. Gynecol.* **169**, 708–12.

Hegele-Hartung, C., Chwalisz, K., Beier, H. M. and Elger, W. (1989) Ripening of the uterine cervix of the guinea-pig after treatment with the progesterone antagonist onapristone (ZK98.299): an electron microscopic study. *Hum. Reprod.* **4**, 369–77.

Hillhouse, E. W., Grammatopoulos, D., Milton, N. G. N. and Quartero, H. W. P. (1993) The identification of a human myometrial corticotrophin releasing hormone receptor that increases in affinity during pregnancy. *J. Clin. Endocrinol. Metab.* **76**, 736–41.

Hillier, K. and Karim, S. M. M. (1970) The human isolated cervix: a study of its spontaneous motility and responsiveness to drugs. *Br. J. Pharmacol.* **40**, 576–7.

Hoffman, B. B., Lavin, T. N., Lefkowitz, R. J. and Ruffolo, R. R. (1981) Alpha adrenergic subtypes in rabbit uterus: mediation of myometrial contraction and regulation by estrogens. *J. Pharmacol. Exp. Ther.* **219**, 290–5.

Honore, J. C., Robert, B., Vacher-Lavenu, M. C. *et al.* (2000) Expression of endothelin receptors in human myometrium during pregnancy and in uterine leiomyomas. *J. Cardiovasc. Pharmacol.* **36**(5 Suppl 1), S386–9

Horton, E. W. and Poyser, N. (1976) Uterine luteolytic hormone: a physiological role for prostaglandin $F_{2\alpha}$. *Physiol. Rev.* **56**, 595–651.

Huang, W. M., Gu, J., Blank, M. A. *et al.* (1984) Peptide-immunoreactive nerves in the mammalian female genital tract. *Histochem. J.* **16**, 1297–310.

Hurwitz, L. (1986) Pharmacology of calcium channels and smooth muscle. *Ann. Rev. Pharmacol. Toxicol.* **26**, 225–58.

Huxley, H. E. (1971) The structural basis of muscular contraction. *Proc. R. Soc. Lond. [series B]* **178**, 131–49.

Inoue, Y., Nakao, K., Obabi, K. *et al.* (1990) Some electrical properties of human pregnant myometrium. *Am. J. Obstet. Gynecol.* **162**, 1090–98.

Ito, A., Kitamura, K., Mori, Y. and Hirakawa, S. (1979) The change in solubility of type 1 collagen in human cervix in pregnancy at term. *Biochem. Med.* **21**, 262–70.

Ito, A., Sato, T., Iga, T. and Mori Y. (1990) Tumor necrosis factor bifunctionally regulates matrix metalloproteinases and tissue inhibitor of metalloproteinases (TIMP) production by human fibroblasts. *FEBS Lett.* **269**(1), 93–5.

Izumi, H., Yallampalli, C. and Garfield, R. E. (1993) Gestational changes in L-arginine-induced relaxation of pregnant rat and human myometrial smooth muscle. *Am. J. Obstet. Gynecol.* **169**, 1327–37.

Jeffcoat, M. K., Geurs, N. C., Reddy, M. S. *et al.* (2001) Periodontal infection and preterm birth: results of a prospective study. *J. Am. Dent. Assoc.* **132**, 875–80.

Jeffcoat, M. K., Hauth, J. C., Geurs, N. C. *et al.* (2003) Periodontal disease and preterm birth: results of a pilot intervention study. *J. Periodontol.* **74**, 1214–18.

Jeffrey, J. J. (1991) Collagen and collagenase: pregnancy and parturition. *Semin. Perinatol.* **15**, 118–12.

Jeffrey, J. J., Coffrey, R. J. and Eizen, A. Z. (1971) Studies of uterine collagenase in tissue culture II. Effect of steroid hormones on enzyme production. *Biochim. Biophys. Acta.* **252**, 143–9.

Jeffrey, J. J. and Koob, T. J. (1980) Endocrine control of collagen degradation in the uterus. In F. Naftolin and P. G. Stubblefield, eds., *Dilatation of the Uterine Cervix*. New York: Raven Press, pp. 135–45.

Johansson, B. and Mellander, S. (1975) Static and dynamic components in the vascular myogenic response to passive changes in length as revealed by electrical and mechanical recordings from the rat portal vein. *Circ Res.* **36**(1), 76–83

Johnson, R. F., Mitchell, C. M., Giles, W. B., Walters, W. A. and Zakar, T. (2002) The in vivo control of prostaglandin H synthase-2 messenger ribonucleic acid expression in the human amnion at parturition. *J. Clin. Endocrinol. Metab.* **87**, 2816–23.

Johnston, T. A., Hodson, S., Greer, I. A., Kelly, R. W. and Calder, A. A. (1993) Plasma glycos-aminoglycan and prostaglandin concentrations before and after the onset of spontaneous labour. In *Prostaglandins in Reproduction*. (Proceedings of the Third European Congress), Edinburgh.

Jones, S. A. and Challis, J. R. G. (1989) Local stimulation of prostaglandin production by corticotrophin releasing hormone in human fetal membranes and placenta. *Biochem. Biophys. Res. Commun.* **159**, 192–4.

Junqueira, L. C. U., Zugaib, M. Montes, G. S. *et al.* (1980) Morphological and histochemical evidence for the occurrence of collagenolysis and for the role of neutrophilic polymorpho-nuclear leukocytes during cervical dilatation. *Am. J. Obstet. Gynecol.* **138**, 273–81.

Karalis, K., Goodwin, G. and Majzoub, J. A. (1996) Cortisol blockade of progesterone: a possible molecular mechanism involved in the initiation of human parturition. *Nature Med.* **2**, 556–60.

Katsura, M., Ito, A., Hirakawa *et al.* (1989). Human recombinant interleukin-1 alpha increases biosynthesis of collagenase and hyaluronic acid in cultured human chorionic cells. *FEBS Lett.* **244**(2), pp.315–18.

Keelan, J. A., Myatt, L. and Mitchell, M. D. (1997) Endocrinology and paracrinology of parturition. In M. G. Elder, R. Romero, and R. F. Lamont, eds., *Preterm Labor*. New York: Churchill Livingstone, pp. 457–91.

Keirse, M. J. N. C. (1979) Endogenous prostaglandins in human parturition. In M. J. N. C. Keirse, A. B. M. Anderson and J. Bennebroek-Gravenhorst, eds., *Human Parturition. New Concepts and Developments*. The Netherlands: Leiden University Press, pp. 101–42.

Keirse, M. J. N. (1990) Progestogen administration in pregnancy may prevent preterm delivery. *BJOG.* **97**, 149–54.

Keirse, M. J. N. C. (1995) New perspectives for the effective treatment of preterm labor. *Am. J. Obstet. Gynecol.* **173**, 618–28.

Kekki, M., Kurki, T., Pelkonen, J. *et al.* (2001) Vaginal clindamycin in preventing preterm birth and peripartal infections in asymptomatic women with bacterial vaginosis: a randomized, controlled trial. *Obstet. Gynecol.* **97**, 643–8.

Kelly, R. W. (1996) Inflammatory mediators and parturition. *J. Reprod. Fertil.* **106**, 89–96.

Kelly, R. W. and Bukman, A. (1990) Antiprogestagenic inhibition of uterine prostaglandin inactivation: a permissive mechanism for uterine stimulation. *J. Steroid Biochem. Mol. Biol.* **37**, 37–101.

Kelly, R. W., Healy, D. L., Cameron, I. T. *et al.* (1986) The stimulation of prostaglandin production by two antiprogesterone steroids in human endometrial cells. *J. Clin. Endocrinol. Metab.* **62**, 1116–23.

Kelly, A. J., Kavanagh, J. and Thomas, J. (2001) Relaxin for cervical ripening and induction of labour. *Cochrane Database Syst. Rev.* 2, CD003103.

Kenyon, S. L., Taylor, D. J. and Tarnow-Mordi, W.; ORACLE Collaborative Group. (2001) Broad-spectrum antibiotics for spontaneous preterm labour: the ORACLE II randomised trial. ORACLE Collaborative Group. *Lancet* **357**(9261), 989–94.

Khan-Dawood, F. S. and Dawood, M. Y. (1984) Estrogen and progesterone receptor and hormone levels in human myometrium and placenta in term pregnancy. *Am. J. Obstet. Gynecol.* **150**, 501–5.

Kinsler, V. A., Thornton, S., Ashford, M. L., Melin, P. and Smith, S. K. (1996) The effect of the oxytocin antagonists F314 and F792 on the in vitro contractility of human myometrium. *BJOG* **103**(4), 373–5.

Klebanoff, M. A., Carey, J. C., Hauth, J. C. *et al.*; National Institute of Child Health and Human Development Network of Maternal-Fetal Medicine Units. (2001) Failure of metronidazole to prevent preterm delivery among pregnant women with asymptomatic *Trichomonas vaginalis* infection. *N. Engl. J. Med.* **345**(7), 487–93.

Kleissl, H. P., van der Rest, M., Naftolin, F., Glorieux, F. H. and De Leon, A. (1978) Collagen changes in human cervix at parturition. *Am. J. Obstet. Gynecol.* **130**, 748–53.

Kokenyesi, R. and Woessner, J. R. (1990) Relationship between dilatation rate of the uterine cervix and a small dermatan sulfate proteoglycan. *Biol. Reprod.* **42**, 87–9.

Krantz, K. E. (1959) Innervation of the human uterus. *Ann. N.Y. Acad. Sci.* **75**, 770–84.

Kupittayanant, S., Luckas, M. J. and Wray, S. (2002) Effect of inhibiting the sarcoplasmic reticulum on spontaneous and oxytocin-induced contractions of human myometrium. *BJOG* **109**, 289–96.

Kurki, T., Laatikainen, T., Salminen-Lappalainen, K. and Ylikorkala, O. (1991) Maternal plasma corticotrophin releasing hormone is elevated in preterm labour but unaffected by indomethacin or nylidrin. *BJOG* **98**, 685–91.

Ledger, W. L., Webster, M., Harrison, L. P. *et al.* (1985) Increase in cervical extensibility during labor induced after isolation of the uterus in the pregnant sheep. *Am. J. Obstet. Gynecol.* **151**, 397–402.

Ledingham, M. A., Denison, F. C., Kelly, R. W., Young, A. and Norman, J. E. (1999) Nitric oxide donors stimulate prostaglandin F(2alpha) and inhibit thromboxane B(2) production in the human cervix during the first trimester of pregnancy. *Mol. Hum. Reprod.* **5**(10), 973–82.

Ledingham, M. A., Thomson, A. J., Greer, I. A. and Norman, J. E. (2000a) Nitric oxide in parturition. *BJOG* **107**(5), 581–93.

Ledingham, M. A., Thomson, A. J., Young, A. *et al.* (2000b) Changes in the expression of nitric oxide synthase in the human uterine cervix during pregnancy and parturition. *Mol. Hum. Reprod.* **6**, 1041–8.

Ledingham, M. A., Thomson, A. J., Jordan, F. *et al.* (2001) Changes in cell adhesion molecule expression in the human uterine cervix and myometrium during pregnancy and parturition. *Obstet. Gynecol.* **97**, 235–42.

Lee, J. H. and Chang, K. C. (1995) Different sensitivity to nitric oxide of human pregnant and non-pregnant myometrial contractility. *Pharmacol. Commun.* **5**, 147–54.

Lees, C., Campbell, S., Jauniaux, E. *et al.* (1994) Arrest of preterm labour and prolongation of gestation with glyceryl trinitrate, a nitric oxide donor. *Lancet* **343**, 1325–6.

Lelaidier, C., Baton, C., Benifla, J. L. *et al.* (1994). Mifepristone for labour induction after previous Caesarean section. *BJOG* **101**, 501–3.

Leppert, P. C. (1992) Cervical softening, effacement and dilatation: A complex biochemical cascade. *J. Mat. Fet. Med.* **1**, 213–23.

   (1995) Anatomy and physiology of cervical ripening. *Clin. Obstet. Gynecol.* **38**, 267–79.

   (1998) Proliferation and apoptosis of fibroblasts and smooth muscle cells in rat uterine cervix throughout gestation and the effect of the antiprogesterone onapristone. *Am. J. Obstet. Gynecol.* **178**, 713–25.

Leppert, P. C. and Yu, S. Y. (1994) Apoptosis in the cervix of pregnant rats in association with cervical softening. *Gynecol. Obstet. Invest.* **37**, 150–4.

Liggins, G. C. (1978) Ripening of the cervix. *Semin. Perinatol.* **2**, 261–71.

   (1981) Cervical ripening as an inflammatory reaction. In D. A. Ellwood and A. B. M. Anderson, eds., The Cervix in Pregnancy and Labour: Clinical and Biochemical Investigations. Edinburgh: Churchill Livingstone, pp. 1–9.

   (1994) Mechanisms of the onset of labor: the New Zealand perspective. *Aust. N. Z. J. Obstet. Gynaecol.* **34**, 338–42.

Lindahl, U. and Hook, M. (1978) Glycosaminoglycans and their binding to biological macro-molecules. *Ann. Rev. Biochem.* **47**, 385–417.

Locksmith, G. J., Clark, P., Duff, P., Saade, G. R. and Schultz, G. S. (2001). Amniotic fluid concentrations of matrix metalloproteinase 9 and tissue inhibitor of metalloproteinase 1 during pregnancy and labor. *Am. J. Obstet. Gynecol.* **184**, 159–64.

Lockwood, C. J., Krikun, G., Aigner, S. and Schatz, F. (1996) Effects of thrombin on steroid-modulated cultured endometrial stromal cell fibrinolytic potential. *J. Clin. Endocrinol. Metab.* **81**, 107–12.

Lye, S. J., Nicholson, B. J., Mascarenhas, M., MacKenzie, L. and Petrocelli, T. (1993) Increased expression of connexin-43 in the rat myometrium during labor is associated with an increase in the plasma estrogen:progesterone ratio. *Endocrinology*, **132**, 2380–6.

McKeown, K. J. and Challis, J. R. (2003) Regulation of 15-hydroxy prostaglandin dehydrogenase by corticotrophin-releasing hormone through a calcium-dependent pathway in human chorion trophoblast cells. *J. Clin. Endocrinol. Metab.* **88**, 1737–41.

McLaren, J., Malak, T. M. and Bell, S. C. (1999) Structural characteristics of term human fetal membranes prior to labour: identification of an area of altered morphology overlying the cervix. *Hum. Reprod.* **14**, 237–41.

McLaren, J., Taylor, D. J. and Bell, S. C. (2000a) Increased concentration of pro-matrix metalloproteinase 9 in term fetal membranes overlying the cervix before labor: implications for membrane remodelling and rupture. *Am. J. Obstet. Gynecol.* **182**(2), 409–16.

   (2000b) Prostaglandin E(2)-dependent production of latent matrix metalloproteinase-9 in cultures of human fetal membranes. *Mol. Hum. Reprod.* **6**(11), 1033–40.

McLean, M., Thompson, D., Zhang, H-P., Brinsmead, M. and Smith, R. (1994) Corticotrophin releasing hormone and beta-endorphin in labour. *Eur. J. Endocrinol.* **131**, 167–72.

McLean, M., Bisits, A., Davis, J. *et al.* (1995) A placental clock controlling the length of human pregnancy. *Nature Med.* **1**, 460–3.

MacLennan, A. H., Green, R. C., Bryant-Greenwood, G. D., Greenwood, F. C. and Seamark, R. F. (1980) Ripening of the human cervix and induction of labour with purified porcine relaxin. *Lancet* **i**, 220–3.

McMurty, J. P., Floerscheim, G. L. and Bryant-Greenwood, G. D. (1980) Characterization of the binding of 125I-labelled succinylated porcine relaxin in human and mouse fibroblasts. *J. Reprod. Fertil.* **58**, 43–9.

McParland, P. C., Bell, S. C., Prinsle, J. H. *et al.* (2001). Regional and cellular localization of osteonectin/SPARC expression in connective tissue and cytotrophoblastic layers of human fetal membranes at term. *Mol. Hum. Reprod.* **7**, 463–74.

Magann, E. F., Perry, K. G., Dockery, J. R. *et al.* (1995) Cervical ripening before medical induction of labor: A comparison of prostaglandin E$_2$, estradiol, and oxytocin. *Am. J. Obstet. Gynecol.* **172**, 1702–8.

Malak, T. M. and Bell, S. C. (1994). Structural characteristics of term human fetal membranes: a novel zone of extreme morphological alteration within the rupture site. *BJOG* **101**(5), 375–86.

Malak, T. M., Ockleford, C. D., Bell, S. C. *et al.* (1993). Confocal immunofluorescence localization of collagen types I, III, IV, V and VI and their ultrastructural organization in term human fetal membranes. *Placenta* **14**(4), 385–406.

Malak, T., Mulholland, G., Bell, S. C. (1994). Morphometric characteristics of the decidua, cytotrophoblast, and connective tissue of the prelabor ruptured fetal membranes. *Ann. NY Acad. Sci.* **734**, 430–2.

Manabe, Y., Yoshimura, S., Mori, T. and Aso, T. (1985) Plasma levels of 13,14-dihydro-15-keto prostaglandin F2 alpha, estrogens, and progesterone during stretch-induced labor at term. *Prostaglandins* **30**(1), 141–52.

Marc, S., Leiber, D. and Harbon, S. (1986) Carbachol and oxytocin stimulate the generation of inositol phosphates in the guinea pig myometrium. *FEBS Lett.* **201**, 9–14.

Matsuo, K., Gokita, T., Karibe, H. and Uchida, M. K. (1989) Calcium independent contraction of uterine smooth muscle. *Biochem. Biophys. Res. Commun.* **155**, 722–7.

Mayer, D. C. and Weeks, S. K. (1992) Antepartum uterine relaxation with nitroglycerin at Caesarean delivery. *Can. J. Anaesth.* **39**, 166–9.

Maymon, E., Romero, R., Pacora, P. *et al.* (2000a). Evidence for the participation of interstitial collagenase (matrix metalloproteinase 1) in preterm premature rupture of membranes. *Am. J. Obstet. Gynecol.* **183**(4), 914–20.

(2000b). Matrilysin (matrix metalloproteinase 7) in parturition, premature rupture of membranes, and intrauterine infection. *Am. J. Obstet. Gynecol.* **182**(6), 1545–53.

(2000c). Evidence of in vivo differential bioavailability of the active forms of matrix metalloproteinases 9 and 2 in parturition, spontaneous rupture of membranes, and intra-amniotic infection. *Am. J. Obstet. Gynecol.* **183**(4), 887–94.

(2000d). Human neutrophil collagenase (matrix metalloproteinase 8) in parturition, premature rupture of the membranes, and intrauterine infection. *Am. J. Obstet. Gynecol.* **183**(1), 94–9.

Mercier, F. J., Dounas, M., Bouaziz, H., Lhuissier, C. and Benhamou, D. (1997) Intravenous nitroglycerin to relieve intrapartum fetal distress related to uterine hyperactivity: a prospective observational study. *Anesth. Analg.* **84**, 1117–20.

Meis, P. J., Klebanoff, M., Thom, E. *et al.* National National Institute of Child Health and Human Development Maternal-Fetal Medicine Units Network. (2003) Prevention of recurrent preterm delivery by 17 alpha-hydroxyprogesterone caproate. *N. Engl. J. Med.* **348**(24), 2379–85.

Mesiano, S., Chan, E. C., Fitter, J. T. *et al.* (2002) Progesterone withdrawal and estrogen activation in human parturition are coordinated by progesterone receptor A expression in the myometrium. *J. Clin. Endocrinol. Metab.* **87**(6), 2924–30.

Millar, L. K., Stollberg, J., DeBuque, L. and Bryant-Greenwood, G. (2000) Fetal membrane distention: determination of the intrauterine surface area and distention of the fetal membranes preterm and at term. *Am. J. Obstet. Gynecol.* **182**, 128–34.

Mitchell, B. F. and Schmid, B. (2001) Oxytocin and its receptor in the process of parturition. *J. Soc. Gynecol. Investig.* **8**, 122–33.

Mitchell, B. F. and Olson, D. M. (2004) Prostaglandin endoperoxide H synthase inhibitors and other tocolytics in preterm labour. *Prostaglandins Leukot. Essent. Fatty Acids* **70** 167–87.

Mitchell, M. D. (1984) The mechanisms of human parturition. *J. Develop. Physiol.* **6**, 107–18.

Monir-Bishty, E., Pierce, S. J., Kupittayanant, S., Shmygol, A. and Wray, S. (2003) The effects of metabolic inhibition on intracellular calcium and contractility of human myometrium. *BJOG*, **110**, 1050–6.

Morrison, J. J. (1996) Physiology and pharmacology of uterine contractility. In P. M. S. O'Brien, ed., *The Yearbook of the RCOG, 1996*. London: RCOG Press, pp. 45–61.

Morrison, J. J. and Smith, S. K. (1994) Prostaglandins and uterine activity. In J. G. Grudinskas and J. L. Yovich, eds., *Cambridge Reviews in Human Reproduction: Uterine Physiology*. Cambridge: Cambridge University Press, pp. 230–51.

Naeye, R. L. and Peters, E. C. (1980) Causes and consequences of premature rupture of fetal membranes. *Lancet.* **1**(8161), 192–4.

Nathan, C. F. (1987) Secretory products of macrophages. *J. Clin. Invest.* **79**, 319–20.

Nathan, C. (1992) Nitric oxide as a secretory product of mammalian cells. *FASEB J.* **6**, 3051–64.

Nathanielsz, P. and Honnebier, M. (1992) Myometrial function. In J. Drife and A. Calder, eds., *Prostaglandins and the Uterus*. London: Springer-Verlag, pp. 161–76.

Negishi, M., Sugimoto, Y. and Ichikawa, A. (1995) Molecular mechanisms of diverse actions of prostanoid receptors. *Biochim. Biophys. Acta* **1259**(1), 109–19.

Nilsson, L., Reinheimer, T., Steinwall, M. and Akerlund, M. (2003) FE 200 440: a selective oxytocin antagonist on the term-pregnant human uterus. *BJOG*. **110**(11), 1025–8.

Nixon, W. C. W. (1951) Uterine activity, normal and abnormal. *Am. J. Obstet. Gynecol.* **62**, 964–84.

Norman, J. E. (1992) Menstrual induction: methods and mechanisms of action. Unpublished M. D. Thesis. University of Edinburgh.

Norman, J. E., Ward, L. M., Martin, W. *et al.* (1997) Effects of cyclic GMP and the nitric oxide donors glyceryl trinitrate and sodium nitroprusside on contractions in vitro of isolated myometrial tissue from pregnant women. *J. Reprod. Fertil.* **110**, 249–54.

Norman, J. E., Thomson, A. J., Telfer, J. F. *et al.* (1999) Myometrial constitutive nitric oxide synthase expression is increased during human pregnancy. *Mol. Hum. Reprod.* **5**, 175–81.

Norman, M., Ekman, G., Ulmsten, U., Barchan, K. and Malmstrom, A. (1991) Proteoglycan metabolism in the connective tissue of pregnant and non-pregnant human cervix. An in vitro study. *Biochem. J.* **275**, 515–20.

Norman, M., Ekman, G. and Malmstrom, A. (1993) Changed proteoglycan metabolism in human cervix immediately after spontaneous vaginal delivery. *Obstet. Gynecol.* **81**, 217–23.

Norstrom, A. (1984) The effects of prostaglandins on the biosynthesis of connective tissue constituents in the non-pregnant human cervix uteri. *Acta Obstet. Gynecol. Scand.* **63**, 169–73.

Norstrom, A., Bergman, I., Lindblom, B. *et al.* (1985) Effects of 9 deoxo- 16, 16 dimethyl-9-methylene PGE$_2$ on muscle contractile activity and collagen synthesis in the human cervix. *Prostaglandins* **29**, 337–46.

Obrink, B. (1973) A study of the interactions between monomeric tropocollagen and glycosaminoglycans. *Eur. J. Biochem.* **33**, 387–400.

Ogawa, M., Hirano, H., Tsubaki, H., Kodama, H. and Tanaka, T. (1998) The role of cytokines in cervical ripening: correlations between the concentrations of cytokines and hyaluronic acid in cervical mucus and the induction of hyaluronic acid production by inflammatory cytokines by human cervical fibroblasts. *Am. J. Obstet. Gynecol.* **179**, 105–10.

Oishi, K., Takano-Ohmuro, H., Minakawa-Matsuo, N. *et al.* (1991) Oxytocin contracts rat uterine smooth muscle in calcium-free medium without any phosphorylation of myosin light chain. *Biochem. Biophys. Res. Commun.* **176**, 122–8.

Olah, K. S. and Gee, H. (1992) The prevention of preterm delivery- can we afford to continue to ignore the cervix? *BJOG.* **99**, 278–80.

Orsino, A., Taylor, C. V. and Lye, S. J. (1996) Connexin-26 and connexin-43 are differentially expressed and regulated in the rat myometrium throughout late pregnancy and with the onset of labor. *Endocrinology* **137**(5), 1545–53.

Osada, K., Tsunoda, H., Miyauchi, T. *et al.* (1997) Pregnancy increases ET-1-induced contraction and changes receptor subtypes in uterine smooth muscle in humans. *Am. J. Physiol..* **272**(2 Pt 2), R541–8.

Osman, I. A. Young, A., Ledingham, M. A. *et al.* (2003) Leukocyte density and pro-inflammatory cytokine expression in human fetal membranes, decidua, cervix and myometrium before and during labour at term. *Mol. Hum. Reprod.* **9**, 41–5

Osmers, R., Rath, W., Adelmann-Grill, B. C. *et al.* (1992) Origin of cervical collagenase during parturition. *Am. J. Obstet. Gynecol.* **166**, 1455–60.

Osmers, R. G. W., Blaser, J., Kuhn, W. and Tschesche, H. (1995) Interleukin-8 synthesis and the onset of labor. *Obstet. Gynecol.* **86**, 223–9.

Ou, C. W., Orsino, A. and Lye, S. J. (1997) Expression of connexin-43 and connexin-26 in the rat myometrium during pregnancy and labor is differentially regulated by mechanical and hormonal signals. *Endocrinology* **138**, 5398–407.

Owman, Ch., Stjernquist, M., Helm, G. *et al.* (1986) Comparative histochemical distribution of nerve fibers storing noradrenaline and neuropeptide Y (NPY) in human ovary, fallopian tube and uterus. *Med. Biol.* **64**, 57–65.

Park, K. H., Chaiworapongsa, T., Kim, Y. M. *et al.* (2003) Matrix metalloproteinase 3 in parturition, premature rupture of the membranes, and microbial invasion of the amniotic cavity. *J. Perinat. Med.* **31**, 12–22

Parry, D. S. and Ellwood, D. A. (1981) Ultrastructural aspects of cervical softening in sheep. In: D. A. Ellwood and A. B. M. Anderson, eds., *The Cervix in Pregnancy and Labour: Clinical and Biochemical Investigations.* Edinburgh: Churchill Livingstone, pp. 74–84.

Petersen, L. K., Skajaa, K. and Uldbjerg, N. (1992) Serum relaxin as a potential marker for preterm labour. *BJOG.* **99**, 292–5.

Petraglia, F., Giardino, L., Coukos, G. *et al.* (1990) Corticotrophin-releasing factor and parturition: plasma and amniotic fluid levels and placental binding sites. *Obstet. Gynecol.* **75**, 784–9.

Price, S. A. and Bernal, A. L. (2001) Uterine quiescence: the role of cyclic AMP. *Exp. Physiol.* **86**, 265–72.

Radestad, A., Bygdeman, M. and Green, K. (1990) Induced cervical ripening with mifepristone (RU486) and bioconversion of arachidonic acid in human pregnant uterine cervix in the first trimester. *Contraception* **41**, 283–92.

Radestad, A., Thyberg, J. and Christensen, N. J. (1993) Cervical ripening with mifepristone (RU486) in first trimester abortion. An electron microscope study. *Hum. Reprod.* **8**, 1136–42.

Ramsay, B., Sooranna, S. R. and Johnson, M. R. (1996) Nitric oxide synthase activities in human myometrium and villous trophoblast throughout pregnancy. *Obstet. Gynecol.* **87**, 249–53.

Rath, W., Adelmann-Girill, B. C., Pieper, U. *et al.* (1987) The role of collagenases and proteases in prostaglandin induced cervical ripening. *Prostaglandins* **34**, 119–27.

Rath, W., Osmers, B. C., Adelmann-Girill, B. C. *et al.* (1988) Biophysical and biochemical changes of cervical ripening. In C. Egarter and P. Husslein, eds., *Prostaglandins for Cervical Ripening and/or Induction of Labour.* Vienna: Facultas, pp. 32–41

Rauk, P. N. and Chiao, J. P. (2000) Interleukin-1 stimulates human uterine prostaglandin production through induction of cyclo-oxygenase-2 expression. *Am. J. Reprod. Immunol.* **43**(3), 152–9.

Reis, F. M., Fadalti, M., Florio, P. and Petraglia, F. (1999) Putative role of placental corticotrophin-releasing factor in the mechanisms of human parturition. *J. Soc. Gynecol. Investig.* **6**(3), 109–19.

Reynolds, S. R. M. (1965) *Physiology of the Uterus.* New York: Hoeber.

Romero, R., Roslansky, P., Oyarzun, E. *et al.* (1988) Labor and infection. II. Bacterial endotoxin in amniotic fluid and its relationship to the onset of preterm labor. *Am. J. Obstet. Gynecol.* **158**, 1044–9.

Romero, R., Gomez, R., Mazor, M., Ghezzi, F. and Yoon, B. H. (1997) The preterm labor syndrome. In M. G. Elder, R. Romero and R. F. Lamont, eds., *Preterm Labor.* New York: Churchill Livingstone, pp. 29–50.

Rosen, T., Kuczynski, E., O'Neill, L. M. *et al.* (2001). Plasma levels of thrombin-antithrombin complexes predict preterm premature rupture of the fetal membranes. *J. Matern. Fetal Med.* **10**(5), 297–300.

Rosselli, M. (1997) Nitric oxide and reproduction. *Mol. Hum. Reprod.* **3**, 639–41.

Rowlands, S., Trudinger, B. and Visva-Lingam, S. (1996) Treatment of preterm cervical dilatation with glyceryl trinitrate, a nitric oxide donor. *Aust. N.Z. J. Obstet. Gynaecol.* **36**, 377–81.

Russell, P. (1979) Inflammatory lesions of the human placenta: clinical significance of acute chorioamnionitis. *Am. J. Obstet. Gynecol.* **2**, 127–37.

Sadovsky, Y., Nelson, D. M., Muglia, L. J. *et al.* (2000) Effective diminution of amniotic prostaglandin production by selective inhibitors of cyclo-oxygenase type 2. *Am. J. Obstet. Gynecol.* **182**(2), 370–6.

Samuelson, U. E., Dalsgaard, C. J., Lundberg, J. M. and Hokfelt, T. (1985) Calcitonin gene-related peptide inhibits spontaneous contractions in human uterus and fallopian tube. *Neurosci. Lett.* **62**, 225–30.

Sato, T., Ito, A. and Mori, Y. (1990) Interleukin 6 enhances the production of tissue inhibitor of metalloproteinases (TIMP) but not that of matrix metalloproteinases by human fibroblasts. *Biochem. Biophys. Res. Commun.* **170**(2), 824–9.

Sawdy, R. J., Slater, D. M., Dennes, W. J., Sullivan, M. H. and Bennett, P. R. (2000) The roles of the cyclo-oxygenases types one and two in prostaglandin synthesis in human fetal membranes at term. *Placenta* **21**(1), 54–7.

Schwartz, L. B. (1997) Understanding human parturition. *Lancet* **350**, 1792–3.

Scott, J. E. and Orford, C. R. (1981) Dermatan sulphate rich proteoglycan associates with rat tail tendon collagen at the d band in the gap region. *Biochem. J.* **197**, 213–16.

Sennstrom, M. B., Ekman, G., Westergren-Thorsson, G. *et al.* (2000) Human cervial ripening, an inflammatory process mediated by cytokines. *Mol. Hum. Reprod.* **6**(4), 375–81.

Sitteri, P. K., Febres, F., Clemens, L. E. *et al.* (1977) Progesterone and maintenance of pregnancy: is progesterone nature's immunosuppressant? *Ann. N.Y. Acad. Sci.* **286**, 384–97.

Slater, D., Berger, L., Newton, R., Moore, G. and Bennett, P. (1994) The relative abundance of type 1 to type 2 cyclo-oxygenase mRNA in human amnion at term. *Biochem. Biophys. Res. Commun.* **198**(1), 304–8.

Slater, D. M., Berger, L., Newton, R., Moore, G. E. and Bennett, P. R. (1995) Changes in the expression of types 1 and 2 cyclo-oxygenase in human fetal membranes at term. *Am. J. Obstet. Gynecol.* **172**, 77–82.

Slater, D., Allport, V. and Bennett, P. (1998) Changes in the expression of the type-2 but not the type-1 cyclo-oxygenase enzyme in chorion-decidua with the onset of labour. *BJOG.* **105**, 745–8.

Slater, D. M., Dennes, W. J., Campa, J. S., Poston, L. and Bennett, P. R. (1999) Expression of cyclo-oxygenase types-1 and -2 in human myometrium throughout pregnancy. *Mol. Hum. Reprod.* **5**(9), 880–4.

Smaill, F. (2002) Antibiotics for asymptomatic bacteriuria in pregnancy (Cochrane Review). In *The Cochrane Library*, Issue 3. Oxford: Update Software.

So, T., Ito, A., Mori, Y. *et al.* (1992). Tumor necrosis factor-alpha stimulates the biosynthesis of matrix metalloproteinases and plasminogen activator in cultured human chorionic cells. *Biol. Reprod.* **46**(5), 772–8.

Somlyo, A.V. (1980) Ultrastructure of vascular smooth muscle. In D. F. Bohr, A. P. Somlyo and H. P. Sparks, eds., *Handbook of Physiology. The Cardiovascular System,* vol. 2. Bethesda: American Physiological Society, pp. 33–70.

Somlyo, A. P., Bond, M., Somlyo, A. V. and Scarpa, A. (1985) Inositol trisphosphate induced calcium release and contraction in vascular smooth muscle. *Proc. Natl. Acad. Sci. U.S.A.* **82**, 5231–5.

Stjernquist, M., Ekblad, E., Owman, Ch. and Sundler, F. (1986) Neuronal localization and motor effects of gastrin releasing peptide (GRP) in rat uterus. *Reg. Peptides* **13**, 197–205.

Stricklin, G. P. and Hibbs, M. S. (1988) Biochemistry and physiology of mammalian collagenases. In M. E. Nimni, ed., *Collagen Biochemistry*, vol. 1. Boca Ranton: CRC Press, pp. 187–205.

Stys, S. J., Clarke, K. E., Clewell, W. M. *et al.* (1980) Hormonal effects on cervical compliance in sheep. In F. Naftolin and P. G. Stubblefield, eds., *Dilatation of the Uterine Cervix*. New York: Raven Press, pp. 147–56.

Swahn, M. L. and Bygdeman, M. (1988) The effect of the antiprogestin RU-486 on uterine contractility and sensitivity to prostaglandin and oxytocin. *BJOG.* **85**, 126–34.

Taggart, M. J. and Wray, S. (1998) Contribution of sarcoplasmic reticular calcium to smooth muscle contractile activation: gestational dependence in isolated rat uterus. *J. Physiol.* **511** (Pt 1): 133–44.

Theobald, G. W., Robards, M. F. and Suster, P. E. N. (1969) Changes in myometrial sensitivity to oxytocin in man during the last six weeks of pregnancy. *Br. J. Obstet. Gynaecol.* **76**, 385–93.

Thomas, J., Kelly, A.J. and Kavanagh, J. (2001) Oestrogens alone or with amniotomy for cervical ripening or induction of labour. *Cochrane Database Syst. Rev.* 4, CD003393.

Thomson, A. J., Lunan, C. B., Cameron, A. D. *et al.* (1997a) Nitric oxide donors induce ripening of the human uterine cervix: a randomised controlled trial. *BJOG.* **104**, 1054–7.

Thomson, A. J., Telfer, J. F., Kohnen, G. (1997b) Nitric oxide synthase activity and localisation do not change in uterus and placenta during human parturition. *Hum. Reprod.* **12**, 2546–52.

Thomson, A. J., Lunan, C. B., Ledingham, M. A. *et al.* (1998) Randomised trial of a nitric oxide donor versus prostaglandin for cervical ripening before first-trimester termination of pregnancy. *Lancet* **352**, 1093–6.

Thomson, A. J., Telfer, J. F., Young, A. *et al.* (1999) Leukocytes infiltrate the myometrium during human parturition: further evidence that labour is an inflammatory process. *Hum. Reprod.* **14**, 229–36.

Thornton, S. and Gillespie, J. I. (1992) Biochemistry of uterine contractions. *Contemp. Rev. Obstet. Gynaecol.* **4**, 121–6.

Tschugguel, W., Schneeberger, C., Lass, H. *et al.* (1999) Human cervical ripening is associated with an increase in cervical inducible nitric oxide synthase expression. *Biol. Reprod.* **60**(6), 1367–72.

Tulchinsky, D., Hobel, C. J., Yeager, E. and Marshall, J. R. (1972) Plasma estrone, estradiol, progesterone, and 17-hydroxyprogesterone in human pregnancy. I. Normal pregnancy. *Am. J. Obstet. Gynecol.* **112**, 1095–100.

Uldbjerg, N. and Malmstrom, A. (1991) The role of proteoglycans in cervical dilatation. *Semin. Perinatol.* **15**, 127–32.

Uldbjerg, N., Ekman, G., Malmstrom, A. *et al.* (1981) Biochemical and morphological changes of human cervix after local application of prostaglandin E_2 in pregnancy. *Lancet* **i**, 267–8.

Uldbjerg, N., Ekman, G. and Malmstrom, A. (1983a) Ripening of the human cervix related to changes in collagen, glycosaminoglycans and collagenolytic activity. *Am. J. Obstet. Gynecol.* **147**, 662–6.

Uldbjerg, N., Ekman, G., Malmstrom, A., Ulmsten, U. and Wingerup, L. (1983b) Biochemical changes in human cervical connective tissue after local application of prostaglandin E$_2$. *Gynecol. Obstet. Invest.* **15**, 291–9.

Uldbjerg, N., Malmstrom, A., Ekman, G. *et al.* (1983c) Isolation and characterization of dermatan sulphate proteoglycan from human uterine cervix. *Biochem. J.* **209**, 497–503.

Uldbjerg, N., Ulmsten, U. and Ekman, G. (1983d) The ripening of the human uterine cervix in terms of connective tissue biochemistry. *Clin. Obstet. Gynecol.* **26**, 14–26.

Ulug, U., Goldman, S., Ben-Shlomo, I. *et al.* (2001). Matrix metalloproteinase (MMP)-2 and MMP-9 and their inhibitor, TIMP-1, in human term decidua and fetal membranes: the effect of prostaglandin F(2alpha) and indomethacin. *Mol. Hum. Reprod.* **7**(12), 1187–93.

Vaisanen-Tommiska, M., Nuutila, M., Aittomaki, K., Hiilesmaa, V. and Ylikorkala, O. (2003) Nitric oxide metabolites in cervical fluid during pregnancy: further evidence for the role of cervical nitric oxide in cervical ripening. *Am. J. Obstet. Gynecol.* **188** (3), 779–85.

Van Meir, C. A., Ramirez, M. M., Matthews, S. G. *et al.* (1997) Chorionic prostaglandin catabolism is decreased in the lower uterine segment with term labour. *Placenta* **18**(2–3), 109–14.

von Maillot, K., Weiss, M., Nagelschmidt, M. *et al.* (1977) Relaxin and cervical dilatation during partuition. *Archiv. Gynakol.* **223**, 323–31.

von Maillot, K., Stuhlsatz, H. W., Mohanaradhkrishan, V. *et al.* (1979) Changes in the glycosaminoglycan distribution pattern in the human uterine cervix during pregnancy and labour. *Am. J. Obstet. Gynecol.* **135**, 503–6.

Wallace, J. L. (1999) Distribution and expression of cyclo-oxygenase (COX) isoenzymes, their physiological roles, and the categorization of nonsteroidal anti-inflammatory drugs (NSAIDs). *Am. J. Med.* **107**(6A), 11S–16S

Watari, M., Watari, H., DiSanto, M. E. *et al.* (1999) Pro-inflammatory cytokines induce expression of matrix-metabolizing enzymes in human cervical smooth muscle cells. *Am. J. Pathol.* **154**(6), 1755–62.

Weiss, G., Goldsmith, L. T., Sachdev, R., von Hagen, S. and Lederer, K. (1993) Elevated first-trimester serum relaxin concentrations in pregnant women following ovarian stimulation predict prematurity risk and preterm delivery. *Obstet. Gynecol.* **82**, 821–31.

Wessen, A., Elowsson, P., Axemo, P. and Lindberg, B. (1995) The use of intravenous nitroglycerin for emergency cervico-uterine relaxation. *Acta Anaesth. Scand.* **39**, 847–9.

Westphal, U., Stroupe, S. D. and Cheng, S. L. (1977) Progesterone binding to serum proteins. *Ann. N.Y. Acad. Sci.* **286**, 10–28.

Wilson, L. Jr. and Parsons, M. (1996) Endocrinology of human gestation. In E. Y. Adashi, J. A. Rock and Z. Rosenwaks, eds., *Reproductive Endocrinology, Surgery and Technology.* Philadelphia: Lippincott-Raven. pp. 452–75.

Winkler, M., Ruck, P., Horny, H. P. *et al.* (1998) Expression of cell adhesion molecules by endothelium in the human lower uterine segment during parturition at term. *Am. J. Obstet. Gynecol.* **178**, 557–61.

Winkler, M., Fischer, D.C., Ruck, P. *et al.* (1999) Parturition at term: parallel increases in interleukin-8 and proteinase concentrations and neutrophil count in the lower uterine segment. *Hum. Reprod.* **14**(4), 1096–100.

Woessner, J. (1994). The family of matrix metalloproteinases. *Ann. N.Y. Acad. Sci.* **732**, 11–21.

Wolff, K., Faxen, M., Lunell, N.O., Nisell, H. and Lindblom, B. (1996) Endothelin receptor type-A and receptor type-B gene-expression in human non-pregnant, term pregnant and pre-eclamptic uterus. *Am. J. Obstet. Gynecol.* **175**, 1295–300.

Wooley, D.E. (1984) Mammalian collagenases. In K.A. Piez and A.H. Reddi, eds., *Extracellular Matrix Biochemistry*. New York: Elsevier, pp. 119–57.

Word, R.A., Kamm, K.E., Stull, J.T. and Casey, M.L. (1990) Endothelin increases cytoplasmic calcium and myosin phosphorylation in human myometrium. *Am. J. Obstet. Gynecol.* **162**, 1103–8.

Worldwide Atosiban versus Beta-Agonists Study Group. (2001) Effectiveness and safety of the oxytocin antagonist atosiban versus beta-adrenergic agonists in the treatment of preterm labour. *BJOG* **108**(2): 133–42.

Wray, S. (1993) Uterine contraction and physiological mechanisms of modulation. *Am. J. Physiol.* **264**, C1–C18.

Xu, P., Alfaidy, N. and Challis, J.R. (2002). Expression of matrix metalloproteinase (MMP)-2 and MMP-9 in human placenta and fetal membranes in relation to preterm and term labor. *J. Clin. Endocrinol. Metab.* **87**, 1353–61.

Yallampalli, C. and Garfield, R.E. (1994) Uterine contractile responses to endothelin-1 and endothelin receptors are elevated during labor. *Biol. Reprod.* **51**, 640–5.

Young, A., Thomson, A.J., Ledingham, M.A. *et al.* (2002) Immunolocalization of pro-inflammatory cytokines in myometrium, cervix and fetal membranes during human parturition at term. *Biol. Reprod.* **66**, 445–9.

Yoshida, M., Sagawa, N., Itoh, H. *et al.* (2001) Nitric oxide increases matrix metalloproteinase-1 production in human uterine cervical fibroblast cells. *Mol. Hum. Reprod.* **7**(10) 979–85.

Zeeman, G.G., Khan-Dawood, F.S. and Dawood, M.Y. (1997) Oxytocin and its receptor in pregnancy and parturition: current concepts and clinical implications. *Obstet. Gynecol.* **89**, 873–83.

3

Transcriptional regulation of labour-associated genes

Tamsin Lindström, Jennifer Loudon and Phillip Bennett

Institute of Reproductive and Developmental Biology, Imperial College, London

Introduction

The clinical onset of labour, characterised by painful uterine contractions leading to cervical dilatation, is a relatively late event in a series of biochemical changes that occur throughout the pregnancy, but particularly in the late third trimester. For most of pregnancy, myometrial contractile activity needs to be repressed, whilst the cervix needs to remain firm and closed to retain the developing fetus within the uterus. Nearer to term, the cervix ripens, a process characterised by dissociation of collagen and a decrease in its concentration and an increase in water content (Osmers *et al.* 1995). This results in a looser matrix so that cervical tissue offers lower resistance to force and its collagen fibres will deform under tension.

In the myometrium, with the onset of labour, fundally dominant contractions begin. Cervical tissue is drawn up into the lower segment of the uterus, in the processes of effacement and dilatation. Eventually with the establishment of labour, the lower segment itself is drawn up towards the upper segment and the fetus is pushed through the birth canal and into the outside world. These changes within the uterus are associated with changes in the expression of a range of genes that Steven Lye in Toronto has termed 'contraction-associated proteins' (CAPs). In the myometrium such proteins include those that form gap junctions (Sparey *et al.* 1999), proteins in the prostaglandins synthetic pathways (Slater *et al.* 1999) and receptors for oxytocin (Fuchs *et al.* 1984) and prostaglandins (Erkinheimo *et al.* 2000).

Clinical experience shows, however, that changes in the fetal membranes and particularly in the cervix are as important as changes in the myometrium. Preterm labour, especially early in the third trimester of pregnancy, is associated with cervical shortening, funnelling and dilatation with little uterine activity. Once preterm labour does begin, often only a few, relatively weak contractions are required to lead to delivery. Cervical change is due to an increase in the synthesis

Preterm Labour Managing Risk in Clinical Practice, eds. Jane Norman and Ian Greer. Published by Cambridge University Press. © Cambridge University Press 2005.

of prostaglandins and inflammatory cytokines, with the cervix itself and the overlying fetal membranes associated with the infiltration of inflammatory cells (Osman *et al.* 2003). The net effect is that biochemical changes associated with labour are very similar to those seen at sites of inflammation, and it follows that they can be prematurely activated by inflammatory stimuli such as infection. The range of proteins involved in the parturition process can therefore be extended to include cytokines, and their functions to include fetal membrane remodelling and rupture and cervical ripening. We therefore prefer the term 'labour-associated proteins'.

Much attention has focused in the past on the inhibition of uterine activity in the prevention of preterm labour, but, with the exception of the inhibition of prostaglandin synthesis, there has been little attention paid to the inhibition of the biochemical processes preceding contractions. There is now growing evidence that there are common factors involved in the regulation of 'labour-associated proteins' and that, it is an increase or decrease in gene expression that mediates changes in their concentrations. Targeting these common factors may represent newer strategies for the prevention of preterm delivery. In this review we will consider the transcriptional regulation of a group of 'labour-associated proteins', the enzymes of the prostaglandin biosynthetic pathway, the chemotactic cytokine interleukin-8 and the oxytocin receptor.

Enzymes of the prostaglandin biosynthetic pathway

Prostaglandins (PGs) are lipid mediators of many different cellular processes. They have an established role in inflammation, making PG biosynthesis a target for non-steroidal anti-inflammatory drugs (NSAIDS) (Vane and Botting 1997). Prostaglandins play a pivotal role in human parturition, during which they act to stimulate myometrial contractility and to promote cervical ripening (Calder and Greer 1992). Non-steroidal anti-inflammatory drugs have been used clinically to prolong pregnancy and labour (Mitchell and Olson 2004), and clinical administration of PGs induces labour and delivery (Calder 1997). Prostaglandins are produced by almost every tissue in the body, including tissues of the human uterus. Concentrations increase in maternal urine, blood (Satoh *et al.* 1979) and in amniotic fluid in association with labour (Keirse and Turnbull 1973; Keirse *et al.* 1974). These elevated PG levels are accompanied by increased expression and activity of key enzymes in PG biosynthesis.

Prostaglandins are derived from arachidonic acid (AA) found in membrane phospholipids of the cell. The PG biosynthetic pathway can be divided into three main stages. The initial step involves the mobilisation of AA from membrane phospholipids by the action of phospholipase (PL) enzymes, PLA_2, PLC and PLD.

Phospholipase C and PLD expression has been demonstrated in fetal membranes and there is some evidence for their involvement in labour (Okazaki *et al.* 1981; Inamori *et al.* 1993). The main body of research has focused on the functions and regulation of the PLA_2 enzymes. Phospholipase-mediated supply of precursor AA is often a rate-limiting step in the arachidonate cascade. In the second stage of PG biosynthesis, the free AA is converted to the PG intermediate, prostaglandin H_2 (PGH_2), in a reaction catalysed by cyclo-oxygenase (COX) enzymes. Since no pathway exists for the re-conversion of PGH_2 to AA, the COX enzymes mediate the committed step of PG biosynthesis. Cyclo-oxygenase activity is also regulated and, despite a net release of AA from fetal membranes during labour, there is sufficient free AA in amniotic fluid and intrauterine tissues for PG biosynthesis to occur before the onset of labour. This demonstrates the importance of the COX enzymes as a major control point in PG biosynthesis in the uterus. Finally, PGH_2 is converted to prostaglandins PGE_2, $PGF_{2\alpha}$, PGI_2, PGD_2 and thromboxane by specific synthase enzymes. The expression and activity of these synthases determines cell type-specific PG production profile. While some regulation of these enzymes has been demonstrated, they are not currently considered to be rate-limiting (Alfaidy *et al.* 2003). Prostaglandin metabolism also plays an important role in altering bioactive PG output in the uterus. Prostaglandin I_2 and thromboxane are spontaneously inactivated, and PGE_2 and $PGF_{2\alpha}$ are metabolically inactivated by the enzyme 15-hydroxyprostaglandin dehydrogenase (PGDH), which is also subject to regulation in uterine tissues (Sangha *et al.* 1994; Patel *et al.* 2003). The net effect of PGs in human labour may be governed by changes at different steps in PG synthesis and metabolism.

PLA_2

The PLA_2 superfamily consists of a broad range of enzymes that catalyse the hydrolysis of the *sn*-2 ester bond of substrate phospholipids to produce lysophospholipids and free fatty acids. Phospholipase A_2 provides precursors for eicosanoid generation (including PGs) when the cleaved fatty acid is arachidonic acid. Phospholipase A_2 enzymes are found in two broad groups, secretory and cytosolic. Secretory Phospholipase A_2s ($sPLA_2$s) are low molecular weight enzymes (13–18 kDa) which function at millimolar concentrations of Ca^{2+} (Chen *et al.* 1994). The $sPLA_2$s are further classified into groups I, II, III, V, X and XII, and the cytosolic PLA_2 ($cPLA_2$s) into groups IV, VI, VII and VIII (Gelb *et al.* 2000; Six and Dennis 2000). The Ca^{2+}-independent $sPLA_2$s play a role in regulating basal phospholipid remodeling reactions and breakdown of dietary phospholipids (Pind and Kuksis 1988). Although $sPLA_2$s lack selectivity for the sn-2 fatty acids of phospholipids and require much higher Ca^{2+} (mM) than normal cellular Ca^{2+} levels (nM–μM) for activation, they too can mediate AA release and PG production depending on the cell type and agonist involved (Kudo *et al.* 1993). The cPLA$_2$, is an 85-kDa enzyme activated by micromolar concentrations of Ca^{2+}. Cytosolic PLA$_2$ shares no homology with other PLA$_2$ enzymes and is the only well-characterised PLA$_2$ that preferentially hydrolyses sn-2 arachidonic acid (Clark *et al.* 1991).

Phospholipase A$_2$s are widely expressed in intrauterine tissues. Cytosolic PLA$_2$ 'knock-out' mice studies suggest a non-redundant role for this enzyme in reproductive physiology. *cpla$_2$-/-* mice fail to go into labour at term and eventually deliver small, unviable litters (Uozumi *et al.* 1997). Both secretory and cytosolic isoenzymes may be involved in phospholipid metabolism in the uterus.

The PLA$_2$ enzymes are differentially expressed in intrauterine tissues. Cytosolic PLA$_2$ is the principal isozyme mediating the liberation of AA in term amnion. Secretory PLA$_2$ isozymes, and in particular Type II sPLA$_2$, are predominant in term placenta (Freed *et al.* 1997; Rice *et al.* 1998). Skannal *et al.* (1997a) showed an increase in total cellular cPLA$_2$ activity in human amnion with gestational age, peaking at term and decreasing after the onset of labour, suggesting that cPLA$_2$ mobilisation of AA is highest just prior to labour onset and becomes depleted during labour. However, Munns *et al.* (1999) found no change in cPLA$_2$ activity in gestational tissues before and during labour. Aitken *et al.* (1992) found a labour-associated increase in the expression of Type II sPLA$_2$ in human placenta, but not in the membranes, while Bennett *et al.* (1994) found no labour-associated difference in expression of Type II sPLA$_2$ in human amnion, chorio-decidua or placenta and suggested that the increased PLA$_2$ activity in fetal membranes and placenta associated with labour is not due to increased sPLA$_2$ expression, but that posttranslational control of sPLA$_2$ may be mediated through changes in expression of annexin I, a member of the annexin protein family known to inhibit PLA$_2$.

Skannal *et al.* (1997b) found protein expression of both sPLA$_2$ and cPLA$_2$ in lower segment human myometrial tissue but found no significant gestational age or labour-associated changes. Slater *et al.* (2000) however, found an increase in the expression of sPLA$_2$, but not of cPLA$_2$, in association with gestational age and labour in both lower and upper segment myometrial tissues, implying a role for sPLA$_2$ in the myometrial PG synthesis associated with labour.

Phospholipase A$_2$s are activated by various stimuli, including hormones, neurotransmitters, endotoxins and cytokines (Clark *et al.* 1995; Murakami *et al.* 1997). The bacterial endotoxin lipopolysaccharide (LPS), which stimulates cytokine release from uterine tissues has been shown to increase the release of Type II sPLA$_2$ and PGE$_2$ from placental and chorio-decidua explants (Nguyen *et al.* 1994; Farrugia *et al.* 1999). Tumow necrosis factor-α (TNFα) and interleukin-1β (1L-1β) induce cPLA$_2$ mRNA and protein expression in amnion-derived WISH cells, and this induction is inhibited by the anti-inflammatory steroid, dexamethasone (Xue *et al.* 1996).

Cytosolic PLA$_2$ is tightly regulated by multiple pathways, employing both posttranslational and transcriptional mechanisms. When cells are stimulated with agents that increase intracellular Ca^{2+} concentrations, cPLA$_2$ translocates from the cytosol to the nuclear membrane where it interacts with its phospholipid substrate, in a process mediated by the N-terminal Ca^{2+}-dependent phospholipid binding regulatory domain of cPLA$_2$. Cytosolic PLA$_2$ contains potential phosphorylation sites for several kinases and can be stimulated by the activation of protein kinases, such as phorbol ester-activated protein kinases C (PKC) and growth factor-activated receptor tyrosine kinase. Phosphorylation appears to be essential for stimulation of cPLA$_2$ enzymatic activity but activation of cPLA$_2$ in intact cells also requires Ca^{2+}-induced translocation of cPLA$_2$ to the nuclear membrane. A secretory-component-like protein found in amniotic fluid has been identified as an inhibitor of cPLA$_2$. This protein is upregulated by progesterone and its levels decrease with labour (Schuster-Woldan *et al.* 1997; Bennett *et al.* 1999).

Rapid cPLA$_2$ responses are mediated through activation of pre-existing enzyme by phosphorylation and intracellular Ca^{2+} fluxes. More prolonged responses can be regulated by changes in cPLA$_2$ mRNA levels. Messenger RNA stabilisation appears to play an important role in cPLA$_2$ expression mediated through an adenosine-uridine-rich sequence in the 3'-untranslated region of cPLA$_2$ (Tay *et al.* 1994). Cytosolic PLA$_2$ activity can also be increased through *de novo* transcription, with significant increases in cPLA$_2$ mRNA and protein levels that occur over hours and result in the prolonged release of AA and eicosanoid production (Dolan-O'Keefe *et al.* 2000).

The cPLA$_2$ promoter resembles a housekeeping gene in that it lacks a TATA box, although in the rat, but not the human, 5' regulatory sequences include nuclear factor-kappaB(NF-κB) and activator protein 1 (AP-1) binding sites. Approximately 150 bp upstream from the transcriptional start site is a 48-bp CA dinucleotide repeat that is conserved in both the human and the rat genes that appears to act as a negative regulator of expression (Naylor and Clark 1990; Wu *et al.* 1994).

Wu *et al.* (1994) identified a number of putative binding sites within the 595-bp 5' of the transcription initiation site of human cPLA$_2$, including five interferon-gamma (IFNγ) response elements (γ-IRE), one interferon-gamma activated sequence (GAS), two potential glucocorticoid response elements (GREs) and two potential octamer binding motifs, as well as a possible CAAT box. The GAS and γ-IRE consensus sequences in the cPLA$_2$ promoter may be involved in IFNγ-induced cPLA$_2$ expression (Wang *et al.* 1993). Glucocorticoids effectively repress cytokine induction of the cPLA$_2$ gene in many different cell types. The presence of putative

GREs in the promoter suggests that steroids may act to suppress $cPLA_2$ synthesis at the transcriptional level, although the GREs identified are hemi-sites that do not allow discrimination of repression and stimulation by the sequence alone. Dolan-O'Keefe et al. (2000) have characterised the entire genomic structure of the human $cPLA_2$ gene, which spans >137-kb region of the human genome and is composed of 18 exons. Deletion studies of a 3.4-kb fragment of the promoter revealed two regions, between bindings sites −3446 and −2271 and between binding sites −543 and −215, responsible for basal expression of $cPLA_2$. The mechanisms of transcriptional regulation of the $cPLA_2$ promoter in human intrauterine tissues have yet to be determined.

Although Type II $sPLA_2$ lacks the Ca^{2+}-dependent membrane association characteristic of $cPLA_2$, it requires Ca^{2+} for catalytic activity. Secretory PLA_2s are classically associated with inflammation and are found both intra- and extracellularly during inflammatory responses. Secretory PLA_2 genes are not expressed under resting conditions in most cell types. Inflammatory cytokines such as IL-1β, IL-6 and TNFα, induce the synthesis and secretion of Type II $sPLA_2$ in various cell types as do agents which elevate cyclic AMP (cAMP) (Crowl et al. 1991; Jacques et al. 1997). The promoter of the rat Type II $sPLA_2$ gene, contains two transcriptional initiation sites, the major one mapped to 25 bp downstream of the TATA box (Ohara et al. 1990). The promoter contains two putative CCAAT/enhancer-binding protein (C/EBP) binding sites (at −295, −282 and −240, −227), and studies in rat vascular smooth muscle cells demonstrate that C/EBPβ and -δ transcription factors mediate induction of the promoter by cAMP elevating agents through one of these sites (Couturier et al. 2000).

The six C/EBP family members identified to date, namely C/EBPα, −β, −γ, −δ, −ε, and −ζ, share a highly-conserved basic region/lencine zipper (bZIP) dimerisation domain by which they form homo- and heterodimers with other family members; C/EBPs are least conserved in their activation domains and vary from strong activators to dominant negative repressors. CCAAT/enhancer-binding protein is a principally nuclear protein that is activated by phosphorylation. It may influence gene expression by binding directly to C/EBP binding sites in the promoters of target genes. CCAAT enhancer-binding proteins have also been shown to interact with transcription factors from other protein families, including the NF-κB.

Nuclear Factor-kappaB is a transcription factor system which classically regulates inflammation associated genes (Baldwin 1996). The NF-κB family of transcription factors comprises five proteins, p65, p50, p52, c-rel and RelB, all of which contain a highly conserved Rel homology domain responsible for dimerisation, nuclear localisation and DNA binding. Nuclear factor-kappaB exists as a homo- or heterodimer sequestered in the cytoplasm in an inactive form by inhibitory proteins (IκBs). Upon stimulation of the cell, an IκB kinase complex (IKK) phosphorylates IκB, which leads to the ubiquitination and subsequent degradation of the IκB protein. Once IκB is degraded, the nuclear localisation signal of NF-κB is unmasked, allowing NF-κB to translocate to the nucleus where it binds to specific NF-κB sites to induce the transcription of a number of genes associated with the inflammatory response. The binding of NF-κB to a recognition site in the sPLA$_2$ promoter has been demonstrated in rat renal mesangial cells, and activation of this transcription factor appears to be an essential component of rat Type II sPLA$_2$ induction in response to IL-1β and TNFα, whereas cAMP triggers a distinct signalling cascade that does not involve NF-κB.

A role for cPLA$_2$ in IL-1β-mediated Type II sPLA$_2$ gene induction has been suggested (Kuwata *et al.* 1998). Balsinde and Dennis (1996) proposed a model in which a rapid cPLA$_2$-generated burst of intracellular AA is required for activation of sPLA$_2$, which produces extracellular AA. Cytosolic PLA$_2$ is thought to activate sPLA$_2$ through the effects of cPLA$_2$-released AA or its metabolites on the sPLA$_2$ promoter mediated by the NF-κB and peroxisome proliferator-activated receptor (PPAR) transcription factors (Desvergne and Wahli 1999).

Peroxisome proliferator-activated receptors belong to the superfamily of ligand-activated nuclear transcription factors, which form heterodimers with the retinoid X receptor (RXR) and bind to peroxisome proliferator response elements (PPREs) to regulate the expression of target genes. Eicosanoids are the natural ligands for PPARs. The rat Type II sPLA$_2$ promoter contains a PPRE binding site. This raises the possibility that eicosanoid production resulting from cPLA$_2$ activation may contribute to PPAR-mediated regulation of the Type II sPLA$_2$ gene. Studies in rat aortic smooth muscle cells showed binding of nuclear factors to PPRE and NF-κB sites in the Type II sPLA$_2$ promoter and demonstrated the involvement of two complementary pathways in IL-1β-induced Type II sPLA$_2$ gene transcription: an NF-κB pathway and a PPARγ-mediated cPLA$_2$ pathway (Couturier *et al.* 2000). Nuclear factor-kappaB and PPARγ are proposed to bind independently to their specific DNA binding sites in the promoter and to cooperate to activate Type II sPLA$_2$ gene expression.

Peroxisome proliferator-activated receptor γ can bind to PPREs to stimulate transcription of target genes, but can also act to inhibit transcription factors that play a role in regulating expression of pro-inflammatory genes, including AP-1, signal transducer and activator of transcription (STAT) and NF-κB (Ricote *et al.* 1998). Alaoui-El-Azher *et al.* (2002) demonstrated that, in guinea pig alveolar macrophages, the NF-κB pathway is essential for the induction of Type II sPLA$_2$ gene expression but that, in contrast to the model proposed by Couturier *et al.* (1999), PPARγ acts to down-regulate Type II sPLA$_2$ synthesis (Alaoui-El-Azher *et al.* 2002). This is likely to be a result of PPARγ interfering with the activity of NF-κB rather than a direct effect of PPARγ on the Type II sPLA$_2$ promoter.

Two distinct mechanisms were postulated depending on the activation state of the cell: in unstimulated cells AA could inhibit sPLA$_2$ by impairing NF-κB translocation as described, whereas in LPS-stimulated cells AA exerted its inhibitory effect via its metabolites, without blocking NF-κB activation, in a mechanism likely to involve PPARγ. Stuhlmeier *et al.* (1997) showed, in porcine aortic endothelial cells, that AA inhibits NF-κB activity by preventing the phosphorylation and degradation of IκBα, and therefore blocking nuclear translocation of NF-κB.

Lappas and Rice have extensively studied the effect of bacterial endotoxin (LPS) upon NF-κB and PLA$_2$ expression in human fetal membranes and placenta. They have found that LPS activates NF-κB and stimulates PLA$_2$ expression, and that NF-κB antagonists inhibit the expression of both cPLA$_2$ and sPLA$_2$ (Lappas *et al.* 2003; Lappas *et al.* 2004). As will be discussed below, at least within the amnion, and possibly also in the myomtrium, there is activation of NF-κB with the onset of labour. It is highly likely that NF-κB plays a major role in the expression of sPLA$_2$, both physiologically at term and in the context of preterm labour associated with infection.

Cyclo-oxygenase (COX)

The COX enzymes catalyse the conversion of AA to PGs. There are three known isoforms of this enzyme, COX-1, COX-2 and COX-3. Cyclo-oxygenase-1 and COX-3 are the products of a single (COX-1) gene with COX-3 being formed by alternative mRNA splicing. Cyclo-oxygenase-2 is the product of a second much smaller COX gene which is homologous to the COX-1 gene within its coding regions but has much smaller introns. The COX enzymes catalyse both a cyclo-oxygenase reaction in which AA is converted to PGG$_2$ and a peroxidase reaction in which PGG$_2$ is reduced to PGH$_2$. The two isozymes are differentially regulated. Cyclo-oxygenase-1 is constitutively expressed in numerous tissue types and its expression is, in general, not regulated (DeWitt *et al.* 1993). Cyclo-oxygenase-2 is typically undetectable in most tissue types under normal physiological conditions but can be expressed at high levels following stimulation by cytokines, growth factors and phorbol esters (DeWitt 1991). Prostaglandin biosynthesis exhibits two kinetically distinct responses, the immediate and delayed phases. In immediate PG biosynthesis, which occurs within several minutes after stimulation with agonists that increase cytoplasmic Ca^{2+} levels, activated cPLA$_2$ supplies AA to COX-1(Murakami *et al.* 1999a). Delayed PG biosynthesis, which occurs gradually over a longer period following a proinflammatory stimulus, requires induction of COX-2 expression with cPLA$_2$ and sPLA$_2$s cooperatively supplying AA to COX-2 (Murakami *et al.* 1997, 1999b).

Studies in COX-1 'knock-out' mice suggest that this isozyme controls the onset of labour by inducing luteolysis. The relevance of these findings for human labour is unclear since there are fundamental differences in the parturition process between mouse and human, including the apparent lack of a role for luteolysis or systemic progesterone withdrawal in the human. The role of COX-2 in labour has been difficult to assess using COX-2 knock-out mice since female knock-outs exhibit impaired ovulation and blastocyst implantation, impeding generation of viable pregnancies for parturition analysis (Lim *et al.* 1997). However, injection of antisense oligonucleotides directed against COX-2 has been shown to inhibit expression of COX-2 mRNA and protein and delay onset of labour in endotoxin-treated pregnant mice.

Most of the current evidence supports a key role for the inducible COX-2, rather than COX-1, in the onset of labour in women. Cyclo-oxygenase-2 mRNA and protein levels increase in intrauterine tissues at term before and during labour (Hirst *et al.* 1995; Slater *et al.* 1995, 1998). The COX-2 transcript has an extensive 3′ untranslated region containing three canonical polyadenylation sites and 22 AUUUA Shaw-Kamen motifs (Appleby *et al.* 1994). The latter sequences are believed to be associated with message instability, translational efficiency and rapid turnover, and are a feature of other inducible, early response genes. The labour-associated increase in COX-2 mRNA levels could be attributable to either an increase in gene transcription rate or a decrease in degradation rate. Both mechanisms have been demonstrated in cell culture models, but Johnson *et al.* (2002) recently demonstrated that, in term amnion in vivo, COX-2 mRNA is transcriptionally regulated and constitutively stable. This suggests that the labour-associated upregulation of COX-2 involves amnion-derived factors that stimulate and maintain COX-2 transcription, leading to accumulation of COX-2 mRNA and increasing enzyme activity throughout the onset and progression of labour until delivery.

Human amnion is a major source of PGs which produces a marked increase in synthesis of PGE_2 with labour onset (Skinner and Challis 1985). This is associated with selective induction of the COX-2 gene, with increased COX-2 activity and mRNA levels reported in amnion following spontaneous delivery, but no changes in COX-1 (Slater *et al.* 1995; Zakar *et al.* 1996). Similarly, chorio-decidual cells increase synthesis of PGE_2 and $PGF_{2\alpha}$ with the onset of labour associated with upregulation of expression of COX-2, but not COX-1 (Slater *et al.* 1998). There is, however, no such COX-2 upregulation with labour onset in placenta in the human (Macchia *et al.* 1997).

Studies on COX-2 expression in myometrium have yielded contradictory results. Zuo *et al.* (1994) reported a decrease in the expression of COX-2 mRNA in women in labour at both preterm and term using *in situ* hybridisation, whereas Erkinheimo *et al.* (2000) found a 15-fold elevation of COX-2 mRNA in myometrium at the onset of labour. Both Sparey *et al.* (1999) and Giannoulias *et al.* (2002) found that COX-2 protein levels in myometrial tissue from both upper and lower uterine segments were unaffected by the onset of parturition. Slater *et al.* (1999) also found no significant change in COX-2 protein or COX-2 mRNA with labour, but did find a significant upregulation in myometrial COX-2 mRNA with advancing gestational age. In contrast, Moore *et al.* (1999), working in collaboration with Slater, found COX-2 mRNA levels to remain unaffected by labour onset or gestational age. Such discrepancies probably reflect methodological differences, the region of myometrium sampled or variation in the proximity to labour of the patients classified as not in labour.

Cyclo-oxygenase-2 gene expression in uterine tissues is induced by pro-inflammatory cytokines. Both IL-1β and TNFα, and LPS have been shown to induce transcription of COX-2 in amnion (Mitchell *et al.* 1993), chorio-decidual (Ishihara *et al.* 1992) and myometrial cells. Induction of COX-2 by oxytocin has been demonstrated in myometrial cell cultures (Molnar *et al.* 1999). Corticotrophin-releasing hormone (CRH) and platelet activating factor (PAF), which also increase in concentration in the uterus near to term, have been shown to stimulate PG synthesis through induction of the COX-2 gene in fetal membrane explants consisting of amnion, chorion and deciduas (Alvi *et al.* 1999).

The stimuli, signal transduction pathways and transcription factors involved in the induction of the COX-2 gene are diversified and cell specific. As a consequence, the role attributed to the different promoter regulatory elements and transcription factors in COX-2 gene transcription is sometimes contradictory. The promoter region of the human COX-2 gene contains several putative regulatory elements, including two C/EBP sites, two NF-κB elements and a cyclic AMP response element (CRE) (which may also function as a C/EBP site) overlapping a non-canonical E box (CRE/E box). Each of these has been implicated in COX-2 induction in different cell types. The CRE/E box site is considered essential for both basal and induced transcription in most cellular systems, although different factors have been reported to bind to the CRE in different cell types.

The C/EBP element of COX-2 promoter appears to play an important role in a number of cell types but not in others. For example Gorgoni *et al.* (2001) found C/EBP to be essential for COX-2 induction in macrophages, but not in fibroblasts. Lipopolysaccharide-induced upregulation of COX-2 mRNA in macrophages involves, in addition to C/EBPβ, the transcription factors cAMP response element-binding protein (CREB), NF-κB and C/EBPδ. Caivano *et al.* (2001) showed this induction to be biphasic, involving initial activation of pre-existing CREB, NF-κB and C/EBPβ followed by new synthesis of C/EBPδ and C/EBPβ. Activated, phosphorylated CREB and NF-κB recruit the intrinsic histone acetylase coactivator

CAMP response element-binding protein-binding protein (CBP)/p300, which acts to make the promoter more accessible to transcription factors and form a bridge to the basal transcription complex.

CCAAT/enhancer-binding protein β has been shown to be involved in COX-2 transcription in human amnion-derived AV3 cells, in which the C/EBP and CRE elements are required for both basal and IL-1β-induced COX-2 expression (Potter *et al.* 2000). It was shown to be involved in the complexes formed with both the C/EBP and CRE response elements and CREB did not appear to participate in the complex at the CRE site. The experiments carried out in these AV3 cells excluded a role for NF-κB. In contrast, Allport *et al.* (2000) showed that NF-κB is involved in the regulation of COX-2 in WISH cells, another human amnion-derived cell line. These studies demonstrated the involvement of both of the NF-κB sites in COX-2 transcription in WISH cells and identified an AP-1 site at −1593 bp that also contributes to promoter activity.

Mestre *et al.* (2001) reported that, in murine macrophages, both the CRE and E box elements can individually mediate COX-2 transcription in response to endotoxin through the binding of c-Jun and CREB to the CRE and of upstream stimulating factor-1 (USF-1) to the E-box. The CRE synergised with other promoter elements, such as NF-κB and C/EBP, to a greater extent than the E box, indicating that the CRE-bound complex was transcriptionally more active. Cyclic AMP response element binding proteins have been shown to be differentially regulated in the myometrium during pregnancy and labour (Bailey *et al.* 2000), implying that the CRE element may also be important in COX-2 expression in uterine tissues during parturition.

Glucocorticoids are potent anti-inflammatory agents that act, in part, through inhibition of PGs. The amnion expresses glucocorticoid receptor (GR) and is exposed to cortisol via conversion from cortisone in the deciduas (Lopez Bernal *et al.* 1982). Cortisol and its synthetic analogues suppress IL-1β- and TNFα-induced COX activity, COX-2 mRNA and protein expression in WISH cells (Albert *et al.* 1994; Trautman *et al.* 1996). Glucocorticoid receptor acts as a mutual antagonist of NF-κB (Almawi and Melemedjian 2002), and so GR may inhibit COX-2 expression by suppressing NF-κB-mediated transcription. Studies in primary amnion cells, however, have produced unexpected results. Glucocorticoids have been shown to inhibit PGE_2 production by freshly dispersed amnion cells, but to stimulate COX-2 activity and PGE_2 production in confluent cultures of amnion cells (Gibb and Lavoie 1990). Using immunohistochemistry and *in situ* hybridisation, Economopoulos *et al.* (1996) demonstrated that dexamethasone increases COX-2, but not COX-1 mRNA and protein levels and that this specific COX-2 induction occurs exclusively in the mesenchymal fibroblasts and not in the epithelial cells present in the amnion culture. This finding may explain the difference between the effect of glucocorticoids on freshly dispersed and on cultured amnion cells, since cultured amnion is likely to contain an increased proportion of fibroblasts. Whittle *et al.* (2000) established amnion epithelial and mesenchymal cells as separate, pure primary cultures and found that PG output by both cell types was increased by dexamethasone.

Prostaglandin synthases

Prostaglandin H_2, formed from PGG_2 by the action of COX-2, is unstable and is converted into more stable metabolites, such as PGD_2, PGE_2 and $PGF_{2\alpha}$, thromboxane (TX) and PGI_2 by the action of the synthases PGDS, PGES and PGFS, TXS and PGIS, respectively (Urade *et al.* 1995). Prostaglandin E synthase expression is higher in placenta compared to myometrium in humans. Two distinct isoforms of PGES have been identified, a cytosolic PGES (cPGES) (Tanioka *et al.* 2000) and a membrane-associated PGES (mPGES) (Jakobsson *et al.* 1999). Cytosolic PGES is constitutively expressed in a wide variety of cells and shows preferential coupling with COX-1 in immediate PGE_2 biosynthesis. Expression of mPGES is strongly induced in inflammatory cells and is preferentially linked with COX-2, promoting delayed and induced immediate PGE_2 biosynthesis (Murakami *et al.* 1999a). Lipopolysaccharide induced-mPGES expression can be blocked by dexamethasone, while cPGES expression remains unaffected. Recent studies have extended the notion of such functional coupling to encompass the other PG synthases. Ueno *et al.* (2001) showed that the PG synthases may be classified into three categories depending on their localisation and COX preference: (i) the perinuclear enzymes that prefer COX-2 (mPGES, PGIS and TXS), (ii) the cytosolic enzyme that prefers COX-1 (cPGES) and (iii) a translocating enzyme that utilises both COX isoforms depending on the stimulus (the secretory PGD synthase isoform, H-PGDS).

Although the roles of PLA_2 and COX in labour have been studied for over a decade, only recently has the role of the prostaglandin synthases been addressed. Alfaidy *et al.* (2003) found immunoreactive mPGES to be highly concentrated in amnion epithelial cells and the chorion laeve trophoblasts, with lower levels in the mesenchymal layers and undetectable in the decidual tissue. Much lower levels of mPGES protein and mRNA were found in placenta than in fetal membranes. The expression of mPGES mRNA did not change with labour in amnion, intact membranes or placenta, but there was an increase in mPGES protein in chorion laeve and a decrease in mPGES protein in placenta during labour. Similarly, Meadows *et al.* (2003) found cPGES immunolocalised in the amnion epithelium, and associated with fibroblasts and macrophages in the chorio-decidual layer, whereas mPGES localised in the amnion epithelium as well as the chorion trophoblast. Both enzymes were found to be associated with lipid particles present in the amnion epithelium, which are more prevalent in term tissues. There were no differences in the amounts of either cPGES or mPGES in amnion and choriodecidua at term or preterm, with or without labour, in either tissue with advancing gestation. Meadows *et al.* (2003) concluded that it does not appear that expression of PGES is the rate-limiting step in PGE_2 synthesis in fetal membranes at labour.

Prostaglandin dehydrogenase

The conversion of PGE_2 and $PGF_{2\alpha}$ to their biologically inactive 15-keto-derivatives is catalysed by 15-Hydroxyprostaglandin dehydrogenase (PGDH). Whilst prostaglandin synthetic enzymes are expressed in the amnion, myometrium, chorion and decidua, PGDH expression predominates in chorion, with low-level activity in decidua and very little activity in amnion. The chorion is therefore a protective barrier preventing the transfer of PGs synthesised within the amnion and chorion to the underlying decidua and myometrium during much of pregnancy. The activity of PGDH decreases in the chorion of some patients in preterm labour (Van Meir *et al.* 1996) as well as term labour (Van Meir *et al.* 1997), leading to a breakdown of the PGDH metabolic barrier and allowing PGs to reach the myometrium and stimulate contractility. This process appears to begin first in the lower segment of the uterus, and may play a role in cervical ripening and fetal membrane remodelling and rupture.

The expression of PGDH, like the enzymes of the PG biosynthetic pathway, is regulated by cytokines but, as might be expected, with generally opposite effects. Intertenkin-1β and TNFα decrease PGDH mRNA levels and PGDH activity in human placental trophoblasts, and these effects can be inhibited by concurrent treatment with the anti-inflammatory cytokine, IL-10 (Pomini *et al.* 1999). It has been postulated that term labour is associated with a decrease in PGDH gene expression and activity in chorion trophoblasts and that this may occur in response to elevated levels of cytokines observed in the inflammatory process of normal labour and/or in association with intrauterine infection (Challis *et al.* 1999). The activity of PGDH is also under hormonal control. Patel *et al.* 2003 demonstrated that progesterone maintains and cortisol decreases PGDH activity and mRNA levels in human chorion and placenta at term.

Treatment of human myometrial cells with a cAMP analogue increases PGDH activity and also enhances progesterone-stimulated promoter activity in the presence of the human progesterone receptor B (PR-B) (Greenland *et al.* 2000). The human progesterone receptor A (PR-A) also confers progesterone responsiveness to the PGDH promoter but, unlike PR-B, its function can not be enhanced by the cAMP analogue. Thus, progesterone exerts its effect on PGDH expression at the transcriptional level.

Three PGDH isoforms have been identified within chorio-decidua and two in placenta, generated by alternative splicing of a single gene. Only the major 824 bp transcript was observed in the myometrium. The mouse PGDH promoter has been shown to contain a putative GRE and oestrogen receptor binding site, as well as potential Sp1, CRE, AP-1, AP-2, and C/EBP elements. Greenland *et al.* (2000) demonstrated striking homology between the proximal promoter region of the mouse and human genes. Conservation of potential binding sites for Myo-D/AP-1 and Sp1/AP-2 suggest functional relevance of these elements. Analysis of 2369 bp of the 5′-flanking region revealed five AP-1 sites, the most proximal of which is neighboured by an Ets site. A clustered region (at −2055/−1964) comprises an AP-1 site adjoined by two adjacent Ets sites, and all three sites are, in turn, flanked by two CREs. Transient transfections showed involvement of AP-1 and Ets in PGDH transcriptional regulation. Cyclic AMP response element-binding protein, c-fos, c-jun and Ets-1 are all capable of interacting with CBP/p300. Therefore, the clustered Ets/AP-1/CRE element could enable multifactorial input to be transduced by a single integrator, the CBP/p300 coactivator. Kirk *et al.* (2003) recently used transient transfection studies to show that the PGDH promoter is more active in prelabour than postlabour amnion cells. Postlabour amnion cells have higher levels of NF-κB activity (see below), and overexpression of NF-κB p65 was found to repress the PGDH promoter. This suggests that, although the PGDH promoter does not carry any consensus NF-κB DNA binding sites, nevertheless cytokines and other stimuli which increase NF-κB activity may decrease PGDH expression. Nuclear factor-kappaB may be acting to downregulate PGDH by direct DNA binding or by its interactions with other transcription factors or cofactors.

Interleukin-8

The changes in structure of the cervix at the time of parturition, with a decrease in the concentration of collagen and its dissociation, a looser matrix and an increase in the water content means that the cervical tissue offers low resistance to force applied and the fibres will move under tension. During myometrial contractions cervical tissue is thus drawn up into the lower segment of the uterus, in the processes of effacement and dilatation. During cervical ripening there is dissociation and degradation of collagen leading to dramatic alterations in collagen structure during this period. These catalytic changes in collagen are mediated by collagenase (a matrix metalloproteinase), the levels of which have been demonstrated to increase both peripherally and in the cervix during labour (Osmers *et al.* 1992, 1995). The principal collagenase is matrix metalloproteinase-8, which is released from the specific granules of neutrophils rather than being synthesised by the cervical stromal fibroblasts (Osmers *et al.* 1992). There is a marked infiltration of neutrophils into the cervical stroma at term whose subsequent degranulation has been demonstrated (Junqueira *et al.* 1980). Interleukin-8 is a chemokine that is known both to attract and to activate neutrophils. The extravasation of neutrophils that it induces takes place by their adherence to and subsequent diapedesis through the endothelial wall of blood vessels. Following the extravasation of neutrophils into tissues IL-8 causes their activation. In rabbits and humans, intradermal injection of IL-8 induces plasma exudation and a massive local infiltration of neutrophils but not infiltration by other leukocytes. This accumulation of neutrophils is particularly marked around the venules and is strongly enhanced by the concomitant administration of PGE$_2$ (Foster *et al.* 1989; Rampart *et al.* 1989). In both guinea pigs and rabbits application of IL-8 to the cervix induces cervical ripening (Chwalisz *et al.* 1994; el Maradny *et al.* 1994).

Interleukin-8 is produced by human endometrium, choriodecidua, decidua placenta and myometrium, and in pregnant and non-pregnant cervices, and by cervical fibroblasts in culture. As with other 'labour associated genes' its expression increases within the uterus with advancing gestational age and with labour (Elliott *et al.* 2000, 2001b). In addition to playing an important role in cervical ripening it probably also acts in the formation of the lower segment of the uterus in late pregnancy and in mediating the inflammatory infiltrate seen in myometrium during labour (Thomson *et al.* 1999; Young *et al.* 2002).

Interleukin-8 is a 77 amino acid protein whose gene is located on chromosome 4q 12–21. It consists of 4 exons and 3 introns and encompasses approximately 5.2 kb generating a single mRNA transcript of 1.8 kb. Its transcription is rapidly inducible, peaking 3 to 4 hours after stimulation with the cytokine IL-1β and rapidly declining thereafter. This transience of expression is attributed to an AT rich sequence in the 3′ untranslated region leading to a destabilisation of the mRNA. The gene contains a TATA and CAAT box, and potential DNA binding sites for the transcription factors AP-1, -2 and -3, NF-κB, hepatocyte nuclear factor-1, glucocorticoid receptor and interferon regulatory protein-1 (Mukaida *et al.* 1994). It also contains an overlapping Oct 1/C/EBP protein site (Wu *et al.* 1997).

Interleukin-8 expression is induced by IL-1β, TNFα, LPS and phorbol esters. In many cell lines it has been shown that NF-κB or C/EBP elements are responsible for transcriptional activation by these stimuli (Harant *et al.* 1996; Wu *et al.* 1997). Members of the NF-κB family bind strongly to the NF-κB binding site of the gene whereas C/EBP binds only weakly to its recognition site. The binding of the NF-κB family members to their binding site, however, results in strong cooperative binding of C/EBP to the adjacent site. It has been shown that the promoter region of the IL-8 gene is regulated in a cell-line specific manner by NF-κB and either an AP-1 or C/EBP element. In a study examining the regulation of IL-8 gene expression in melanoma cells transfected with part of the IL-8 promoter (−101 to +40 from transcription start) it was found that the NF-κB binding site was essential for transcriptional activation by all-*trans* retinoic acid, IL-1β or TNFα (Harant *et al.* 1996).

Elliott *et al.* (2001a) used site-directed mutagenesis of each of the IL-8 promoter DNA binding sites for the transcription factors NF-κB, AP-1 and C/EBP, which are in close proximity to each other and to the coding region of the gene. They found that the NF-κB site was essential for basal and IL-1β-stimulated gene expression in cervical and amnion cells. Neither of the other binding sites appeared to be essential for gene expression but did play an additive role in promoter activity.

Progesterone and dexamethasone have been shown in several cell culture systems and in explants of various uterine tissues to inhibit IL-8 expression. Dexamethasone has also been shown to reduce the formation of NF-κB complexes composed of p50 (NF-κB1) and p65 (RelA). This may be due to a direct interaction between the glucocorticoid receptor and NF-κB. It has been shown that the glucocorticoid and progesterone receptors can physically associate with RelA causing mutual repression (Mukaida *et al.* 1994; Kalkhoven *et al.* 1996). Nuclear Factor-kappaB activation involves degradation of the cytoplasmic inhibitor of NF-κB, IκB. Dexamethasone has been found to cause transcriptional activation of the IκBα gene resulting in an increase in its synthesis. This IκBα associates with NF-κB in the cytoplasm resulting in a reduced rate of translocation of NF-κB to the nucleus (Auphan *et al.* 1995). However, other work suggests that dexamethasone may inhibit NF-κB by targeting active NF-κB through an IκBα-independent mechanism (Adcock *et al.* 1999). Inhibition of IL-8 production by dexamethasone, and/or progesterone, may therefore occur by the glucocorticoid or progesterone receptor binding either to the IL-8 gene, to the RelA element of NF-κB and/or by the induction of the cytoplasmic inhibitor of NF-κB, IκB. In human bone marrow stromal cell cultures, dexamethasone and hydrocortisone inhibit IL-1β-stimulated IL-8 expression. The addition of cycloheximide to these cultures, however, abolished this effect, suggesting that the formation of new protein, which may be IκBα, is required for the glucocorticoid inhibition of production to be observed.

Interleukin-8 production by the term human placenta is increased during labour and by treatment with the antiprogesterone onapristone. Similarly, in biopsies of first trimester cervix, IL-8 production is increased if the woman is pretreated with the progesterone antagonist mifepristone prior to collection of the biopsy (Denison *et al.* 2000). Production of IL-8 by placenta was also shown to be reduced by culture of tissue explants with progesterone and dexamethasone, the former effect being reversible by antigestagens such as mifepristone (Elliott *et al.* 1998). Loudon *et al.* (2003) examined the effects of IL-1β and progesterone on IL-8 synthesis, mRNA and promoter activity in amnion cells and lower segment fibroblast cells (used as a model for cervical fibroblasts). In both cell types, progesterone had no effect on basal IL-8 synthesis. In lower segment fibroblast cells, IL-1β significantly increased IL-8 protein and mRNA expression, but progesterone significantly attenuated these effects. In amnion cells, IL-1β also increased IL-8 synthesis, mRNA and promoter expression; however, progesterone significantly attenuated these effects only in cells collected before and not after the onset of labour. This supports the concept that progesterone may play a role in maintenance of cervical competence. The lack of effect of progesterone on IL-8 in postlabour cells may be the result of downregulation of the progesterone receptor (PR) during labour or because of increased NF-κB activity which acts to repress PR (see below).

Oxytocin Receptor

The increased oxytocin sensitivity of myometrial tissue at term is due to increased oxytocin receptor (OTR) expression. There is a 300-fold increase in the human OTR mRNA in the myometrium of the term uterus, compared with the non-pregnant uterus (Fuchs *et al.* 1984; Kimura *et al.* 1996). Within the uterus, OTRs are present in myometrial cells where they mediate contractions and in epithelial endometrial and amnion cells where they mediate prostaglandin release. The oxytocin receptor is a cell surface membrane receptor with seven transmembrane domains which belongs to the class I G protein-coupled receptor (GPCR) family. The OTR gene encodes 389 amino acids and is present as a single copy in the human genome mapped to the gene locus 3p25–3p26.2. The gene spans 17 kb and contains three introns and four exons. Deletion experiments show that approximately 1000 bp upstream of the coding region are needed for OTR expression (Inoue *et al.* 1994). In other species such as the rat, OTR is upregulated by oestrogen and downregulated by progesterone (Soloff 1975, 1983; Murata *et al.* 2000). The human OTR promoter does not, however, contain any full consensus oestrogen or progesterone response elements (ERE, PRE) and there is no evidence of direct action of steroids on the OTR gene promoter. In the tammar wallaby, which has a double uterine system but only becomes pregnant in one uterus, OTR expression only increases in the pregnant uterus at term and remains unchanged on the non-pregnant horn. This suggests that OTR is modulated by local rather than by circulating factors (Parry *et al.* 1997).

The OTR promoter contains putative transcription factor binding sites for C/EBP and NF-κB. These transcription factors are activated by cytokines such as IL-1β and IL-6. Expression of IL-1β and IL-6 increases with labour. However the effect of cytokines on OTR activity is conflicting. Schmid *et al.* (2001) and Helmer *et al.* (2002) reported a decrease in OTR mRNA in an immortalised human myometrial cell line after treatment with IL-1β. Schmidt *et al.* (2001) used an immortalised cell line derived from non-pregnant human myometrium and expressed IL-1β effects as a ratio of the pre-treatment OTR mRNA without controls for each time point. This approach does not enable correction for mRNA degradation occurring during the 24 hours of the study. Helmer *et al.* (2002) used a commercially available smooth muscle cell line whose origin is unclear. They used only long incubations with IL-1β ranging from 6 to 48 hours and only 6 hour data was presented. It is doubtful that immortalised cell lines from nonpregnant myometrium represent good models for the pregnant uterus.

Rauk *et al.* (Rauk and Friebe-Hoffmann 2000; Rauk *et al.* 2001) reported a downregulation of OTR mRNA after treatment with IL-1β and an upregulation after treatment with IL-6 in primary human uterine smooth muscle cells. This study measured OTR mRNA concentrations by Southern analysis of agarose gels. Although the study did show an increase in OTR expression at earlier time points the authors concentrated on the downregulation seen at 25 hours. In a study which used quantitative reverse transcriptase-polymerase chain reaction (RT-PCR) a more accurate method to measure mRNA concentrations, and with controls at each time point Terzidou *et al.* (2002) found that IL-1β induces an increase in OTR mRNA that is maximal at 4 hours and is associated with nuclear translocation and an increase in the DNA binding of transcription factors C/EBPβ and NF-κB. In co-transfection experiments they found that OTR promoter activity is increased by C/EBPβ and NF-κB p65 but that there was a more dramatic induction of OTR promoter activity if C/EBPβ and NF-κB p65 were coexpressed. This suggests that OTR, like COX-2 and IL-8, can be induced within the uterus by inflammatory cytokines and that NF-κB acting together with C/EBP plays an important role in its transcription. The concept that OTR is positively, not negatively, regulated by inflammatory mediators is intuitive given the 'inflammatory' nature of the biochemistry of parturition, but how NF-κB and C/EBP interact, and how important they are in vivo remains to be seen.

Transcription factor activity and the onset of labour

The genes associated with labour, including OTR, the enzymes controlling PG synthesis and IL-8, are, at least in part, regulated at the transcriptional level, involving transcription factors such as AP-1, C/EBP and NF-κB. Many labour associated genes also contain CREs. Several recent studies have examined changes in levels and activity of these transcription factors in uterine tissues in association with pregnancy and labour.

Cyclic AMP signalling

Components of the cAMP signalling pathway are differentially regulated in myometrium during pregnancy to promote uterine quiescence until the onset of labour (Europe-Finner *et al.* 1993, 1994). Increases in cAMP changes gene expression through phosphorylation of the transcription factors CRE modulator protein (CREM) and the activating transcription factor family (ATF), which bind to the CRE element in the regulatory regions of responsive genes. Cyclic AMP response element-binding protein, CREM and ATF2 are members of a large class of transcription factors known as bZIP proteins. There are major changes in the expression of protein isoforms of CREB, CREM and ATF2 in the human myometrium during pregnancy (Bailey *et al.* 2000). Cyclic AMP response element binding-protein is primarily expressed in non-pregnant myometrium. The CREMt2α isoform decreases in myometrial tissue during pregnancy and labour, whereas the CREMα isoform is elevated several-fold in pregnant tissue compared to non-pregnant. The CREMα isoform functions as a transrepressor and can also dimerise with CREB, the resulting dimers binding strongly to CREs and, in most cases, acting as potent transrepressors. A novel small variant of ATF2 (ATF2-sm) has recently been identified by Bailey *et al.* (2002). In reporter studies, the repressive effect of CREMα alone appears to be cancelled out by the activating effect of ATF2-sm. Expression of this ATF2 isoform in the myometrium is greater in the upper compared to the lower uterine region during gestation/labour. This raises the possibility that ATF2-sm may promote the expression of genes that propagate fundally dominant contractions before and at the onset of labour. Such genes may include those encoding the OTR, connexin-43 (Cx-43) and COX-2, all of which have CRE motifs in their promoter regions and whose expression within the myometrium during pregnancy/labour is co-localised with this ATF2 isoform.

Activator protein-1 and nuclear factor kappa B

The AP-1 family of transcription factors consists of the proteins c-Jun, JunB, JunD, c-Fos, FRA-1, FRA-2, and FosB, which bind to DNA as either homodimers of the Jun family members or heterodimers of Fos and Jun family proteins. These different dimers have different DNA-binding and transcriptional activation characteristics. In rat myometrium, oestrogen induces the expression of c-fos, c-jun, junD, and junB (Cicatiello *et al.* 1992), while progesterone reduces c-fos, fra-1, fra-2 and junB, but not junD, mRNA levels. c-fos, fosB and fra-1 mRNA levels in rat myometrium are significantly higher during labour, while fra-2 mRNA levels rise earlier and peak during labour (Mitchell and Lye 2002). The OTR and Cx-43 genes, whose expression in the myometrium is required specifically at the time of labour, contain AP-1 binding sites in their promoter, so an increase in AP-1 members during labour may induce expression of these genes. A temporal correlation has been demonstrated between the expression of c-fos and Cx-43 in rat myometrium during labour (Piersanti and Lye 1995) and overexpression of c-fos and c-jun in myometrial cells activates the Cx-43 promoter through the AP-1 site (Mitchell and Lye 2001).

Stretch is imposed on the myometrium by the growing fetus throughout pregnancy and more acutely at the time of labour, and may act together with endocrine stimuli to regulate expression of labour-associated genes. In vitro, stretching of human myometrial cells results in increased COX-2 mRNA levels that are associated with increased activation of AP-1, as assessed by DNA binding studies (Sooranna *et al.* 2004). In rat smooth muscle cells, stretch induces c-fos, fosB, fra-1, c-jun and junB with varying kinetics, while junD and fra-2 levels do not change (Mitchell and Lye 2002). Thus AP-1 proteins may mediate the transduction of mechanical, as well as endocrine, signals during labour.

Activator Protein-1 proteins may also interact with other transcription factors, and cross-coupling between AP-1 and NF-κB proteins has been reported, which results in a synergistic increase in activity at both AP-1 and NF-κB sites (Stein *et al.* 1993). Nuclear factor-kappaB has been shown to be essential for the induction of the human COX-2 and the rat Type II sPLA$_2$ genes (Antonio *et al.* 2002) in many cell types, and may also be involved in AA-mediated signalling (Alaoui-El-Azher *et al.* 2002). Yan *et al.* (2002) found no increase in nuclear NF-κB levels in chorion and amnion at term or after labour, and reported an increase in the nuclear localisation of NF-κB in decidua at term whether or not labour had occurred, suggesting that NF-κB may be important in the activation phase, rather than the stimulation phase, of parturition. However, this study examined only changes in protein levels in the nucleus, so increases in NF-κB activity independent of nuclear translocation may have gone undetected since phosphorylation status and DNA-binding of NF-κB was not assessed.

Using DNA-binding assays and transfection studies, Allport *et al.* (2001) demonstrated constitutive activation of NF-κB in human amnion in association with labour, at a time when COX-2 mRNA and protein levels are known to increase. This activation of NF-κB appears to occur despite a large increase in the synthesis of the inhibitory IκBα protein. Lee *et al.* (2003) showed that, in amnion at the time of labour, there is an increase in the expression of the IkBβ protein. The IκBβ protein acts, like IκBα, to bind to NF-κB but, unlike IκBα, does not cause NF-κB to be exported from the nucleus and allows it to remain transcriptionally active. Similar studies in myometrium are more difficult to perform since myometrial cell cultures take several weeks to grow but it is clear that IL-1β, TNFα, and IL-6 can stimulate NF-κB in myometrium suggesting a probable role for NF-κB in myometrial gene expression (Lindstrom *et al.* 2002). Nuclear factor-kappaB has been reported to interact with members of the C/EBP family and as discussed above, NF-κB may act in synergy with C/EBPβ to regulate expression of the OTR in the myometrium (Terzidou *et al.* 2002).

Steroid hormones

Progesterone inhibits uterine contractions and cervical ripening, promoting pregnancy maintenance (Meis *et al.* 2003), and such a 'progesterone block' must be overcome for labour to occur. Unlike in many other species, in humans labour is not preceded by a detectable withdrawal of progesterone. However, many labour-associated genes, which are normally repressed by progesterone, such as interleukin-1β (Morishita *et al.* 1999), connexin-43 (Kilarski *et al.* 2000) and matrix metalloproteinose-8 (Shimonovitz *et al.* 1998), are upregulated in association with human labour and it is postulated that such a process may be mediated by changes in the function of the PR. The PR protein structure contains a DNA-binding domain (DBD), a hormone-binding domain (HBD) and a variable N-terminal domain. The progesterone receptor is unique within its family group as it exists as two isoforms PR-B (116 kDa) and PR-A (94 kDa). Progesterone receptor-A is a truncated form of PR-B lacking the first 164 N-terminal amino acids. Two distinct promoters within the single copy gene for PR have been described that independently regulate the expression of the two isoforms of PR. The expression of pure homodimers of PR-B has shown that this receptor functions as an activator of transcription. Pure PR-A act as a repressor of transcription (Vegeto *et al.* 1993). An inhibitory function region (IF) has also been characterised lying in a 292 amino-acid segment upstream of activation function-1 (AF1). Inhibitory function region inhibits the activation of transcription directed by both AF1 and AF2 but does not affect AF3 (Hovland *et al.* 1998). This may explain the functional difference between these two receptor isoforms. Heterodimers of PR-A/B also function as transcriptional repressors, therefore PR-A is a dominant negative inhibitor of the transcriptional regulation due to PR-B.

There are changes in the expression of PR in myometrium and amnion leading to an increase in the PR-A:PR-B ratio. Peiber *et al.* (2001) have shown that PR-A inhibits PR-B-mediated transactivation in human amnion and myometrium and suggested that an increase in the PR-A:PR-B ratio may be a cause of 'functional progesterone withdrawal' in myometrium. Mesiano *et al.* (2002) showed that this does occur, at least at the level of mRNA. Kalkhoven *et al.* (1996) reported a mutual negative interaction between the PR and NF-κB that has also been demonstrated in human amnion and myometrium (Allport *et al.* 2001).

Inhibition of NF-κB in the prevention of preterm delivery?

Several lines of evidence suggest a key role for NF-κB in human labour. Many labour-associated genes, including those encoding IL-8 and enzymes of the PG cascade, contain NF-κB elements in their promoters and require NF-κB for their transcription; NF-κB is activated in response to LPS and pro-inflammatory cytokines known to be involved in labour onset; NF-κB in turn stimulates cytokine production, which may result in a positive feed-forward loop with further activation of NF-κB and pro-labour gene upregulation; NF-κB activity is increased in amnion in association with labour. Nuclear factor-kappaB may negatively interact with the PR and thus contribute to a 'functional' progesterone withdrawal. Nuclear factor-kappaB synergistically interacts with AP-1 and C/EBP proteins that are also involved in regulation of labour-associated genes. Nuclear factor-kappaB therefore potentially constitutes a therapeutic target in the prevention of preterm delivery. It is currently a target for drug development in inflammation-associated disorders as diverse as brain injury (Williams *et al.* 2003), inflammatory bowel disease (Segain *et al.* 2003) and cancer. Several strategies have been used to block NF-κB by targeting different steps leading to its activation.

The most direct approach is to block the binding of NF-κB to its cognate site on DNA. A popular strategy uses transcription factor decoys, double-stranded oligodeoxynucleotides (ODN), which bind and compete for the same DNA sites as a specific transcription factor and prevent the binding and transcriptional activity of the factor itself. Such NF-κB ODNs have been shown to inhibit TNFα-induced cytokine and adhesion molecule in an in vivo mouse model of nephritis (Tomita *et al.* 2000). Further upstream in the signalling cascade, the components that normally inhibit NF-κB activation can be targeted. Proteasome inhibitors block the TNFα-induced expression of intercellular adhesion molecule-1(ICAM-1) by inhibiting degradation of the inhibitory IκB protein (Jobin *et al.* 1998). In addition, since phosphorylation of IκBα leads to its ubiquitination and subsequent degradation, compounds that inhibit this phosphorylation, such as sodium salicylate (aspirin) and ibuprofen, prevent activation of NF-κB. Other compounds, including glucocorticoids and IL-10, inhibit NF-κB activity by upregulating IκBα levels (Auphan *et al.* 1995). Glucocorticoids may also inhibit NF-κB by another mechanism, since the GR may physically interact with NF-κB, and thus interfere with its DNA binding or transactivation ability, or it may compete for common coactivator proteins. Interleukin-10 can also operate through multiple mechanisms. It has been shown to repress the activity of the IKK complex and impede IκBα degradation, and also to directly block NF-κB DNA binding (Schottelius *et al.* 1999). Interleukin-10 has been shown to selectively inhibit the activation of NF-κB in stimulated human monocytes, while having no effect on several other transcription factors, including

C/EBP, AP-1, GR and CREB, and clinical trials have established the tolerability and clinical efficacy of a systemic IL-10 therapy for the treatment of Crohn's disease.

Over the years, enzymes involved in PG biosynthesis and metabolism have been the targets for pharmacotherapy with varied success. The recent characterisation of the genes encoding these enzymes and continuing elucidation of their transcriptional control will enable the development of more specific prostanoid inhibitors that target transcription factor activity. Nuclear factor-kappaB is emerging as a potential transcriptional target but, while several agents already in use utilise modulation of NF-κB as part of their therapeutic effect (e.g. glucocorticoids, NSAIDS), NF-κB is also important in other pathways that are required for the normal functioning of the body. Therefore modulation of NF-κB must be selective and specific to prevent toxicity. Further in vivo studies are needed to determine the relative importance and potential interdependence of the different transcription factors (e.g. NF-κB, AP-1, C/EBP, CREB, PPARγ) involved in the regulation of labour-associated pathways.

REFERENCES

Adcock, I. M., Nasuhara, Y., Stevens, D. A. *et al.* (1999) Ligand-induced differentiation of glucocorticoid receptor (GR) trans-repression and transactivation: preferential targetting of NF-kappaB and lack of I-kappaB involvement. *Br. J. Pharmacol.* **127**, 1003–11.

Aitken, M. A., Rice, G. and Brennecke, S. (1992) Relative abundance of human placental phospholipase A2 messenger RNA in late pregnancy. *Prostaglandins* **43**, 361–70.

Alaoui-El-Azher, M., Wu, Y., Havet, N. *et al.* (2002) Arachidonic acid differentially affects basal and lipopolysaccharide-induced sPLA(2)-IIA expression in alveolar macrophages through NF-kappaB and PPAR-gamma-dependent pathways. *Mol. Pharmacol.* **61**, 786–94.

Albert, T. J., Su, H. C., Zimmerman, P. D. *et al.* (1994) Interleukin-1 beta regulates the inducible cyclo-oxygenase in amnion-derived WISH cells *Prostaglandins* **48**, 401–16.

Alfaidy, N., Sun, M., Challis, J. *et al.* (2003) Expression of membrane prostaglandin E synthase in human placenta and fetal membranes and effect of labour. *Endocrine* **20**, 219–26.

Allport, V. C., Slater, D. M., Newton, R. *et al.* (2000) NF-kappaB and AP-1 are required for cyclo-oxygenase 2 gene expression in amnion epithelial cell line (WISH) *Mol. Hum. Reprod.* **6**, 561–5.

Allport, V. C., Pieber, D., Slater, D. M. *et al.* (2001) Human labour is associated with nuclear factor-kappaB activity which mediates cyclo-oxygenase-2 expression and is involved with the 'functional progesterone withdrawal'. *Mol. Hum. Reprod.* **7**, 581–6.

Almawi, W. Y. and Melemedjian, O. K. (2002) Negative regulation of nuclear factor-kappaB activation and function by glucocorticoids. *J. Mol. Endocrinol.* **28**, 69–78.

Alvi, S. A., Brown, N. L., Bennett, P. R. *et al.* (1999) Corticotrophin-releasing hormone and platelet-activating factor induce transcription of the type-2 cyclo-oxygenase gene in human fetal membranes. *Mol. Hum. Reprod.* **5**, 476–80.

Antonio, V., Brouillet, A., Janvier, B. *et al.* (2002) Transcriptional regulation of the rat type IIA phospholipase A2 gene by cAMP and interleukin-1beta in vascular smooth muscle cells: interplay of the CCAAT/enhancer binding protein (C/EBP), nuclear factor-kappaB and Ets transcription factors. *Biochem. J.* **368**, 415–24.

Appleby, S. B., Ristimaki, A., Neilson, K. *et al.* (1994) Structure of the human cyclo-oxygenase-2 gene. *Biochem. J.* **302** (**Pt 3**) 723–7.

Auphan, N., DiDonato, J. A., Rosette, C. *et al.* (1995) Immunosuppression by glucocorticoids: inhibition of NF-kappa B activity through induction of I kappa B synthesis. *Science* **270**, 286–90.

Bailey, J., Sparey, C., Phillips, R. J. *et al.* (2000) Expression of the cyclic AMP-dependent transcription factors, CREB, CREM and ATF2, in the human myometrium during pregnancy and labour. *Mol. Hum. Reprod.* **6**, 648–60.

Bailey, J., Phillips, R. J., Pollard, A. J. *et al.* (2002) Characterisation and functional analysis of cAMP response element modulator protein and activating transcription factor 2 (ATF2) isoforms in the human myometrium during pregnancy and labour: identification of a novel ATF2 species with potent transactivation properties. *J. Clin. Endocrinol. Metab.* **87**, 1717–28.

Baldwin, A. S., Jr. (1996) The NF-kappa B and I kappa B proteins: new discoveries and insights. *Annu. Rev. Immunol.* **14**, 649–83.

Balsinde, J. and Dennis, E. A. (1996) The incorporation of arachidonic acid into triacylglycerol in P388D1 macrophage-like cells. *Eur. J. Biochem.* **235**, 480–5.

Bennett, P., Slater, D., Berger, L. *et al.* (1994) The expression of phospholipase A2 and lipocortins (annexins) I, II and V in human fetal membranes and placenta in association with labour. *Prostaglandins* **48**, 81–90.

Bennett, W. A., Allbert, J. R., Brackin, M. N. *et al.* (1999) Secretory component in human amniotic fluid and gestational tissues: a potential endogenous phospholipase A2 inhibitor. *J. Soc. Gynecol. Investig.* **6**, 311–17.

Caivano, M., Gorgoni, B., Cohen, P. *et al.* (2001) The induction of cyclo-oxygenase-2 mRNA in macrophages is biphasic and requires both CCAAT enhancer-binding protein beta (C/EBP beta) and C/EBP delta transcription factors. *J. Biol. Chem.* **276**, 48693–701.

Calder, A. A. (1997) Review of prostaglandin use in labour induction. *BJOG* **104 Suppl 15**, 2–7; discussion 20–5.

Calder, A. A. and Greer, I. A. (1992) Prostaglandins and the cervix. *Baillieres Clin. Obstet. Gynaecol.* **6**, 771–86.

Challis, J. R., Patel, F. A. and Pomini, F. (1999) Prostaglandin dehydrogenase and the initiation of labour. *J. Perinat. Med.* **27**, 26–34.

Chen, J., Engle, S. J., Seilhamer, J. J. *et al.* (1994) Cloning and recombinant expression of a novel human low molecular weight Ca(2+)-dependent phospholipase A2. *J. Biol. Chem.* **269**, 2365–8.

Chwalisz, K., Benson, M., Scholz, P. *et al.* (1994) Cervical ripening with the cytokines interleukin 8, interleukin 1 beta and tumour necrosis factor alpha in guinea-pigs. *Hum. Reprod.* **9**, 2173–81.

Cicatiello, L., Ambrosino, C., Coletta, B. *et al.* (1992) Transcriptional activation of jun and actin genes by oestrogen during mitogenic stimulation of rat uterine cells. *J. Steroid Biochem. Mol. Biol.* **41**, 523–8.

Clark, J. D., Lin, L. L., Kriz, R. W. *et al.* (1991) A novel arachidonic acid-selective cytosolic PLA$_2$ contains a Ca(2 +)-dependent translocation domain with homology to PKC and GAP. *Cell*, **65**, 1043–51.

Clark, J. D., Schievella, A. R., Nalefski, E. A. *et al.* (1995) Cytosolic phospholipase A2. *J. Lipid. Mediat. Cell Signal.* **12**, 83–117.

Couturier, C., Antonio, V., Brouillet, A. *et al.* (2000) Protein kinase A-dependent stimulation of rat type II secreted phospholipase A(2) gene transcription involves C/EBP-beta and -delta in vascular smooth muscle cells. *Arterioscler. Thromb. Vasc. Biol.* **20**, 2559–65.

Couturier, C., Brouillet, A., Couriaud, C. *et al.* (1999) Interleukin 1beta induces type II-secreted phospholipase A(2) gene in vascular smooth muscle cells by a nuclear factor kappaB and peroxisome proliferator-activated receptor-mediated process. *J. Biol. Chem.* **274**, 23085–93.

Crowl, R. M., Stoller, T. J., Conroy, R. R. *et al.* (1991) Induction of phospholipase A2 gene expression in human hepatoma cells by mediators of the acute phase response. *J. Biol. Chem.* **266**, 2647–51.

Denison, F. C., Riley, S. C., Elliott, C. L. *et al.* (2000) The effect of mifepristone administration on leukocyte populations, matrix metalloproteinases and inflammatory mediators in the first trimester cervix. *Mol. Hum. Reprod.* **6**, 541–8.

Desvergne, B. and Wahli, W. (1999) Peroxisome proliferator-activated receptors: nuclear control of metabolism. *Endocr. Rev.* **20**, 649–88.

DeWitt, D. L. (1991) Prostaglandin endoperoxide synthase: regulation of enzyme expression. *Biochim. Biophys. Acta* **1083**, 121–34.

DeWitt, D. L., Meade, E. A. and Smith, W. L. (1993) PGH synthase isoenzyme selectivity: the potential for safer nonsteroidal antiinflammatory drugs. *Am. J. Med.* **95**, 40S–44S.

Dolan-O'Keefe, M., Chow, V., Monnier, J. *et al.* (2000) Transcriptional regulation and structural organization of the human cytosolic phospholipase A(2) gene. *Am. J. Physiol. Lung Cell Mol. Physiol.* **278**, L649–57.

Economopoulos, P., Sun, M., Purgina, B. *et al.* (1996) Glucocorticoids stimulate prostaglandin H synthase type-2 (PGHS-2) in the fibroblast cells in human amnion cultures. *Mol. Cell. Endocrinol.* **117**, 141–7.

el Maradny, E., Kanayama, N., Halim, A. *et al.* (1994) Interleukin-8 induces cervical ripening in rabbits. *Am. J. Obstet. Gynecol.* **171**, 77–83.

Elliott, C. L., Kelly, R. W., Critchley, H. O. *et al.* (1998) Regulation of interleukin 8 production in the term human placenta during labour and by antigestagens. *Am. J. Obstet. Gynecol.* **179**, 215–20.

Elliott, C. L., Slater, D. M., Dennes, W. *et al.* (2000) Interleukin 8 expression in human myometrium: changes in relation to labour onset and with gestational age. *Am. J. Reprod. Immunol.* **43**, 272–7.

Elliott, C. L., Allport, V. C., Loudon, J. A. *et al.* (2001a) Nuclear factor-kappa B is essential for upregulation of interleukin-8 expression in human amnion and cervical epithelial cells. *Mol. Hum. Reprod.* **7**, 787–90.

Elliott, C. L., Loudon, J. A., Brown, N. *et al.* (2001b) IL-1beta and IL-8 in human fetal membranes: changes with gestational age, labour, and culture conditions. *Am. J. Reprod. Immunol.* **46**, 260–7.

Erkinheimo, T. L., Saukkonen, K., Narko, K. *et al.* (2000) Expression of cyclo-oxygenase-2 and prostanoid receptors by human myometrium. *J. Clin. Endocrinol. Metab.* **85**, 3468–75.

Europe-Finner, G. N., Phaneuf, S., Watson, S. P. *et al.* (1993) Identification and expression of G-proteins in human myometrium: upregulation of G alpha s in pregnancy. *Endocrinology* **132**, 2484–90.

Europe-Finner, G. N., Phaneuf, S., Tolkovsky, A. M. *et al.* (1994) Down-regulation of G alpha s in human myometrium in term and preterm labour: a mechanism for parturition. *J. Clin. Endocrinol. Metab.* **79**, 1835–9.

Farrugia, W., Nicholls, L. and Rice, G. E. (1999) Effect of bacterial endotoxin on the in vitro release of Type II phospholipase-A2 and prostaglandin E2 from human placenta. *J. Endocrinol.* **160**, 291–6.

Foster, S. J., Aked, D. M., Schroder, J. M. *et al.* (1989) Acute inflammatory effects of a monocyte-derived neutrophil-activating peptide in rabbit skin. *Immunology* **67**, 181–3.

Freed, K. A., Moses, E. K., Brennecke, S. P. *et al.* (1997) Differential expression of type II, IV and cytosolic PLA$_2$ messenger RNA in human intrauterine tissues at term. *Mol. Hum. Reprod.* **3**, 493–9.

Fuchs, A. R., Fuchs, F., Husslein, P. *et al.* (1984) Oxytocin receptors in the human uterus during pregnancy and parturition. *Am. J. Obstet. Gynecol.* **150**, 734–41.

Gelb, M. H., Valentin, E., Ghomashchi, F. *et al.* (2000) Cloning and recombinant expression of a structurally novel human secreted phospholipase A2. *J. Biol. Chem.* **275**, 39823–6.

Giannoulias, D., Patel, F. A., Holloway, A. C. *et al.* (2002) Differential changes in 15-hydroxyprostaglandin dehydrogenase and prostaglandin H synthase (types I and II) in human pregnant myometrium. *J. Clin. Endocrinol. Metab.* **87**, 1345–52.

Gibb, W. and Lavoie, J. C. (1990) Effects of glucocorticoids on prostaglandin formation by human amnion. *Can. J. Physiol. Pharmacol.* **68**, 671–6.

Gorgoni, B., Caivano, M., Arizmendi, C. *et al.* (2001) The transcription factor C/EBPbeta is essential for inducible expression of the cox-2 gene in macrophages but not in fibroblasts. *J. Biol. Chem.* **276**, 40769–77.

Greenland, K. J., Jantke, I., Jenatschke, S. *et al.* (2000) The human NAD + -dependent 15-hydroxyprostaglandin dehydrogenase gene promoter is controlled by Ets and activating protein-1 transcription factors and progesterone. *Endocrinology* **141**, 581–97.

Harant, H., de Martin, R., Andrew, P. J. *et al.* (1996) Synergistic activation of interleukin-8 gene transcription by all-trans-retinoic acid and tumor necrosis factor-alpha involves the transcription factor NF-kappaB. *J. Biol. Chem.* **271**, 26954–61.

Helmer, H., Tretzmuller, U., Brunbauer, M. *et al.* (2002) Production of oxytocin receptor and cytokines in primary uterine smooth muscle cells cultivated under inflammatory conditions. *J. Soc. Gynecol. Investig.* **9**, 15–21.

Hirst, J. J., Teixeira, F. J., Zakar, T. *et al.* (1995) Prostaglandin endoperoxide-H synthase-1 and -2 messenger ribonucleic acid levels in human amnion with spontaneous labour onset. *J. Clin. Endocrinol. Metab.* **80**, 517–23.

Hovland, A. R., Powell, R. L., Takimoto, G. S. *et al.* (1998) An N-terminal inhibitory function, IF, suppresses transcription by the A-isoform but not the B-isoform of human progesterone receptors. *J. Biol. Chem.* **273**, 5455–60.

Inamori, K., Sagawa, N., Hasegawa, M. *et al.* (1993) Identification and partial characterization of phospholipase D in the human amniotic membrane. *Biochem. Biophys. Res. Commun.* **191**, 1270–7.

Inoue, T., Kimura, T., Azuma, C. *et al.* (1994) Structural organization of the human oxytocin receptor gene. *J. Biol. Chem.* **269**, 32451–6.

Ishihara, O., Khan, H., Sullivan, M. H. *et al.* (1992) Interleukin-1 beta stimulates decidual stromal cell cyclo-oxygenase enzyme and prostaglandin production. *Prostaglandins* **44**, 43–52.

Jacques, C., Bereziat, G., Humbert, L. *et al.* (1997) Posttranscriptional effect of insulin-like growth factor-I on interleukin-1beta-induced type II-secreted phospholipase A2 gene expression in rabbit articular chondrocytes. *J. Clin. Invest.* **99**, 1864–72.

Jakobsson, P. J., Thoren, S., Morgenstern, R. *et al.* (1999) Identification of human prostaglandin E synthase: a microsomal, glutathione-dependent, inducible enzyme, constituting a potential novel drug target. *Proc. Natl. Acad. Sci. U. S. A.* **96**, 7220–5.

Jobin, c., Hellerbrand, c., Licato, L. L., Brenner, D. A. and Sartor, R. B. (1998) Mediation by NF-KappaB of cytokine induced expression of intercellular adhesion molecule 1 (ICAM-1) in an intestinal epithelial cell line, a process blocked by proteasome inhibitors. *Gut* **42**, 779–87.

Johnson, R. F., Mitchell, C. M., Giles, W. B. *et al.* (2002) The in vivo control of prostaglandin H synthase-2 messenger ribonucleic acid expression in the human amnion at parturition. *J. Clin. Endocrinol. Metab.* **87**, 2816–23.

Junqueira, L. C., Zugaib, M., Montes, G. S. *et al.* (1980) Morphologic and histochemical evidence for the occurrence of collagenolysis and for the role of neutrophilic polymorphonuclear leukocytes during cervical dilation. *Am. J. Obstet. Gynecol.* **138**, 273–81.

Kalkhoven, E., Wissink, S., van der Saag, P. T. *et al.* (1996) Negative interaction between the RelA(p65) subunit of NF-kappaB and the progesterone receptor. *J. Biol. Chem.* **271**, 6217–24.

Keirse, M. J. and Turnbull, A. C. (1973) E prostaglandins in amniotic fluid during late pregnancy and labour. *J. Obstet. Gynaecol. Br. Commonw.* **80**, 970–3.

Keirse, M. J., Flint, A. P. and Turnbull, A. C. (1974) F prostaglandins in amniotic fluid during pregnancy and labour. *J. Obstet. Gynaecol. Br. Commonw.* **81**, 131–5.

Kilarski, W. M., Hongpaisan, J., Semik, D. *et al.* (2000) Effect of progesterone and oestradiol on expression of connexin43 in cultured human myometrium cells. *Folia. Histochem. Cytobiol.* **38**, 3–9.

Kimura, T., Takemura, M., Nomura, S. *et al.* (1996) Expression of oxytocin receptor in human pregnant myometrium. *Endocrinology* **137**, 780–5.

Kirk, R. E., Slater, D. M., Gellerson, B. *et al.* (2003) Regulation of NAD + -dependent 15-hydroxyprostaglandin dehydrogenase in human term amnion with response to labour. *J. Soc. Gynecol. Investig.* **10**, 145A.

Kudo, I., Murakami, M., Hara, S. *et al.* (1993) Mammalian non-pancreatic phospholipases A2. *Biochim. Biophys. Acta* **1170**, 217–31.

Kuwata, H., Nakatani, Y., Murakami, M. *et al.* (1998) Cytosolic phospholipase A2 is required for cytokine-induced expression of type IIA secretory phospholipase A2 that mediates optimal cyclo-oxygenase-2-dependent delayed prostaglandin E2 generation in rat 3Y1 fibroblasts. *J. Biol. Chem.* **273**, 1733–40.

Lappas, M., Permezel, M., Georgiou, H. M. *et al.* (2002) Regulation of proinflammatory cytokines in human gestational tissues by peroxisome proliferator-activated receptor-gamma: effect of 15-deoxy-delta(12,14)-PGJ(2) and troglitazone. *J. Clin. Endocrinol. Metab.* **87**, 4667–72.

Lappas, M., Permezel, M., Georgiou H. M. *et al.* (2004) Regulation of phospholipase isozymes by nuclear factor-kappaB in human gestational tissues in vitro. *J. Clin. Endocrinol. Metab.* **89**, 2365–72.

Lappas, M., Permezel, M. and Rice, G. E. (2003) *N*-Acetyl-cysteine inhibits phospholipid metabolism, proinflammatory cytokine release, protease activity, and nuclear factor-kappaB deoxyribonucleic acid-binding activity in human fetal membranes in vitro. *J. Clin. Endocrinol. Metab.* 2003 **88**, 1723–9.

Lee, Y., Allport, V., Sykes, A. *et al.* (2003) The effects of labour and of interleukin 1 beta upon the expression of nuclear factor kappa B related proteins in human amnion. *Mol. Hum. Reprod.* **9**, 213–18.

Lim, H., Paria, B. C., Das, S. K. *et al.* (1997) Multiple female reproductive failures in cyclo-oxygenase 2-deficient mice. *Cell* **91**, 197–208.

Lindstrom, T. L. Y. S., Allport, V. C. and Bennett P. R. (2002) The pattern of increased NF-kappaB activity in the myometrium in association with labour differs from that stimulated by IL-1beta but both stimulate the COX-2 promoter. *J. Soc. Gynecol. Investig.* **9**, 132A.

Lopez Bernal, A., Anderson, A. B. and Turnbull, A. C. (1982) Cortisol:cortisone interconversion by human decidua in relation to parturition: effect of tissue manipulation on 11 beta-hydroxysteroid dehydrogenase activity. *J. Endocrinol.* **93**, 141–9.

Loudon, J. A., Elliott, C. L., Hills, F. *et al.* (2003) Progesterone represses interleukin-8 and cyclo-oxygenase-2 in human lower segment fibroblast cells and amnion epithelial cells. *Biol. Reprod.* **69**, 331–7.

Macchia, L., Di Paola, R., Guerrese, M. C. *et al.* (1997) Expression of prostaglandin endoperoxide H synthase 1 and 2 in human placenta at term. *Biochem. Biophys. Res. Commun.* **233**, 496–501.

Matsuo, M., Ensor, C. M. and Tai, H. H. (1997) Characterization of the genomic structure and promoter of the mouse NAD + -dependent 15-hydroxyprostaglandin dehydrogenase gene. *Biochem. Biophys. Res. Commun.* **235**, 582–6.

Meadows, J. W., Eis, A. L., Brockman, D. E. *et al.* (2003) Expression and localization of prostaglandin E synthase isoforms in human fetal membranes in term and preterm labour. *J. Clin. Endocrinol. Metab.* **88**, 433–9.

Meis, P. J., Klebanoff, M., Thom, E. *et al.* (2003) Prevention of recurrent preterm delivery by 17 alpha-hydroxyprogesterone caproate. *N. Engl. J. Med.* **348**, 2379–85.

Mesiano, S., Chan, E. C., Fitter, J. T. *et al.* (2002) Progesterone withdrawal and oestrogen activation in human parturition are coordinated by progesterone receptor A expression in the myometrium. *J. Clin. Endocrinol. Metab.* **87**, 2924–30.

Mestre, J. R., Rivadeneira, D. E., Mackrell, P. J. *et al.* (2001) Overlapping CRE and E-box promoter elements can independently regulate COX-2 gene transcription in macrophages. *FEBS. Lett.* **496**, 147–51.

Mitchell, J. A. and Lye, S. J. (2001) Regulation of connexin43 expression by c-fos and c-jun in myometrial cells. *Cell. Commun. Adhes.* **8**, 299–302.

Mitchell, J. A. and Lye, S. J. (2002) Differential expression of activator protein-1 transcription factors in pregnant rat myometrium. *Biol. Reprod.* **67**, 240–6.

Mitchell, B. F. and Olson, D. M. (2004) Prostaglandin endoperoxide H synthase inhibitors and other tocolytics in preterm labour. *Prostaglandins Leukot. Essent. Fatty Acids.* **70**, 167–87.

Mitchell, M. D., Edwin, S. S., Lundin Schiller, S. *et al.* (1993) Mechanism of interleukin-1 beta stimulation of human amnion prostaglandin biosynthesis: mediation via a novel inducible cyclo-oxygenase. *Placenta* **14**, 615–25.

Molnar, M., Rigo, J., Jr, Romero, R. *et al.* (1999) Oxytocin activates mitogen-activated protein kinase and up-regulates cyclo-oxygenase-2 and prostaglandin production in human myometrial cells. *Am. J. Obstet. Gynecol.* **181**, 42–9.

Moore, S. D., Brodt-Eppley, J., Cornelison, L. M. *et al.* (1999) Expression of prostaglandin H synthase isoforms in human myometrium at parturition. *Am. J. Obstet. Gynecol.* **180**, 103–9.

Morishita, M., Miyagi, M. and Iwamoto, Y. (1999) Effects of sex hormones on production of interleukin-1 by human peripheral monocytes. *J. Periodontol.* **70**, 757–60.

Mukaida, N., Morita, M., Ishikawa, Y. *et al.* (1994) Novel mechanism of glucocorticoid-mediated gene repression. Nuclear factor-kappa B is target for glucocorticoid-mediated interleukin 8 gene repression. *J. Biol. Chem.* **269**, 13289–95.

Munns, M. J., Farrugia, W., King, R. G. *et al.* (1999) Secretory type II PLA_2 immunoreactivity and PLA_2 enzymatic activity in human gestational tissues before, during and after spontaneous-onset labour at term. *Placenta* **20**, 21–6.

Murakami, M., Nakatani, Y., Atsumi, G. *et al.* (1997) Regulatory functions of phospholipase A2. *Crit. Rev. Immunol.* **17**, 225–83.

Murakami, M., Kambe, T., Shimbara, S. *et al.* (1999a) Functional coupling between various phospholipase A2s and cyclo-oxygenases in immediate and delayed prostanoid biosynthetic pathways. *J. Biol. Chem.* **274**, 3103–15.

Murakami, M., Kambe, T., Shimbara, S. *et al.* (1999b) Different functional aspects of the group II subfamily (Types IIA and V) and type X secretory phospholipase A(2)s in regulating arachidonic acid release and prostaglandin generation. Implications of cyclo-oxygenase-2 induction and phospholipid scramblase-mediated cellular membrane perturbation. *J. Biol. Chem.* **274**, 31435–44.

Murata, T., Murata, E., Liu, C. X. *et al.* (2000) Oxytocin receptor gene expression in rat uterus: regulation by ovarian steroids. *J. Endocrinol.* **166**, 45–52.

Naylor, L. H. and Clark, E. M. (1990) d(TG)n.d(CA)n sequences upstream of the rat prolactin gene form Z-DNA and inhibit gene transcription. *Nucleic. Acids. Res.* **18**, 1595–601.

Nguyen, H. T., Rice, G. E., Farrugia, W. *et al.* (1994) Bacterial endotoxin increases type II phospholipase A2 immunoreactive content and phospholipase A2 enzymatic activity in human choriodecidua. *Biol. Reprod.* **50**, 526–34.

Ohara, O., Ishizaki, J., Nakano, T. *et al.* (1990) A simple and sensitive method for determining transcription initiation site: identification of two transcription initiation sites in rat group II phospholipase A2 gene. *Nucleic Acids Res.* **18**, 6997–7002.

Okazaki, T., Casey, M. L., Okita, J. R. *et al.* (1981) Initiation of human parturition. XII. Biosynthesis and metabolism of prostaglandins in human fetal membranes and uterine decidua. *Am. J. Obstet. Gynecol.* **139**, 373–81.

Osman, I., Young, A., Ledingham, M. A. *et al.* (2003) Leukocyte density and pro-inflammatory cytokine expression in human fetal membranes, decidua, cervix and myometrium before and during labour at term. *Mol. Hum. Reprod.* **9**, 41–5.

Osmers, R., Rath, W., Adelmann-Grill, B. C. *et al.* (1992) Origin of cervical collagenase during parturition. *Am. J. Obstet. Gynecol.* **166**, 1455–60.

Osmers, R. G., Adelmann-Grill, B. C., Rath, W. *et al.* (1995) Biochemical events in cervical ripening dilatation during pregnancy and parturition. *J. Obstet. Gynaecol.* **21**, 185–94.

Parry, L. J., Bathgate, R. A., Shaw, G. *et al.* (1997) Evidence for a local fetal influence on myometrial oxytocin receptors during pregnancy in the tammar wallaby (Macropus eugenii). *Biol. Reprod.* **56**, 200–7.

Patel, F. A., Funder, J. W. and Challis, J. R. (2003) Mechanism of cortisol/progesterone antagonism in the regulation of 15-hydroxyprostaglandin dehydrogenase activity and messenger ribonucleic acid levels in human chorion and placental trophoblast cells at term. *J. Clin. Endocrinol. Metab.* **88**, 2922–33.

Pieber, D., Allport, V. C., Hills, F. *et al.* (2001) Interactions between progesterone receptor isoforms in myometrial cells in human labour. *Mol. Hum. Reprod.* **7**, 875–9.

Piersanti, M. and Lye, S. J. (1995) Increase in messenger ribonucleic acid encoding the myometrial gap junction protein, connexin-43, requires protein synthesis and is associated with increased expression of the activator protein-1, c-fos. *Endocrinology* **136**, 3571–8.

Pind, S. and Kuksis, A. (1988) Solubilization and assay of phospholipase A2 activity from rat jejunal brush-border membranes. *Biochim. Biophys. Acta* **938**, 211–21.

Pomini, F., Caruso, A. and Challis, J. R. (1999) Interleukin-10 modifies the effects of interleukin-1beta and tumor necrosis factor-alpha on the activity and expression of prostaglandin H synthase-2 and the NAD + -dependent 15-hydroxyprostaglandin dehydrogenase in cultured term human villous trophoblast and chorion trophoblast cells. *J. Clin. Endocrinol. Metab.* **84**, 4645–51.

Potter, S., Mitchell, M. D., Hansen, W. R. *et al.* (2000) NF-IL6 and CRE elements principally account for both basal and interleukin-1 beta-induced transcriptional activity of the proximal 528bp of the PGHS-2 promoter in amnion-derived AV3 cells: evidence for involvement of C/EBP beta. *Mol. Hum. Reprod.* **6**, 771–8.

Rampart, M., Van Damme, J., Zonnekeyn, L. *et al.* (1989) Granulocyte chemotactic protein/interleukin-8 induces plasma leakage and neutrophil accumulation in rabbit skin. *Am. J. Pathol.* **135**, 21–5.

Rauk, P. N. and Friebe-Hoffmann, U. (2000) Interleukin-1 beta down-regulates the oxytocin receptor in cultured uterine smooth muscle cells. *Am. J. Reprod. Immunol.* **43**, 85–91.

Rauk, P. N., Friebe-Hoffmann, U., Winebrenner, L. D. *et al.* (2001) Interleukin-6 up-regulates the oxytocin receptor in cultured uterine smooth muscle cells. *Am. J. Reprod. Immunol.* **45**, 148–53.

Rice, G. E., Wong, M. H., Farrugia, W. *et al.* (1998) Contribution of type II phospholipase A2 to in vitro phospholipase A2 enzymatic activity in human term placenta. *J. Endocrinol.* **157**, 25–31.

Ricote, M., Li, A. C., Willson, T. M. *et al.* (1998) The peroxisome proliferator-activated receptor-gamma is a negative regulator of macrophage activation. *Nature* **391**, 79–82.

Sangha, R. K., Walton, J. C., Ensor, C. M. *et al.* (1994) Immunohistochemical localization, messenger ribonucleic acid abundance, and activity of 15-hydroxyprostaglandin dehydrogenase in placenta and fetal membranes during term and preterm labour. *J. Clin. Endocrinol. Metab.* **78**, 982–9.

Satoh, K., Yasumizu, T., Fukuoka, H. *et al.* (1979) Prostaglandin F2 alpha metabolite levels in plasma, amniotic fluid, and urine during pregnancy and labour. *Am. J. Obstet. Gynecol.* **133**, 886–90.

Schmid, B., Wong, S. and Mitchell, B. F. (2001) Transcriptional regulation of oxytocin receptor by interleukin-1beta and interleukin-6. *Endocrinology* **142**, 1380–5.

Schottelius, A. J., Mayo, M. W., Sartor, R. B. *et al.* (1999) Interleukin-10 signalling blocks inhibitor of kappaB kinase activity and nuclear factor kappaB DNA binding. *J. Biol. Chem.* **274**, 31868–74.

Schuster-Woldan, N., Hilton, M. and Wilson, T. (1997) RU486 inhibits synthesis of an endogenous inhibitor of cell arachidonate release from choriodecidua tissue. *Mol. Hum. Reprod.* **3**, 743–7.

Segain, J. P., Raingeard de la Bletiere, D., Sauzeau, V. *et al.* (2003) Rho kinase blockade prevents inflammation via nuclear factor kappa B inhibition: evidence in Crohn's disease and experimental colitis. *Gastroenterology* **124**, 1180–7.

Shimonovitz, S., Hurwitz, A., Hochner-Celnikier, D. *et al.* (1998) Expression of gelatinase B by trophoblast cells: down-regulation by progesterone. *Am. J. Obstet. Gynecol.* **178**, 457–61.

Six, D. A. and Dennis, E. A. (2000) The expanding superfamily of phospholipase A(2) enzymes: classification and characterization. *Biochim. Biophys. Acta* **1488**, 1–19.

Skannal, D. G., Brockman, D. E., Eis, A. L. *et al.* (1997a) Changes in activity of cytosolic phospholipase A2 in human amnion at parturition. *Am. J. Obstet. Gynecol.* **177**, 179–84.

Skannal, D. G., Eis, A. L., Brockman, D. *et al.* (1997b) Immunohistochemical localization of phospholipase A2 isoforms in human myometrium during pregnancy and parturition. *Am. J. Obstet. Gynecol.* **176**, 878–82.

Skinner, K. A. and Challis, J. R. (1985) Changes in the synthesis and metabolism of prostaglandins by human fetal membranes and decidua at labour. *Am. J. Obstet. Gynecol.* **151**, 519–23.

Slater, D. M., Berger, L. C., Newton, R. *et al.* (1995) Expression of cyclo-oxygenase types 1 and 2 in human fetal membranes at term. *Am. J. Obstet. Gynecol.* **172**, 77–82.

Slater, D., Allport, V. and Bennett, P. (1998) Changes in the expression of the type-2 but not the type-1 cyclo-oxygenase enzyme in chorio-decidua with the onset of labour. *BJOG* **105**, 745–8.

Slater, D. M., Dennes, W. J., Campa, J. S. *et al.* (1999) Expression of cyclo-oxygenase types-1 and -2 in human myometrium throughout pregnancy. *Mol. Hum. Reprod.* **5**, 880–4.

Slater, D. M., Myles, L., Sykes, A. *et al.* (2000) Expression of secretory and cytosolic phospholipase A2 in human myometrium: changes in relation to gestational age and labour onset. *J. Soc. Gynecol. Investig.* **7**, 129A.

Soloff, M. S. (1975) Uterine receptor for oxytocin: effects of oestrogen. *Biochem. Biophys. Res. Commun.* **65**, 205–12.

Soloff, M. S., Fernstrom, M. A., Periyasamy, S. *et al.* (1983) Regulation of oxytocin receptor concentration in rat uterine explants by oestrogen and progesterone. *Can. J. Biochem. Cell Biol.* **61**, 625–30.

Sooranna, S. R., Lee, Y., Kim, L. U. *et al.* (2004) Mechanical stretch activates type 2 cyclo-oxygenase via activator protein-1 transcription factor in human myometrial cells. *Mol. Hum. Reprod.* **10**, 109–13.

Sparey, C., Robson, S. C., Bailey, J. *et al.* (1999) The differential expression of myometrial connexin-43, cyclo-oxygenase-1 and -2, and Gs alpha proteins in the upper and lower segments of the human uterus during pregnancy and labour. *J. Clin. Endocrinol. Metab.* **84**, 1705–10.

Stein, B., Baldwin, A. S., Jr, Ballard, D. W. *et al.* (1993) Cross-coupling of the NF-kappa B p65 and Fos/Jun transcription factors produces potentiated biological function. *EMBO. J.* **12**, 3879–91.

Stuhlmeier, K. M., Kao, J. J. and Bach, F. H. (1997) Arachidonic acid influences proinflammatory gene induction by stabilizing the inhibitor-kappaBalpha/nuclear factor-kappaB (NF-kappaB) complex, thus suppressing the nuclear translocation of NF-kappaB. *J. Biol. Chem.* **272**, 24679–83.

Tanioka, T., Nakatani, Y., Semmyo, N. *et al.* (2000) Molecular identification of cytosolic prostaglandin E2 synthase that is functionally coupled with cyclo-oxygenase-1 in immediate prostaglandin E2 biosynthesis. *J. Biol. Chem.* **275**, 32775–82.

Tay, A., Maxwell, P., Li, Z. G. *et al.* (1994) Cytosolic phospholipase A2 gene expression in rat mesangial cells is regulated post-transcriptionally. *Biochem. J.* **304** (Pt 2), 417–22.

Terzidou, V., Christian, M., Lee, Y. *et al.* (2002) Regulation of Human Oxytocin Receptor by C/EBP and NF-κB. *J. Soc. Gynecol. Investig.* **9**, 90A.

Thomson, A. J., Telfer, J. F., Young, A. *et al.* (1999) Leukocytes infiltrate the myometrium during human parturition: further evidence that labour is an inflammatory process. *Hum. Reprod.* **14**, 229–36.

Tomita, N., Morishita, R., Tomita, S. *et al.* (2000) Transcription factor decoy for NFkappaB inhibits TNF-alpha-induced cytokine and adhesion molecule expression in vivo. *Gene. Ther.* **7**, 1326–32.

Trautman, M. S., Edwin, S. S., Collmer, D. *et al.* (1996) Prostaglandin H synthase-2 in human gestational tissues: regulation in amnion. *Placenta* **17**, 239–45.

Ueno, N., Murakami, M., Tanioka, T. *et al.* (2001) Coupling between cyclo-oxygenase, terminal prostanoid synthase, and phospholipase A2. *J. Biol. Chem.* **276**, 34918–27.

Uozumi, N., Kume, K., Nagase, T. *et al.* (1997) Role of cytosolic phospholipase A2 in allergic response and parturition. *Nature* **390**, 618–22.

Urade, Y., Watanabe, K. and Hayaishi, O. (1995) Prostaglandin D, E, and F synthases. *J. Lipid. Mediat. Cell Signal.* **12**, 257–73.

Van Meir, C. A., Sangha, R. K., Walton, J. C. *et al.* (1996) Immunoreactive 15-hydroxyprostaglandin dehydrogenase (PGDH) is reduced in fetal membranes from patients at preterm delivery in the presence of infection. *Placenta* **17**, 291–7.

Van Meir, C. A., Ramirez, M. M., Matthews, S. G. *et al.* (1997) Chorionic prostaglandin catabolism is decreased in the lower uterine segment with term labour. *Placenta* **18**, 109–14.

Vane, J. R. and Botting, J. M. (1997) Mechanism of aspirin-like drugs. *Semin. Arth. Rheum.* **26**, 2–10.

Vegeto, E., Shahbaz, M. M., Wen, D. X. *et al.* (1993) Human progesterone receptor A form is a cell- and promoter-specific repressor of human progesterone receptor B function. *Mol. Endocrinol.* **7**, 1244–55.

Wang, I. M., Mehta, V. and Cook, R. G. (1993) Regulation of TL antigen expression. Analysis of the T18d promoter region and responses to IFN-gamma. *J. Immunol.* **151**, 2646–57.

Whittle, W. L., Gibb, W. and Challis, J. R. (2000) The characterization of human amnion epithelial and mesenchymal cells: the cellular expression, activity and glucocorticoid regulation of prostaglandin output. *Placenta* **21**, 394–401.

Williams, A. J., Hale, S. L., Moffett, J. R. *et al.* (2003) Delayed treatment with MLN519 reduces infarction and associated neurologic deficit caused by focal ischemic brain injury in rats via antiinflammatory mechanisms involving nuclear factor-kappaB activation, gliosis, and leukocyte infiltration. *J. Cereb. Blood Flow Metab.* **23**, 75–87.

Wu, G. D., Lai, E. J., Huang, N. *et al.* (1997) Oct-1 and CCAAT/enhancer-binding protein (C/EBP) bind to overlapping elements within the interleukin-8 promoter. The role of Oct-1 as a transcriptional repressor. *J. Biol. Chem.* **272**, 2396–403.

Wu, T., Ikezono, T., Angus, C. W. *et al.* (1994) Characterization of the promoter for the human 85 kDa cytosolic phospholipase A2 gene. *Nucleic Acids Res.* **22**, 5093–8.

Xue, S., Slater, D. M., Bennett, P. R. *et al.* (1996) Induction of both cytosolic phospholipase A2 and prostaglandin H synthase-2 by interleukin-1 beta in WISH cells inhibited by dexamethasone. *Prostaglandins* **51**, 107–24.

Yan, X., Sun, M. and Gibb, W. (2002) Localization of nuclear factor-kappa B (NF kappa B) and inhibitory factor-kappa B (I kappa B) in human fetal membranes and decidua at term and preterm delivery. *Placenta* **23**, 288–93.

Young, A., Thomson, A. J., Ledingham, M. *et al.* (2002) Immunolocalization of proinflammatory cytokines in myometrium, cervix, and fetal membranes during human parturition at term. *Biol. Reprod.* **66**, 445–9.

Zakar, T., Olson, D. M., Teixeira, F. J. *et al.* (1996) Regulation of prostaglandin endoperoxide H2 synthase in term human gestational tissues. *Acta Physiol. Hung.* **84**, 109–18.

Zuo, J., Lei, Z. M., Rao, C. V. *et al.* (1994) Differential cyclo-oxygenase-1 and -2 gene expression in human myometria from preterm and term deliveries. *J. Clin. Endocrinol. Metab.* **79**, 894–9.

4

Fetal outcome following preterm delivery

Malcom Levene and Lawrence Miall

The General Infirmary at Leeds

Introduction

Severe prematurity is the commonest cause of death and disability in perinatal medicine. It is essential to provide parents whose baby is at risk of being delivered extremely prematurely with an accurate and honest assessment of their baby's chance of survival and, if the child does survive to go home, inform them of the risk of severe disability in later life. With increasing survival of very immature babies the focus has shifted, to an extent, to discussions with the parents of whether the child is likely to be disabled and the severity of any subsequent disability. Predictions of severe disability, including cerebral palsy, severe learning problems, blindness and deafness, are reasonably accurate on a statistical basis, but in recent years it has become increasingly apparent that babies who survive into childhood with no severe neurological disability may show significant problems at school age, and these may, in turn, cause considerable distress to the family. This chapter reviews the best evidence on risk of death and disability in severely prematurely born babies.

The chapter is divided into five sections including a general critique of preterm delivery outcome studies, as well as reviews of mortality, severe disability, less severe short-term morbidity and long-term outcome into adolescence.

Methodology of outcome reviews

The medical literature on survival and disability rates varies considerably and this variation is dependent on a number of methodological factors. Table 4.1 lists some of the potential confounding variables, and these will be discussed in detail here in order to develop actuarial tables, which give the best evidence for outcome in the perinatal period, so that the parents may be most accurately advised.

Description of immaturity

In the past, estimation of the duration of pregnancy has been based on maternal dates. For obvious reasons these may be unreliable and consequently in many

Preterm Labour Managing Risk in Clinical Practice, eds. Jane Norman and Ian Greer. Published by Cambridge University Press. © Cambridge University Press 2005.

Table 4.1. Important factors to be considered which may bias mortality and morbidity statistical data

Description of immaturity
Regional vs. hospital specific outcome
Time period of study
Denominator
Age at death
Growth restriction
Multiple births
Racial characteristics
Lethal congenital malformations
Low follow-up compliance

follow-up studies, authors have chosen to refer to outcome by birthweight, which is considered to be the most objective descriptor of maturity. There is an obvious limitation in defining survival by birth weight in that obstetricians who advise families prior to delivery may have little ability to precisely estimate fetal weight. Additionally, growth restriction may have an independent effect on outcome. With early ultrasound imaging, a more accurate assessment of gestational age (or verification of the maternal dates) is possible. Consequently, mortality and disability rates expressed by gestational age are likely to be more valuable from both the obstetric and paediatric point of view.

The description of outcome by birth weight is also confounded by variations in the way that the birth weight-specific categories are determined. Some reports take very low birth weight babies as 1500 g and below, whilst others refers to those babies of up to 1499 g. As it is common practice to round up weight to the nearest 10 g when weighing newborn babies, it is likely that there will be a systematic bias as a result of this practice. For these reasons, the best evidence for outcome as a result of immaturity is described by gestational age (in completed weeks of pregnancy) and the data within this chapter will give prognostic information using gestational age wherever possible.

Regional versus hospital-specific outcome

Follow-up studies from referral centres, often based on teaching hospitals, may be biased in selection criteria. If the referral centre is a recognised centre of excellence, then the sickest babies may be referred, whilst less sick infants may be retained in the base hospital. This may cause a significant bias towards higher mortality amongst the sickest babies in the referral centre. Equally, unreliable access to cots for all very sick babies within referral centres may bias the population sampled. For these reasons, regionally-based studies are less likely to be associated with bias, as all babies within a geographically-defined area will be included irrespective of which hospital they are looked after. The larger the geographical area, the more reliable and generalisable the information becomes. It is for this reason that we have concentrated in this chapter on reporting data derived from regional studies. Where data are not available from regional studies, it is made clear that these data may be less reliable.

The most reliable outcome and follow-up data are those based on national cohorts. There are now a number of studies describing the national outcome of all babies born in a one year period from Holland (Verloove-Vanhorick *et al.* 1986), Britain (Costeloe *et al.* 2000), Finland (Tommiska *et al.* 2001), and Canada (Kramer *et al.* 2000). Other good studies report more localised geographically-based data from the United States (Gould *et al.* 2000; Hernandez *et al.* 2000) and Sweden (Holmgren and Hogberg 2001). The Dutch study (Verloove-Vanhorick *et al.* 1986) refers to babies of birthweight 1500 g and below, born in 1983 and, as such, reflects an era of neonatal medicine that is less relevant to modern practices. More recently, a British study (Costeloe *et al.* 2000) has reported the survival and outcome of all extremely immature babies of 25 weeks' gestation and below born in the UK in 1997. This study is particularly valuable, as it is a recent cohort and describes a very large group of babies. Other studies are based on the collection of national statistics, which may not accurately reflect gestational age.

Time period of study

An obvious criticism of outcome studies in groups of premature babies is that the older the children are at the time that survival and neurodevelopmental outcome is reported, so the longer ago the time that they were born. Differences in neonatal management may have occurred between the time that they were born and the present era. The two most important innovations in perinatal medicine that have affected mortality and morbidity in recent years are the widespread use of antenatal corticosteroids and the introduction of surfactant therapy for ventilated babies. Although the beneficial effect of antenatal steroids was first recognised over 30 years ago, it was only in the 1990s that this form of treatment became relatively widespread. Surfactant therapy, for babies with respiratory distress syndrome, became increasingly available from 1990 and mortality rates in infants of 23–26 weeks' gestation fell significantly after the introduction of surfactant therapy, but not in the most immature subgroup of 23 and 24 weeks' gestation babies (Jacobs *et al.* 2000). It is therefore most appropriate to consider the modern era for perinatal medicine to be from 1990 onwards, and this chapter has selectively given particular emphasis to studies reporting babies who were born from 1990 onwards. It has been shown that the gestational age of babies born in the 1990s is lower than cohorts born in the 1980s, and that the survival rates for these very immature babies in the more recent era is significantly higher than those born in the 1980s (O'Shea *et al.* 1997; Emsley *et al.* 1998; Gould *et al.* 2000).

Denominator

It has been shown that there is a potential for selection bias in preterm cohort studies, dependent on when the babies were admitted to the study. Some outcome studies refer only to babies admitted to the Neonatal Intensive Care Unit, whilst others refer to all babies born alive, and yet others include stillbirths within the same gestational age range as well as those born alive. There is clearly a continuum of mortality from those babies who die in labour, those who are born alive but in whom resuscitation is unsuccessful or not offered and who are never admitted to a Neonatal Intensive Care Unit, and those who die despite intensive care.

A recently-published systematic review has shown clear evidence of selection bias in preterm survival studies (Evans and Levene 2001). For infants of 23–27 weeks of gestation there was a significant trend towards increased survival in cohorts where outcome was reported for those babies who were admitted alive to the neonatal unit (Grade C studies), compared with all babies born alive, including those deaths prior to admission (Grade B studies) and of outcome of all pregnancies where both stillbirths and livebirths were included (Grade A studies). Grade C studies exaggerated survival compared to Grade A studies by 100% at 23 weeks (20% vs. 10%) and by 56% at 24 weeks (42% vs. 27%). Even at 26 weeks comparison of these two types of studies showed a difference of 13% (62% vs. 55%).

It is clear that if survival figures based on admission to a neonatal unit are used by medical staff counselling parents prior to the birth of their very preterm baby, then there may be an overestimation of the survival statistics for each gestational age group. This will not provide parents with the best information, and for this reason the survival figures described in this chapter refer mainly to those studies that report stillbirths and deaths prior to admission to the neonatal unit, as well as outcome of babies admitted to a neonatal unit.

Age at death

Official government mortality rates in perinatal and neonatal deaths are defined by an arbitrary census age such as 7 days for perinatal deaths and 28 days for neonatal deaths. Depending on how mortality rates are expressed, reports on mortality of very premature babies may be distorted by the manner in which time of death is registered. Most deaths in extremely low birth weight babies occur in the first 3–4 days of life (Meadow *et al.* 1996; O'Shea *et al.* 1997). In babies born with birthweight <750 g, if death occurs, the majority (88.5%) die on the first day of

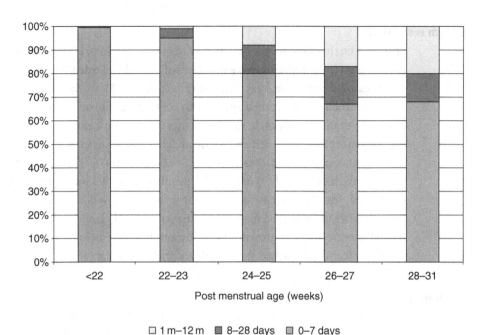

Figure 4.1   Time of death for a national Canadian cohort born 1992–4 (Joseph *et al.* 2000).

life, with more than one half of those deaths occurring in the first hour of life (57%) (Hernandez *et al.* 2000) and there has been no change in the time of death in this subgroup in recent years (Gould *et al.* 2000).

There is evidence that with reducing mortality amongst these very premature infants in more recent years, the time to death has been prolonged. Gould *et al.* (2000) studied time to death in subgroups of very low birthweight infants when two timed cohorts (1993 vs. 1987) representing all births in California were compared. There was a significant increase in both average and median times until death between the two cohorts when a subgroup of babies 750–999 g (8 day increase) and 1000–1499 g (11 day increase) were compared. In one study of mortality rates in infants born at 22–25 weeks, reporting mortality at 28 days after birth would only have included 92% of those who survived until 180 days of beyond (discharge from hospital) (El-Metwally *et al.* 2000).

Figure 4.1 shows the timing of death in a group of very immature babies (<32 weeks' gestation) born 1992–4 in Canada. Almost all of the most immature die in the first week of life, but with increasing gestational age the time of death is shifted to the right, with 20% of deaths occurring after the first month of life in babies of 28–31 weeks (Joseph *et al.* 2000).

Growth restriction

Studies referring to outcome based on either birth weight or gestational age may be confounded by unrepresentative numbers of growth-retarded babies. A study of a large national cohort of very immature babies (25–31 weeks of gestation) who were also small for gestational age (<10th centile) has shown a significantly higher mortality than appropriately grown infants (25th–75th centile) when gestational age, singleton/multiple birth and mode of delivery is adjusted for (odds ratio (OR) 2.38, 95% confidence interval (CI) 1.25–4.54 $p = 0.007$). The outcome for very severe growth-restricted ($\leq$ 1st centile) premature infants was worse than a group controlled for gestational age without growth-restriction. The outcome for severely growth-restricted infants < 550 g was dismal (Lee *et al.* 2001). The additional adverse effect of growth restriction on mortality is supported by a number of other recently published studies (Piper *et al.* 1996; Bernstein *et al.* 2000).

Multiple births

There has been a marked increase in the numbers of multiple births in recent years largely due to assisted reproductive technologies. Multiple birth is associated with a fivefold increase in the rate of prematurity compared with singletons (Alexander *et al.* 1998, Demissie *et al.* 2001) and babies comprising multiple birth cohorts make a significant contribution to the burden of neonatal intensive care offered to very immature babies. Surprisingly, survival rates for very immature twins appear to be higher than those of singletons of the same gestation or birthweight (Cheung *et al.* 2000; Glinianaia *et al.* 2000).

In a survey of all babies born in the northern Region of England (approximately 40 000 births per year), the extended perinatal mortality rate (EPMR), defined as the total number of stillbirths and neonatal deaths up to 28 days per 1000 livebirths and stillbirths, for the years 1988–94 was higher for multiple births weighing <1000 g than in a comparable group of singletons (753.5 vs. 631/1000) (Glinianaia *et al.* 2000). Interestingly, for each higher birthweight category up to 2499 g there was an increase in the EPMR in singletons compared with twins. Another geographically-based study of all births in Sweden 1982–95 showed that singletons born between 28–36 weeks had higher perinatal, neonatal and infant mortality than did twins born in the same period (Cheung *et al.* 2000).

Racial characteristics

Survival rates for White and Black babies have been compared in studies from the United States. Preterm birth rates for Whites increased from 8.8% in 1989 to 10.2% in 1997, but for Black babies the rates fell from 19% to 17.5% over the same period of time (Demissie *et al.* 2001). The main factors in this increasing trend in White babies was Obstetric intervention comprising increases in both preterm induction of labour and preterm Caesarean section rates. Despite this, in 1997 the mortality rate for preterm infants was considerably higher in both the neonatal and infant periods for Black babies compared with Whites (Demissie *et al.* 2001).

In very low birth weight infants born in the USA there was a greater reduction in mortality rates amongst White babies than Black babies in the years 1988–91 with the introduction of surfactant therapy. The improvement in survival was contributed predominately by a reduction in death from respiratory disorders that appeared to have a more beneficial effect on White than Black infants (Ranganathan *et al.* 2000). The rates of decline in neonatal mortality from all respiratory causes were twice as great in White infants than African American infants.

Lethal congenital malformations

Many studies reporting outcome of prematurely born babies exclude those with "lethal" congenital malformations and most studies acknowledge this in their description. Each outcome study should be carefully scrutinised to ascertain whether this correction was made.

Follow-up compliance

Many follow-up studies are weakened by low follow-up compliance with only one half or less of children who survived being seen at the follow-up age. It has been shown quite convincingly that those children that are hardest to find for follow-up may be the ones with the most disability (Tin *et al.* 1998; Callanan *et al.* 2001). Thus careful attention to compliance is essential in order to reduce the risk of bias. We have chosen not to review follow-up studies in the section on severe disability where compliance is less than 85%.

Mortality

It is clear from the above that observer bias may significantly influence the result of outcome studies of the premature infants. We have reviewed studies of babies born in 1990 or beyond where mortality is expressed by gestational age groups. These studies largely report a defined geographical location where the denominator data are given and includes stillbirths or deaths in labour. Ten such studies have been identified (see Table 4.2) and Figure 4.2 shows the mortality rates by gestational age 22–31 weeks inclusive. There is a stepwise increase in the proportion of surviving babies when these studies are pooled together. This represents the best data currently available.

Table 4.2. Details of ten studies describing neonatal mortality in the modern era

Author	Date babies born	Region	Age at ascertainment
Tin *et al.* (1997)	1991–4	Northern Region, UK	1 year
Kramar *et al.* (2000)	1989–3	Canada (single centre)	6 months
Kilpatrick *et al.* (1997)	1990–4	USA (single centre)	Discharge from hospital
Lefebvre *et al.* (1996)	1987–92	Canada (single centre)	Discharge from hospital
Holmgren and Hogberge (2001)	1991–6	Sweden, Northern	1 year
Doyle (2001)	1991–2	Victoria, Australia	5 years
Sutton and Bajuk (1999)	1992–3	NSW, Australia	1 year
Cartlidge and Stewart (1997)	1993–4	Wales, UK	1 year
El-Metwally *et al.* (2000)	1993–7	USA (single centre)	Discharge from hospital

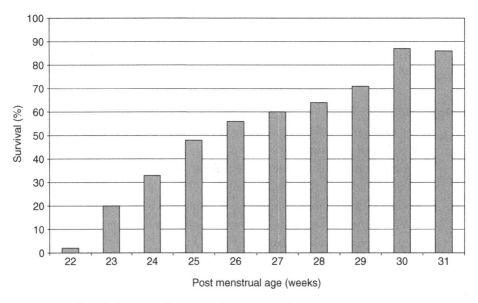

Figure 4.2.   Overall survival by gestational age after preterm birth.

Major disabilities

Although the question of survival will be most parents' first concern, the fear of
irreversible brain injury usually increases rapidly once survival looks increasingly
likely. It is therefore very important to be able to give the most accurate estimate of
adverse outcome in these very immature babies. Severely abnormal outcome is
usually defined as intellectual impairment (IQ or developmental quotient below
two standard deviations from the mean), severe cerebral palsy (inability to walk

Table 4.3. Details of three studies describing major disability

Author	Date babies born	Region	Follow-up age
Jacobs et al. (2000)	1990–4	Canada (3 centres)	18–24 months
Doyle (2001)	1991–2	Victoria, Australia	5 years
Tin et al. (1997)	1991–4	Northern Region, UK	12 months

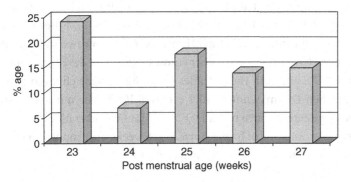

Figure 4.3.   Incidence of major disability amongst survivors.

independently), severe visual impairment or deafness requiring hearing amplification. To date there are very few reports that describe severely adverse outcome based on geographical populations in the era of modern neonatal intensive care (1990 onwards).

Overall severe disability

In a UK national survey of babies born at gestational age 25 weeks and less, 22.6% of those surviving to 30 months of age had severe disability based on the definition above (Wood et al. 2000). Two further recent studies of babies born in the modern neonatal era and reporting a cohort of survivors delivered at 23–28 weeks (Lefebvre et al. 1996) and 23–27 weeks (Sutton and Bajuk 1999), surviving to 18 months and 12 months respectively had a near identical proportion of survivors with major disability; 15% and 14.5%. It was not possible from these studies to determine the proportion severely disabled by gestational age group.

Three outcome studies of babies born in 1990 and beyond report major disability by gestational age groups (Table 4.3, Figure 4.3) and, although the numbers in each group are small, there appears to be a high risk of severe disability at 23 and 24 weeks (approximately 25%), with a reduction at 25 weeks and above in the order of 14%–18%. (Tin et al. 1997; Jacobs et al. 2000; Doyle 2001). This supports the suggestion from the three papers described above that the most immature survivors had the highest risk of serious adverse outcome. With the exception of the study from the state of Victoria, Australia where the follow-up period was 5 years, the other two studies only reported follow-up to one year (Tin *et al.* 1997) and 18–24 months (Jacobs *et al.* 2000). Some caution is necessary in interpreting these data as major disability may later emerge which is not apparent when the children are assessed at a very young age.

Intellectual impairment

Only one geographically-based study has reported IQ levels in survivors born in 1991–3 and who survived to 5 years of age (Doyle 2001). Fifteen per cent were found to be significantly intellectually impaired (IQ below two standard deviations from the mean (>-2SD)). Two other studies report low developmental quotients (DQ) (>-2SD), but both these studies only followed the children to a relatively young age when DQ may not predict eventual IQ. In the most immature group (<26 weeks' gestation) 30% had a DQ > -2SDs (Wood *et al.* 2000). In the other study reporting outcome of babies born 24–26 weeks the proportion with a similar significantly low DQ was 23% (Piecuch *et al.* 1997).

Cerebral palsy (CP)

Six studies report the proportion of severely preterm infants who survived with cerebral palsy (Lefebvre *et al.* 1996; Piecuch *et al.* 1997; Sutton and Bajik 1999; Jacobs *et al.* 2000; Wood *et al.* 2000; Doyle 2001). The overall rate of CP in these studies varies from 11%–18%. Overall 188 (15%) babies survived to develop CP out of 1243 survivors. Severe or major cerebral palsy was reported in four studies (Lefebvre *et al.* 1996; Jacobs *et al.* 2000; Wood *et al.* 2000; Doyle 2001) and the proportion of survivors with this type of CP was 4%–10%. Overall, 71 (7%) of 995 survivors of severe prematurity developed major cerebral palsy.

Blindness

The major cause of blindness in very premature surviving infants is severe retinopathy of prematurity (ROP) with stages four and five of the disease representing retinal detachment. The other important cause is cortical blindness usually associated with severe periventricular leukomalacia involving the optic radiations within the occipital region.

Severe ROP occurs almost exclusively in infants of <1000 g birthweight. There is a clear association with low gestational age, low birthweight and high levels of supplemental oxygen, as described in the 1950s (Lanman *et al.* 1954), though other factors, especially retinal immaturity and genetic predisposition may be important. With increased awareness of the risks of hyperoxia, the incidence of ROP has fallen (Blair *et al.* 2001). The risk of blindness due to ROP fell from 6/89 (6.7%) in

Table 4.4. Blindness due to ROP

Reference	Population	Blindness due to ROP
Wood *et al.* (2000)	$< =25$ weeks	6/283 (2.1%)
Emsley *et al.* (1998)	23–25 weeks	7/40 (18%)
Sutton & Bajuk (1999)	<28 weeks	5/255 (2%)
Finnstrom *et al.* (1997)	<1000 g	11/370 (3%)
Victorian Infant Study (1997)	<1000 g	5/237 (2.1%)
O'Shea *et al.* (1997)	<800 g	5/129 (3.8%)

1979 to 5/237 (2.1%) in 1991 (OR for blindness 0.24 (95% CI 0.06–0.93)) amongst a cohort of ELBW (extremely low birthweight) infants in Victoria, Australia (Victorian Infant Collaborative Study Group 1997). In the UK EpiCure study 7/283 (2%) infants $< =25$ weeks were blind at 30 months and six of these were due to ROP (Wood *et al.* 2000).

Blindness is a relatively rare sequelae of severe prematurity and has been reported to occur in 0.9%–2.5% of very immature infants (Lefebvre *et al.* 1996; Jacobs *et al.* 2000; Wood *et al.* 2000; Doyle 2001). The highest incidence of blindness occurred in the most immature follow-up group (Wood *et al.* 2000). Table 4.4 summarises recent studies reporting the incidence of blindness due to ROP.

Severe hearing impairment

Deafness severe enough to require hearing amplification was a relatively rare outcome in very prematurely born infants. In four recent studies the incidence of severe deafness was reported to be 0.9%–3.6% (Lefebvre *et al.* 1996; Jacobs *et al.* 2000; Wood *et al.* 2000; Doyle 2001).

Short-term morbidity

Where possible we have tried to concentrate on studies which collected data on geographically-defined populations. Some single centre studies are described where the centre was likely to have provided a comprehensive tertiary service to a defined geographical region. All the studies mentioned collected data prospectively over a period of time. Where possible we have included studies based on gestational age. However, many of the large longer-term follow-up studies are based on cohorts defined on the basis of birthweight, and where necessary we have included these. Information on gestation within these studies is provided where possible. For school-age outcomes we only considered studies with greater than five years' follow-up. For long-term outcomes into adulthood we have only considered studies where follow-up was at least 18 years. Where studies include data from the pre-surfactant era we have made this clear.

Chronic lung disease and home oxygen

Preterm infants surviving neonatal intensive care are at increased risk of chronic lung disease (CLD). Northway's original definition of bronchopulmonary dysplasia (BPD), which relied on radiological abnormality at 28 days of life (Northway *et al.* 1967), has largely been replaced by a clinical definition of CLD. This term is now used to refer to infants requiring supplemental oxygen at 36 weeks' postconception age (PCA) and has a higher positive predictive value for poor respiratory outcome than oxygen dependency at 28 days (63% vs. 38%) (Shennan *et al.* 1988). However, a recent study showed that oxygen dependency at 28 days is independently associated with respiratory symptoms to the age of 5 years and respiratory morbidity (Kinali *et al.* 1999).

The prevalence of CLD is inversely related to gestational age, but also seems to be reducing in frequency, with a significant reduction between 1980 and 1990 (OR of 0.88 for each successive year) (Corcoran *et al.* 1993). Rates of CLD for preterm infants born in the era of antenatal steroid therapy and postnatal surfactant use vary between 14% and 43% (Greenough 2000). In a recent Finnish national cohort study 83/211 (39%) ELBW infants were oxygen dependent at 36 weeks (Tommiska *et al.* 2001), and in a Swedish national prospective study of 633 ELBW infants the rate was 28% (Finnstrom *et al.* 1997). The prevalence of CLD is still high amongst infants born in the modern era at the extremes of prematurity. Chronic lung disease occurs in 57% to 70% of survivors at 23 weeks, 33%–89% at 24 weeks and 16%–71% at 25 weeks' gestational age (Hack and Fanaroff 1999). In a large national cohort of infants $<=25$ weeks' gestational age, 231/314 (74%, 95% CI 68%–78%) were receiving supplemental oxygen at 36 weeks and 51% at 40 weeks' post-menstrual age, despite nearly three-quarters receiving postnatal corticosteroid treatment for CLD (Costeloe *et al.* 2000). Oxygen dependency at 36 weeks' post-menstrual age in all VLBW (very low birth weight) infants in a large cohort was 23%, but rose to 52% in the subgroup of infants <750 g (Lemons *et al.* 2001).

Whilst CLD has implications for long-term respiratory morbidity, one of the major short-term implications for parents is the need for supplemental oxygen at discharge. Increasing numbers of infants with CLD are now able to be cared for at home, as part of a home-oxygen therapy programme. Few studies, however, document the rates of home-oxygen treatment. In the EPICure study, 32% of infants $<=25$ weeks were discharged on oxygen (Costeloe *et al.* 2000). In a US cohort 15% of 4438 VLBW infants surviving to discharge were sent home on oxygen, compared to 34% in the smallest infants <750 g (Lemons *et al.* 2001).

Table 4.5. Oxygen dependency at 36 weeks

Reference	$<=23$ weeks	24 weeks	25 weeks	Total
Costeloe *et al.* (2000)	86%	77%	70%	74%
Hack *et al.* (2002)	57%–70%	38%–89%	16%–71%	
Tommiska *et al.* (2001)			ELBW ($<$1000 g)	39%
Finnstrom *et al.* (1997)			ELBW ($<$1000 g)	28%
Lemons *et al.* (2001)			$<$750 g	52%

Amongst a geographically-defined cohort of infants at the limit of viability (BW< 500 g), 9/18 (50%) infants surviving to discharge were sent home on supplemental oxygen, for a mean duration of 15 (range 4–33) months (Sauve *et al.* 1998).

Retinopathy of prematurity

Blindness due to severe ROP is considered above in the section on major disability. Retinopathy of prematurity is due to abnormal proliferation of blood vessels in the developing retina. Less severe degrees of visual impairment still cause considerable morbidity. Mild visual impairment was present in 5% of infants 23–25 weeks, myopia in 6 (15%) and strabismus (squint) in 5 (13%) (Emsley *et al.* 1998). In the EPICure study of infants $<=25$ weeks, squint was present at 30 months in 71/283 (25%) infants and ten per cent wore eye-glasses. Ten per cent had some useful vision but this was not fully correctable. Eighty-two per cent had normal visual function (Wood *et al.* 2000). Amongst 2449 infants <1251 g enrolled in the Multicentre Trial of Cryotherapy for Retinopathy of Prematurity (CRYO-ROP), 289/2449 (11.8%) showed strabismus at 3 and 12 month follow-up, and the overall prevalence of strabismus during the first year of life was 14.7%. These infants were born between 1986 and 1987 (Bremer *et al.* 1998).

Necrotising enterocolitis and feeding difficulties

Necrotising enterocolitis (NEC) can occur in infants of any gestation, though it is more common in preterm infants. In extremely preterm infants there are often no particular risk factors, other than prematurity, but in term and moderately preterm infants it is associated with gut ischaemia secondary to perinatal asphyxia and intra-uterine growth retardation. Necrotising enterocolitis usually develops after the introduction of enteral feeding. It carries a mortality of around 22% and complications in those who survive include recurrence of NEC, stricture formation and malabsorption due to short bowel syndrome.

The incidence of proven NEC in a large prospective cohort of 4438 VLBW infants born in the mid 1990s in the USA was 7%. In a subgroup of infants with birthweight 501–600 g the incidence of proven NEC was 15% (Lemons *et al.* 2001) and in infants <500 g an incidence of 22% has been reported (Sauve *et al.* 1998).

The incidence of NEC in ELBW infants in Finland was 14% based on clinical signs and 9% based on bowel perforation (Tommiska *et al.* 2001). Many studies report NEC rates in survivors, rather than live born infants, which leads to an apparently lower incidence. In Sweden only 2% of ELBW infants *surviving to discharge* had suffered NEC (Finnstrom *et al.* 1997). In the EPICure cohort (infants $< = 25$ weeks), the incidence of surgical intervention for suspected NEC amongst survivors was 13/308 (4%). In a further 497 infants who died, NEC was the stated cause of death in 17 (3.6%) (Costeloe *et al.* 2000).

Feeding problems are common in extremely preterm infants, for a variety of reasons including poor swallowing, gastro-oesophogeal reflux and brain injury. In one study 5/13 (38%) infants with BW <500 g were gastrostomy fed at 3 years of age (Sauve *et al.* 1998).

Rehospitalisation

Premature infants commonly require rehospitalisation after discharge home. Rehospitalisation within the first year of life ranges from 53% to 69% for ELBW infants (O'Shea *et al.* 1997; Sauve *et al.* 1998).

One of the common reasons for rehospitalisation is lower respiratory tract infection, especially respiratory syncitial virus (RSV) infection in winter months. A study of 1721 preterm infants (23–36 weeks) showed 3.2% were rehospitalised in their first year of life due to RSV infection. The risk of rehospitalisation was increased for gestational age <32 weeks (OR 2.6), CLD (OR 3.7) and being discharged during winter (OR 2.7) (Joffe *et al.* 1999).

School age outcomes

By definition prospective studies, which have assessed very long-term neurodevelopmental and respiratory outcomes, relate to cohorts of infants born prior to the era of antenatal steroid and postnatal surfactant therapy. However, several large geographically-defined cohort studies are now reporting long-term outcomes into school age (i.e. > five years).

Chronic respiratory symptoms

Lung function tests are abnormal in 11 years-olds born prematurely. Very low birthweight infants with a history of chronic lung disease show hyperexpansion with a significantly higher residual volume/total lung capacity than either preterm infants without CLD or infants who were not ventilated (Doyle *et al.* 1996). Similar results were obtained in a cohort of preterm infants <32 weeks, where preterm infants with CLD had significantly reduced forced expiratory volume in 1 second (FEV1) and significantly reduced forced vital capacity (FVC) at age 7 years compared with both term controls and aged matched controls without BPD (Gross *et al.* 1998). An obstructive respiratory function pattern may persist into adolescence, although some improvement has been seen between the ages of 8 and 15 years (Koumbourlis *et al.* 1996).

Half of all VLBW infants will wheeze recurrently through infancy and approximately 33% will continue to wheeze throughout their pre-school years. This is more likely if there is a family history of atopy or if they were oxygen dependent at 28 days (Greenough *et al.* 1996; Kinali *et al.* 1999). Amongst a large cohort of 5–11 year olds, wheezing most days was associated with a history of prematurity, and each additional week of gestation reduced the risks of subsequent wheezing at school age by 10% (Rona *et al.* 1993).

Dyspraxia

Cerebral palsy as a major disability is described above. Less severe forms of movement disorder such as dyspraxia (clumsiness) are nevertheless potentially disabling conditions. Preterm infants are at increased risk of on-going motor impairment into adolescence even if they are free of major neurodevelopmental disabilities and attend mainstream school. In a cohort of 12–13 year old VLBW (<1250 g) survivors in the Mersey region of the UK, 51% showed clinically important or borderline motor impairment; of these 34% had significant motor impairment vs. 5% of controls. Test of motor function included manual dexterity, ball skills and balance. Boys fared significantly worse than girls (Powls *et al.* 1995).

Extremely low birthweight infants score significantly worse than term controls for fine motor and gross motor function at the age of eight. The majority of these children show problems in more than one area of fine motor control. Even amongst those children free of disability the rate of fine motor problems is three times higher than controls (32% vs. 10%) (Whitfield *et al.* 1997). An increase in left handedness and fine motor incoordination is commoner in low birthweight children (Elliman *et al.* 1991). In a cohort of infants <35 weeks' gestation from a single hospital, 44% of survivors without a major disability scored badly (<15th percentile) on a test of fine and gross motor function and 17% were <15th percentile in tests of visual-motor integration skills (Jongmans *et al.* 1997).

Cognitive ability

A cohort of 400 ELBW (<800 g) infants born in British Columbia between 1974 and 1985 have been followed prospectively. Ninety-six per cent follow-up was obtained amongst the 120 surviving children at a mean age of 8.6 years. Severe or multiple neurosensory disabilities (any of blindness, deafness, non-ambulatory CP IQ < 69) was present in 14% of the ELBW group and 13% had borderline IQ (Global IQ score 70–84) versus none in the term control group. Extremely low birth weight infants were three times more likely to have learning disorders (47% vs. 18%) than controls. Overall 26% of the ELBW group were free of disability vs. 82% of controls. As in most studies, outcome was significantly better in girls than boys (35% free of disability vs. 12%) (Whitfield *et al.* 1997).

Impaired cognitive and neurosensory function inevitably leads to school difficulties. Amongst a regional cohort of ELBW infants followed to between 12 and 16 years of age, neurosensory impairments were present in 28% versus 1% of controls. The ELBW group scored 13 to 18 points lower on psychometric testing and had a higher need for special educational assistance or had to repeat a grade (OR = 9.0) compared to controls (Saigal *et al.* 2001). Teachers rated VLBW 12 year olds lower in all curriculum areas than controls, and their maths and reading-comprehension scores were lower even after correction for IQ differences. There was no evidence of catch-up between 6 and 12 years of age (Botting, *et al.* 1998).

In the Victorian cohort (median gestation 27 weeks) 46% had an IQ at aged 14 years within one SD of the control mean. Ten per cent had an IQ 2 to 3 SD below and 10% > 3 SD below the mean, (Doyle and Casalaz 2001).

Whilst many studies have focused on the extremely low birthweight or extremely premature infant, one recent study examined the educational and behavioural outcomes at 7 years amongst a geographical cohort of children born between 32 and 35 weeks' gestational age. Of these 3% attended a special school and 25% required extra educational support. Poor outcome was reported in 32% for writing, 29% in mathematics, 31% in fine motor skills but only 12% in physical education (Huddy *et al.* 2001). As the numbers of infants born with this degree of prematurity are considerable, there is clearly a large 'hidden' disability attributable to premature birth amongst children attending normal schools.

A recently published meta-analysis of 15 case-control studies reporting cognitive outcome beyond 5 years of age analysed data on over 3000 preterm infants (<37 weeks) and controls, born over a 20 year period. Weighted mean differences showed a 10.9 points difference (95% CI 9.2–12.5) in mean cognitive score, in favour of controls. Mean cognitive score correlated with both gestational age ($R^2 = 0.49$, $p < 0.001$) and birthweight ($R^2 = 0.51$, $p < 0.001$) (see Figure 4.4).

Behaviour

Very low birthweight children are at increased risk of psychiatric symptoms, especially attention deficit hyperactivity disorder (ADHD). Amongst VLBW 12 year olds, 23% meet the diagnostic criteria for ADHD versus 6% of peers.

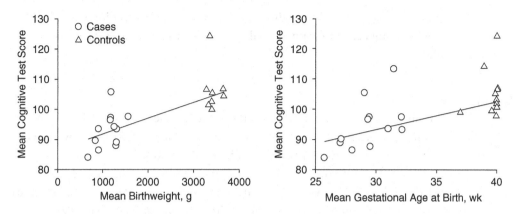

Figure 4.4. Correlations between mean cognitive scores, birthweight and gestational age. Reprinted with permission from Bhutta *et al.* (2002).

A psychiatric disorder was present in 28% compared with 9% in the control group (Botting *et al.* 1997). A recent population-based study found 40% of 11 year olds born <2000 g had behavioural problems versus 7% of controls (OR 8.2, 95% CI 3–25). A psychiatric disorder was present in 27% (OR 3.1, 95% CI 1.5–6.5), and these children tended to increased inattention, low self-esteem and increased social problems (Elgen *et al.* 2002).

Behavioural outcomes at age eight are significantly worse in ELBW infants than controls, with worse social skills, psychotic behaviours, poor social integration and attention to task. Whilst ELBW survivors were more distractable, the British Columbia study showed no significant increase in hyperactivity (Whitfield *et al.* 1997).

An increase in hyperactivity was described in 9% of ELBW adolescents versus 2% of term controls (Saigal *et al.* 2001). Behavioural problems appear to be commoner even in children born only slightly preterm; amongst 7 year olds born between 32–35 weeks 19% showed an abnormal hyperactivity score compared to a background rate of 10% (Huddy *et al.* 2001).

In a recent meta-analysis of 16 case-control studies reporting behavioural outcomes beyond 5 years of age, the pooled relative risk of developing ADHD was 2.64 (95% CI 1.85–3.78) for infants born pre-term (<37 weeks) compared with term infants (Bhutta *et al.* 2002). They also demonstrated an increase in abnormal internalising or externalising behaviour in preterm infants in over 80% of the studies. Whilst this meta-analysis includes data from 1556 cases and 1720 controls, the infants were born over a wide range of time chronologically, with the earliest born in 1974.

There is some evidence that children with blindness due to ROP are at increased risk of autistic symptoms. One study showed 15 of 27 infants blind due to ROP had autistic disorder versus 2 of 14 control children who were congenitally blind due to other disorders. The authors speculate that this association may be due to other associated cerebral damage, rather than due to the blindness per se (Ek *et al.* 1998).

Quality of life

A number of studies have tried to ascertain whether the poor neurodevelopmental outcome of preterm infants leads to a reduction in their actual or perceived quality of life in later years. Health-related quality of life (HRQOL) at 8 years of age was significantly lower amongst ELBW Canadian children born in the late 1970s than controls (HRQOL 0.82 vs. 0.95, $p < 0.0001$) (Saigal *et al.* 1994). A Danish study interviewed a group of VLBW young adults (18–20 years) born in 1980–2. They were compared with term controls and LBW infants (1500–2300 g). Objective quality of life (QoL) was lower in the VLBW group, even amongst those who did not have a handicap or a chronic health problem (0.79 vs. 0.84). Interestingly, subjective QoL was not significantly different amongst the three groups. In all groups objective QoL had improved since a previous cohort of VLBW infants born in 1971–4 (Dinesen and Greisen 2001).

Growth

It is virtually impossible to replicate in utero growth rates in preterm infants and, consequently, poor growth is very common. Growth failure, defined as weight <10th centile at 36 weeks was present in 97% of VLBW infants born in the mid 1990s (Lemons *et al.* 2001). Clearly these data are confounded by the fact that they are based on birthweight and may include a proportion of infants with intra-uterine growth restriction.

Whilst some 'catch-up' growth occurs during childhood, extremely preterm and ELBW infants remain smaller and lighter than their peers at school age. Significantly more 7 year olds born <750 g had a weight and height measurement >2 SD below the population mean, compared with term controls (relative risk 2.3, 95% CI 0.9–6.1) for weight and 7.1 (95% CI 2–25.5) for height) (Hack *et al.* 1994). In a cohort of ELBW infants followed up at 12–16 years, mean height and weight z-scores (SD scores) were –0.55 and –0.35 (approximately one half to one third of a SD below the mean) respectively compared with controls. Significant catch-up growth had occurred in this group even after 8 years of age (Saigal *et al.* 2001).

Very low birthweight 11–13 year olds are an average of 4.1cm (z-score –0.48) shorter than normal birthweight peers, despite a normal bone age. They also have significantly lower weight and head circumference. By using the bone age to predict final adult height, the authors predicted that 33% of the VLBW children would achieve a final adult height < 10th centile and 17% would be < 3rd centile (Powls *et al.* 1996).

Adolescent and adult outcomes

Only a very few studies have followed up cohorts of preterm infants into adulthood. These babies were obviously born before the modern era of neonatal intensive care. Very low birthweight adults (median gestation at birth of 29 weeks) are more likely to have chronic health problems, lower IQ and lower academic achievement than normal birthweight peers (OR for severe cognitive impairment (IQ < 70) 4.0, 95% CI 1.3–12.2). Overall IQ score was 4.6 points lower in the VLBW group (Hack *et al.* 2002). Interestingly, at age 20 the VLBW group showed reduced rates of substance abuse and reduced offending behaviour compared with term controls. The authors speculate that this decrease in risk taking behaviour may be due to increased parental monitoring of VLBW children (Hack *et al.* 2002). Long-term growth remains impaired. These VLBW adults were significantly shorter than controls, with 10% having a height <3rd centile, vs. 5% of controls.

Most young adults and adolescents who had BPD in infancy have some degree of pulmonary dysfunction. Lung function tests show increased airway hyper-reactivity, airway obstruction and hyperinflation. It is not known whether these lung function abnormalities are clinically significant in terms of impaired respiratory function (Northway *et al.* 1990).

Summary

The predicted outcome for fetuses born prematurely is dependent predominantly on their gestational age at birth. The long-term outcomes reported in the literature reflect neonatal practice a decade ago. However, we can say that on the basis of the current published evidence, a fetus delivered at less than 26 weeks' gestation and less than 1000 g will have a 39% chance of survival to 1 year (Costeloe *et al.* 2000), an 11%–18% chance of developing cerebral palsy, a 0.9%–3.6% chance of deafness, a 32%–34% chance of being discharged home on supplemental oxygen, a 2%–4% chance of blindness due to retinopathy, a 25% chance of squint and a 4%–9% chance of requiring surgery for NEC. Of those discharged home over half will be rehospitalised during their first year and a third will have recurrent wheeze in their pre-school years. Slightly less than 50% of these infants will be free of any disability and approximately a quarter will have significant cognitive or developmental problems. A quarter will have psychiatric symptoms and they are at increased risk of attention deficit. As young adults they will be shorter and have a four to ten point lower IQ than their peers but their quality of life will not be subjectively worse.

REFERENCES

Alexander, G. R., Kogan, M., Martin, J. and Papiernik, E (1998) What are the fetal growth patterns of singletons, twins and triplets in the United States? *Clin. Obstet. Gynecol.*, **41**, 114–25.

Bernstein, I. M., Horbar, J. D., Badger, G. J., Ohlsson, A. and Golan, A. (2000) Morbidity and mortality among very-low-birthweight neonates with intrauterine growth restriction. *Am. J. Obstet. Gynecol.* **182**, 198–206.

Bhutta, A. T., Cleves, M. A., Casey, P. H., Cradock, M. M. and Anand, K. J. (2002) Cognitive and behavioral outcomes of school-aged children who were born preterm: a meta-analysis. *JAMA* **288**, 728–37.

Blair, B. M., O'halloran, H. S., Pauly, T. H. and Stevens, J. L.(2001) Decreased incidence of retinopathy of prematurity, 1995–1997. *J AAPOS* **5**, 118–22.

Botting, N., Powls, A., Cooke, R. W. and Marlow, N. (1997) Attention deficit hyperactivity disorders and other psychiatric outcomes in very low birthweight children at 12 years. *J. Child Psychol. Psychiatry* **38**, 931–41.

(1998) Cognitive and educational outcome of very-low-birthweight children in early adolescence. *Dev. Med. Child Neurol.* **40**, 652–60.

Bremer, D. L., Palmer, E. A., Fellows, R. R. *et al.* (1998) Strabismus in premature infants in the first year of life. Cryotherapy for Retinopathy of Prematurity Cooperative Group. *Arch. Ophthalmol.* **116**, 329–33.

Callanan, C., Doyle, L. W., Rickards, A. L. *et al.* (2001) Children followed with difficulty: How do they differ? *J. Paediatr. Child Health* **37**, 152–6.

Cartlidge, P. H. T. and Stewart, J. H. (1997) Survival of very low birthweight and very preterm infants in a geographically defined population. *Acta Paediatr.* **86**, 105–10.

Cheung, Y. B., Yip, P. and Karlberg, J. (2000). Mortality of twins and singletons by gestational age: a varying-coefficient approach. *Am. J. Epidemiol.* **152**, 1107–16.

Corcoran, J. D., Patterson, C. C., Thomas, P. S. and Halliday, H. L. (1993) Reduction in the risk of bronchopulmonary dysplasia from 1980–1990: results of a multivariate logistic regression analysis. *Eur. J. Pediatr.* **152**, 677–81.

Costeloe, K., Hennessy, E., Gibson, A. T., Marlow, N. and Wilkinson, A. R. for the EPICure Study Group. (2000) The EPICure study: outcomes to discharge from hospital for infants born at the threshold of viability. *Pediatrics* **106**, 659–71.

Demissie, K., Rhoads, G. G., Ananth, C. V. *et al.* (2001) Trends in preterm birth and neonatal mortality among blacks and whites in the United States from 1989 to 1997. *Am. J. Epidemiol.* **154**, 307–15.

Dinesen, S. J. and Greisen, G. (2001) Quality of life in young adults with very low birth weight. *Arch. Dis. Child Fetal Neonatal Ed.* **85**, F165–9.

Doyle, L. W., Ford, G. W., Olinsky A., Knoches, A. M. and Callanan, C. (1996) Bronchopulmonary dysplasia and very low birthweight: lung function at 11 years of age. *J. Paediatr. Child Health* **32**, 339–43.

Doyle, L. W. and Casalaz, D. Victorian Infant Collaborative Study Group (2001) Outcome at 14 years of extremely low birthweight infants: a regional study. *Arch. Dis. Child Fetal Neonatal Ed.* **85**, F159–64.

Doyle, L. W. Victorian Infant Collaborative Study Group (2001) Outcome at 5 years of age of children 23 to 27 weeks' gestation: refining the prognosis. *Pediatrics* **108**, 134–41.

Ek, U., Fernell, E., Jacobson, L. and Gillberg, C. (1998) Relation between blindness due to retinopathy of prematurity and autistic spectrum disorders: a population-based study. *Dev. Med. Child Neurol.* **40**, 297–301.

Elgen, I., Sommerfelt, K. and Markestad, T. (2002) Population based, controlled study of behavioural problems and psychiatric disorders in low birthweight children at 11 years of age. *Arch. Dis. Child. Fetal Neonatal Ed.* **87**, F128–32.

Elliman, A. M., Bryan, E. M., Elliman, A. D., Walker, J. and Harvey, D. R. (1991) Coordination of low birthweight seven-year-olds. *Acta Paediatr. Scand.* **80**, 316–22.

El-Metwally, D., Vohr, B. and Tucker, R. (2000) Survival and neonatal morbidity at the limits of viability in the mid 1990s: 22 to 25 weeks. *J. Pediatr.* **137**, 616–22.

Emsley, H. C., Wardle, S. P., Sims, D. G., Chiswick, M. L. and D'Souza, S. W. (1998) Increased survival and deteriorating developmental outcome in 23 to 25 week old gestation infants, 1990–4 compared with 1984–9. *Arch. Dis. Child. Fetal Neonatal Ed.* **78**, F99–104.

Evans, D. J. and Levene, M. I. (2001) Evidence of selection bias in preterm survival studies: a systematic review. *Arch. Dis. Child. Fetal Neonatal Ed.* **84**, F79–84.

Finnstrom, O., Olausson, P. O., Sedin, G. *et al.* (1997) The Swedish national prospective study on extremely low birthweight (ELBW) infants. Incidence, mortality, morbidity and survival in relation to level of care. *Acta Paediatr.* **86**, 503–11.

Glinianaia, S. V., Pharoah, P. and Sturgiss, S. (2000) Comparative trends in cause-specific fetal and neonatal mortality in twin and singleton births in the North of England, 1982–1994. *BJOG* **107**, 452–60.

Gould, J. B., Benitz W. E. and Liu, H. (2000) Mortality and time to death in very low birth weight infants: California, 1987 and 1993. *Pediatrics* **105**, E37.

Greenough, A. (2000) Measuring respiratory outcome. *Semin. Neonatol.* **5**, 119–26.

Greenough, A., Giffin, F. J., Yuksel, B. and Dimitriou, G. (1996) Respiratory morbidity in young school children born prematurely – chronic lung disease is not a risk factor? *Eur. J. Pediatr.* **155**, 823–6.

Gross, S. J., Iannuzzi, D. M., Kveselis, D. A and Anbar, R. D. (1998). Effect of preterm birth on pulmonary function at school age: a prospective controlled study. *J. Pediatr.* **133**, 188–92.

Hack, M. and Fanaroff, A. A. (1999) Outcomes of children of extremely low birthweight and gestational age in the 1990's. *Early Hum. Dev.* **53**, 193–218.

Hack, M., Taylor, H. G., Klein, N. *et al.* (1994) School-age outcomes in children with birth weights under 750 g. *N. Engl. J. Med.* **331**, 753–9.

Hack, M., Flannery, D. J., Schluchter, M. *et al.* (2002) Outcomes in young adulthood for very-low-birthweight infants. *N. Engl. J. Med.* **346**, 149–57.

Hernandez, J. A., Hall, D. M., Goldson, E. J., Chase, M. and Garrett, C. (2000) Impact of infants born at the threshold of viability on the neonatal mortality rate in Colorado. *J. Perinatol.* **1**, 21–6.

Holmgren, P. A. and Hogberg, U. (2001) The very preterm infant – a population-based study. *Acta Obstet. Gynecol. Scand.* **80**, 525–31.

Huddy, C. L., Johnson, A. and Hope P. L. (2001) Educational and behavioural problems in babies of 32–35 weeks gestation. *Arch. Dis. Child. Fetal Neonatal Ed.* **85**, F23–8.

Jacobs, S. E., O'Brien, K., Inwood, S., Kelly, E. N. and Whyte, H. E. (2000) Outcome of infants 23–26 weeks' gestation pre and post surfactant. *Acta Paediatr.* **89**, 959–65.

Joffe, S., Escobar, G. J., Black, S. B., Armstrong, M. A. and Lieu, T. A. (1999) Rehospitalisation for respiratory syncytial virus among premature infants. *Pediatrics* **104**, 894–9.

Jongmans, M., Mercuri, E., de Vries, L., Dubowitz, L. and Henderson, S. E.(1997) Minor neurological signs and perceptual-motor difficulties in prematurely born children. *Arch. Dis. Child. Fetal Neonatal Ed.* **76**, F9–14.

Joseph, K. S., Kramer, M. S., Allen, A. C. *et al.* (2000) Gestational age- and birthweight-specific declines in infant mortality in Canada. *Paediatr. Perinat. Epidemiol.* **14**, 332–9.

Kilpatrick, S. J., Schlueter, M. A., Piecuch, R. *et al.* (1997) Outcome of infants born at 24–26 weeks' gestation: I. Survival and cost. *Obstet. Gynecol.* **90**, 803–8.

Kinali, M., Greenough, A., Dimitriou, G., Yuksel, B. and Hooper, R. (1999) Chronic respiratory morbidity following premature delivery–prediction by prolonged respiratory support requirement? *Eur. J. Pediatr.* **158**, 493–6.

Koumbourlis, A. C., Motoyama, E. K., Mutich, R. L. *et al.* (1996) Longitudinal follow-up of lung function from childhood to adolescence in prematurely born patients with neonatal chronic lung disease. *Pediatr. Pulmonol.* **21**, 28–34.

Kramer, M. S., Demissie, K., Yang, H. *et al.* (2000) The contribution of mild and moderate preterm birth to infant mortality. *JAMA* **284**, 843–9.

Lanman, J. T., Guy, L. P. and Danus, I. (1954) Retrolental fibroplasia and oxygen therapy. *JAMA* **55**, 223–6.

Lee, M. J., Conner, E. L., Charafeddine, L., Woods, J. R. Jr and Priore, G. D. (2001) A critical birth weight and other determinants of survival for infants with severe intrauterine growth restriction. *Ann. NY Acad Sci.* **943**, 326–39.

Lefebvre, F., Glorieux, J. and St-Laurent-Gagnon, T. (1996) Neonatal survival and disability rate at age 18 months for infants born between 23 and 28 weeks of gestation. *Am. J. Obstet. Gynecol.* **174**, 833–8.

Lemons, J. A., Bauer, C. R., Oh, W. *et al.* (2001) Very low birth weight outcomes of the National Institute of Child Health and Human Development Neonatal Research Network, January 1995 through December 1996. NICHD Neonatal Research Network. *Pediatrics* **107**, E1.

Meadow, W., Reimshisel, T. and Lantos, L. (1996) Birth weight-specific mortality for extremely low birth weight infants vanishes by four days of life: epidemiology and ethics in the neonatal intensive care unit. *Pediatrics* **97**, 636–43.

Northway, W. H., Jr, Rosan, R. C. and Porter, D. Y. (1967) Pulmonary disease following respirator therapy of hyaline-membrane disease. Bronchopulmonary dysplasia. *N. Engl. J. Med.* **276**, 357–68.

Northway, W. H. Jr, Moss, R. B., Carlisle, K. B. *et al.* (1990) Late pulmonary sequelae of bronchopulmonary dysplasia. *N. Engl. J. Meda.* **323**, 1793–9.

O'Shea, T. M., Klinepeter, K. L., Goldstein, D. J., Jackson, B. W. and Dillard, R. G. (1997) Survival and developmental disability in infants with birthweights of 501 to 800 grams, born between 1979 and 1994. *Pediatrics* **100**, 982–6.

Piecuch, R. E., Leonard, C. H., Cooper, B. A. *et al.* (1997) Outcome of infants born at 24–26 weeks' gestation: II. Neurodevelopmental outcome. *Obstet. Gynecol.* **90**, 809–14.

Piper, J. M., Xenakis, E. M., McFarland, M. *et al.* (1996) Do growth retarded premature infants have different rates of perinatal morbidity and mortality than appropriately grown premature infants? *Obstet. Gynecol.* **87**, 169–74.

Powls. A., Botting, N., Cooke, R. W. and Marlow, N. (1995) Motor impairment in children 12 to 13 years old with a birthweight of less than 1250 g. *Arch. Dis. Child. Fetal Neonatal Ed.* **73**, F62–6.

Powls, A., Botting, N., Cooke, R. W., Pilling, D. and Marlow, N. (1996) Growth impairment in very low birthweight children at 12 years: correlation with perinatal and outcome variables. *Arch. Dis. Child. Fetal Neonatal Ed.* **75**, F152–7.

Ranganathan, D., Wall, S., Khoshnood, B., Singh, J. K. and Lee, K. S. (2000) Racial differences in respiratory-related neonatal mortality among very low birth weight infants. *J. Pediatr.* **136**, 454–9.

Rona, R. J., Gulliford, M. C. and Chinn, S. (1993) Effects of prematurity and intrauterine growth on respiratory health and lung function in childhood. *BMJ.* **306**, 817–20.

Saigal, S., Feeny, D., Furlong, W. *et al.* (1994) Comparison of the health-related quality of life of extremely low birth weight children and a reference group of children at age eight years. *J. Pediatr.* **125**, 418–25.

Saigal, S., Stoskopf, B. L., Streiner, D. L. and Burrows, E. (2001) Physical growth and current health status of infants who were of extremely low birth weight and controls at adolescence. *Pediatrics* **108**, 407–15.

Sauve, R. S., Robertson, C., Etches, P., Byrne, P. J. and Dayer-Zamora, V. (1998) Before viability: a geographically based outcome study of infants weighing 500 grams or less at birth. *Pediatrics* **101**, 438–45.

Shennan, A. T., Dunn, M. S., Ohlsson, A., Lennox, K. and Hoskins, E. M. (1988) Abnormal pulmonary outcomes in premature infants: prediction from oxygen requirement in the neonatal period. *Pediatrics* **82**, 527–32.

Sutton, L. and Bajuk, B. (1999) Population-based study of infants born at less than 28 weeks' gestation in New South Wales, Australia, in 1992–3. New South Wales Neonatal Intensive Care Unit Study Group. *Paediatr. Perinat. Epidemiol.* **13**, 288–301.

The Victorian Infant Collaborative Study Group. (1997). Improved outcome into the 1990s for infants weighing 500–999 g at birth. *Arch. Dis. Child. Fetal Neonatal Ed.* **77**, F91–4.

Tin, W., Fritz, S., Wariyar, U. and Hey E. (1998) Outcome of very preterm birth: children reviewed with ease at 2 years differ from those followed up with difficulty. *Arch. Dis. Child. Fetal Neonatal Ed.* **79**, F83–7.

Tin, W., Wariyar, U. and Hey, E. (1997) Changing prognosis for babies of less than 28 weeks' gestation in the north of England between 1983 and 1994. Northern Neonatal Network. *Br. Med. J.* **314**, 107–11.

Tommiska, V., Heinonen, K., Ikonen, S. *et al.* (2001) A national short-term follow-up study of extremely low birth weight infants born in Finland in 1996–1997. *Pediatrics* **107**, E2.

Verloove-Vanhorick, S. P., Verwey R. A., Brand, R. *et al.* (1986) Neonatal mortality risk in relation to gestational age and birthweight. Results of a national survey of preterm and very-low birthweight infants in the Netherlands. *Lancet* **333**, 55–7.

Whitfield, M. F., Grunau, R. V. and Holsti, L. (1997) Extremely premature (< or = 800 g) schoolchildren: multiple areas of hidden disability. *Arch. Dis. Child. Fetal Neonatal Ed.* **77**, F85–90.

Wood, N. S., Marlow, N., Costeloe, K., Gibson, A. T. and Wilkinson, A. R. (2000) The EPICure Study Group. Neurologic and developmental disability after extremely preterm birth. *N. Eng. J. Med.* **343**, 378–84.

5

The prediction of preterm labour

Philip Owen and Fiona Mackenzie

Princess Royal Maternity, Glasgow

Risk scoring

Accurate prospective identification of a subgroup of pregnancies at increased risk of preterm labour and delivery permits the rational use of interventions aimed at prolonging gestation. Several epidemiological and obstetric associations are well recognised (Chapter 1) including low socioeconomic status, young age and primiparity, ethnic group and previous preterm delivery or mid-trimester loss (Lumley 1993).

In an effort to provide a useful screening test for preterm delivery risk, several scoring systems have evolved that quantify a variety of epidemiological and pregnancy features, together with digital assessment of the cervix. By applying the scoring system described by Creasy et al. (1980) to a San Fransisco population, Holbrook et al. (1989) found that gestational age at delivery was inversely correlated with risk score. However, in this series in which 15.8% of women were classified as high risk, the positive predictive value (PPV) of a high score was only 22.8%. Other studies have also found risk scoring to perform poorly, particularly in primigravidae since there is no past obstetric performance upon which to assign risk. This is illustrated by the study of Mercer et al. (1996) who constructed a scoring system using over 100 clinical variables obtained at 23–24 weeks' gestation in nearly 3000 women. Women were considered to be at high risk if their risk for spontaneous preterm delivery was >20%. Less than a quarter of those subsequently delivering preterm were correctly identified; the PPV were low at 29% and 33% for nulliparous and multiparous women respectively (Mercer et al. 1996).

The limitations of formal risk scoring in the prediction of preterm delivery means that it lacks many of the characteristics required of an effective screening test (Keirse 1989). Alternative methods such as detecting fetal fibronectin in cervico-vaginal secretions, quantifying preterm uterine activity, measuring circulating endocrine and inflammatory markers and the ultrasonic measurement of cervical length have been explored and will be described.

Preterm Labour Managing Risk in Clinical Practice, eds. Jane Norman and Ian Greer. Published by Cambridge University Press. © Cambridge University Press 2005.

Cervical/vaginal secretions

Fetal fibronectin

Fetal fibronectin (fFn) is a protein found in amniotic fluid, placental tissue and the extracellular substance of the decidua basalis next to the placental intervillous space. The virtual disappearance of fFn from the vaginal secretions by 22 weeks coincides with fusion of the chorion and decidua capsularis with the decidua parietalis of the uterine wall; the reappearance of fibronectin before labour may represent the separation of the chorion from the decidua prior to the onset of labour. In women with uncomplicated pregnancies ending in term delivery, fFn can be detected in the cervical secretions of up to 50% of pregnancies in the first trimester and 30% beyond 37 weeks' gestation but is present in only 4% of normal pregnancies between 21 and 37 weeks (Lockwood *et al.* 1991). In their study of 117 women presenting with preterm uterine activity and intact membranes, Lockwood *et al.* (1991) found that the presence of fFn in the cervico-vaginal secretions was a good indicator of those who subsequently went on to deliver prematurely and a negative result was highly predictive of the pregnancy going to term.

Bedside testing without the need for laboratory involvement makes fFn in vaginal secretions an attractive test for management of the symptomatic woman (Senden and Owen 1996), but ruptured membranes, recent (< 24 hours) sexual intercourse, antepartum haemorrhage or vaginal examination may invalidate the test result (McKenna *et al.* 1999), so it is not applicable to all women presenting with preterm uterine activity.

Promising early results have stimulated a large number of studies into the predictive value of fFn testing in low-risk and high risk asymptomatic women and also in symptomatic (contracting) women but the results of different studies are often conflicting. Systematic reviews of the published literature (Chien *et al.* 1997; Honest *et al.* 2002) find that fFn testing in asymptomatic women (low-risk and high-risk) is not a clinically useful procedure. Fibronectin testing amongst asymptomatic twin pregnancies does not predict spontaneous preterm birth before 35 weeks' gestation (Gibson *et al.* 2004). However, in women experiencing preterm uterine activity, a negative test reduces the likelihood of delivery within 7–10 days of presentation from 3% to less than 1%; a positive test increases the likelihood of delivery within 7–10 days from 3% to 14% (Honest *et al.* 2002). A negative test therefore implies a low risk for delivery in the near future and might form the basis for withholding interventions with subsequent reductions in hospital admissions, inter-hospital transfers and costs (Joffe *et al.* 1999).

The potential clinical utility of fFn testing in symptomatic women presenting with uterine activity at 31 weeks' gestation is illustrated in Table 5.1 below (from Honest *et al.* 2002). This highlights the clinical implications of introducing a test

Table 5.1. Clinical utility of Ffn testing

Test result	Probability of SPB within 7–10 days of testing (%)	Risk of RDS at 32 weeks' gestation	Rate of RDS at 32 weeks' gestation (%)	Number needed to treat
No testing	4.5	0.53	2.0	109
Test positive	20.6	0.53	11.0	17
Test negative	1.0	0.53	0.4	509

that has some discriminative power in differentiating true from false preterm labour. Without testing, over one hundred women will receive antenatal corticosteroids in order to prevent one case of respiratory distress syndrome (RDS); if corticosteroids are only administered to fFn test positive women, only 17 women will receive treatment to prevent one case of RDS. The high negative predictive value (NPV) of fFn testing for delivery within 7 days (99%) results in a low likelihood of an infant developing potentially avoidable RDS as a consequence of withholding steroids following a false negative fFn test result; at 32 weeks' gestation, the risk is approximately 0.5%

Uterine activity monitoring

In an effort to detect preterm labour before cervical dilatation becomes too advanced to institute tocolytic therapy, patient education and self-palpation of the uterus have been proposed. The development of an ambulatory method of home uterine activity monitoring (HUAM) in the mid eighties resulted in a more objective assessment of the value of uterine activity measurement in the prediction of preterm labour and delivery. The self-detection of uterine activity underestimates the true frequency of contractions even amongst those specifically asked to record it in a hospital setting, with the result that objective monitoring provides an earlier diagnosis of labour onset (Newman *et al.* 1990).

Several randomised trials have evaluated the use of HUAM in the early prediction of preterm labour and the subsequent influence on preterm delivery rates. Most did not control for the intensive nursing input involved with HUAM and so it is not possible to separate any benefit accruing from HUAM to the monitoring alone. Bearing this and other limitations in mind, the trials suggest that, although preterm labour is not diagnosed more frequently by HUAM, the incidence of preterm delivery is significantly reduced, but data on eventual neonatal outcomes is generally lacking (Keirse 1992). The presumed explanation is that the HUAM groups present at a stage in labour where tocolysis by whatever means is more successful. Despite these apparently encouraging findings, the US Preventive Services Task Force (1993) considered there to be insufficient evidence to recommend for or against HUAM as a screening test in high-risk pregnancies. More recently, a large observational study (Iams *et al.* 2002) demonstrated that whilst the likelihood of delivering before 35 weeks' gestation increased with the frequency of uterine activity, it was unable to identify a threshold frequency of contractions that was clinically useful for predicting preterm delivery.

Cervical ultrasound

The inverse relationship between cervical length on digital examination and risk of preterm delivery is long established and digital cervical examination has previously been a central component of some preterm labour prevention programmes. Digital examination is subject to considerable inter and intra-observer variation, which limits its use as a diagnostic test, and has been superseded by ultrasound evaluation. The assessment of cervical length using ultrasound has been shown to be superior to digital examination as a predictor of preterm birth in both asymptomatic high- and low-risk women (Iams *et al.* 1996; Berghella *et al.* 1997).

The precise mechanisms whereby the length of the cervix influences the risk of preterm delivery are not fully established. It is likely that cervical length at least influences the mechanical resistance of the cervix to delivery and may influence the immune competence or resistance to the ascent of micro-organisms offered by the cervical mucus plug.

Early ultrasound studies of the cervix were performed transabdominally, but transvaginal ultrasound (TVS) assessment of the cervix is superior since there is better visualisation of the cervix. Transvaginal ultrasound also avoids the artefactual elongation of the cervix that is sometimes seen in the presence of a full maternal bladder (Andersen 1991; To *et al.* 2000b).

The appropriate technique for transvaginal cervical ultrasound measurement is well described (Iams *et al.* 1996). The ultrasound probe is placed in the anterior fornix of the vagina in women with an empty bladder. Care is taken to avoid exerting undue pressure on the cervix, which could increase it's apparent length. A sagittal view of the cervix is obtained demonstrating the external os as a triangular area of echodensity, a V-shaped notch at the internal os and a faint line of echolucency between the two (Figure 5.1 and photos). Each examination should be performed over a three-minute period in order to note any dynamic changes in the cervix. For the purposes of preterm delivery prediction, cervical length is the measurement of choice with inter and intra-observer variability reported to be between 5% and 10% (Iams *et al.* 1996, Berghella *et al.* 1997).

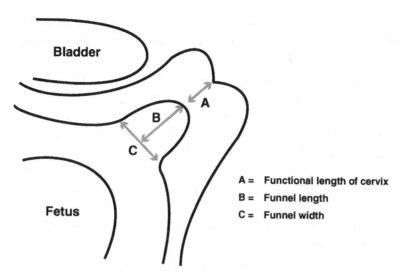

A = Functional length of cervix
B = Funnel length
C = Funnel width

Figure 5.1   Schematic diagram of transvaginal ultrasound of cervix.
Photos
Transvaginal ultrasound of cervix demonstrating
a.   long closed cervix
b.   shorter cervix with evidence of funnelling

Other sonographic cervical parameters have also been described and assessed, including the presence or not of funnelling, funnel length and width, percent funnelling (funnel length/(funnel length plus cervical length) × 100) and cervical index (1 + funnel length/cervical length) (Figure 5.1). The funnel appearance describes dilatation of the internal cervical os creating the appearance of a funnel. In the presence of internal os dilatation it has been suggested that percentage funnelling is more accurate than the functional length of the cervix (Berghella *et al.* 1997). However, in a large study involving 6334 women attending for routine antenatal care, the presence of funnelling (defined as dilatation of the internal os of > or = 5 mm in width) did not significantly improve accuracy beyond cervical length measurement alone in the prediction of spontaneous delivery before 33 weeks (To *et al.* 2001). Similarly, amongst high-risk pregnancies cervical length alone was equal to other sonographic cervical parameters for the prediction of spontaneous preterm birth (Guzman *et al.* 2001).

The change in appearance of the cervix in response to transfundal or suprapubic pressure has been proposed as a method of evaluating the competence of the cervix in high-risk cases. Macdonald *et al.* (2001) reported cervical shortening in response to such pressure and proposed that opening of the cervical internal os at rest or with fundal pressure was the earliest feature of cervical incompetence.

However, after controlling for cervical length, neither funnelling nor dynamic shortening with fundal pressure were found to be significant independent predictors of preterm birth (Owen *et al.* 2001).

With the advent of 3D ultrasound, there are some recent reports of its application to cervical assessment. Bega *et al.* (2000) compared 2D and 3D cervical assessments in a pilot study on high-risk women; the interrater reliability of the 3D ultrasound measurements was high and multiplanar evaluation of the cervix showed that the standard 2D sagittal view may under or overestimate cervical length. It remains to be seen whether cervical length determined by 3D, or additional information such as cervical volume measurement, improves the predictive ability of ultrasonographic cervical assessment.

The range of cervical length measurements before 20 weeks is much wider than after this gestation. After 20 weeks' gestation, the cervix appears to shorten or efface slightly with increasing gestation, with median values falling from 35–40 mm at 24–28 weeks to 30–35 mm after 32 weeks. At 24 weeks the cervical length amongst singleton pregnancies has a normal distribution, with the 50th centile at 35 mm and the 10th and 90th at 25 mm and 45 mm, respectively (Iams *et al.* 1996) (Figure 5.2). The median cervical length is similar in twin pregnancies at 38 mm at 23 weeks' gestation, but the 5th and 1st centiles are lower at 19 mm and 7 mm compared to 23 mm and 12 mm respectively (Heath *et al.* 1998; Souka *et al.* 1999). Twin pregnancies are twice as likely as singletons to have a short cervix ($< = 25$ mm) at both 24 and 28 weeks (Goldenberg *et al.* 1996). The rate of change of cervical length amongst twin pregnancies is described (Fujita *et al.* 2002) but does not identify pregnancies destined to deliver before 35 weeks' gestation any more accurately than a single measurement of cervical length (Gibson *et al.* 2004). In triplet pregnancies the distribution of cervical length at 23 weeks' gestation is further skewed to the left, with a median of 34 mm and a 5th centile of 15 mm (To *et al.* 2000a).

The relationship between mid-trimester cervical length and subsequent risk of preterm delivery amongst singleton pregnancies has been examined in a number of large, observational studies. A short cervix detected by ultrasound has been shown to be an independent predictor of preterm delivery and transvaginal assessment of the cervix demonstrates an inverse correlation between cervical length and the risk of preterm delivery (Figure 5.2) (Iams *et al.* 1996, Heath *et al.* 1998).

There are many published studies but they are heterogeneous with variations in the patient populations, the gestational age at the time of measurement, the frequency of measurements, the cervical length cut-off used to evaluate predictive ability, whether information gained from cervical sonography was used to alter patient management or not and the gestational age at delivery used

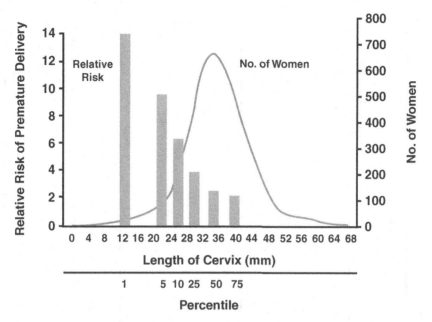

Figure 5.2   Distribution of subjects among percentiles for cervical length measured by transvaginal ultrasonography at 24 weeks of gestation (blue line) and the relative risk of spontaneous preterm delivery before 35 weeks of gestation according to percentiles for cervical length (green bars). The risks among women with values at or below the 1st, 5th,10th, 25th, 50th and 75th percentiles for cervical length are compared with the risk among women with values above the 75th percentile (adapted from Iams *et al*. 1996).

to define preterm delivery. For these reasons, the available data does not readily lend itself to systematic review, although such a review has been reported (Leitich *et al.* 1999).

The predictive ability will be influenced by the population studied, with most available information being available for low-risk or non-selected populations, high-risk singleton populations, multiple pregnancies and symptomatic women. The findings of the most relevant published studies are presented in Tables 5.2–5.5.

As one might expect in any diagnostic or predictive test in an obstetric population, the specificities and NPVs are high, often approaching 100%. However, with the possible exception of testing in the symptomatic population, this is unlikely to be useful since the clinician is principally interested in identifying women who will deliver preterm and not those who will not. For this reason, the sensitivity (proportion of all cases delivering preterm having a short cervix) and PPV (the proportion of cases with a short cervix subsequently delivering preterm) are more relevant.

Table 5.2. Cervical length and spontaneous preterm birth (SPB) in general obstetric populations

Study	Number of subjects	Country	Gestational age at testing (weeks)	Clinician blinded Y/N	Cervical length cut-off (mm)	Incidence SPB (%)	Definition of SPB (weeks)	Sensitivity	Specificity	PPV	NPV
Iams et al. (1996)	2915	USA	24	Y	<=25	4.3	<35	37	92	18	97
					<=20		<35	23	97	26	97
Heath et al. (1998)	2567	UK	23	N	<=15	1.5	<32	58		52	
Taipale and Hiilesmaa (1998)	3694	Finland	18–22	Y	<=25	0.8	<35	7	100	15	
Hassan et al. (2000)	6877	USA	14–24	N	<=15	3.6	<32	8	99	48	97

Table 5.3. Cervical length and spontaneous preterm birth (SPB) in high-risk women

Study	Number of cases	Gestational age at testing (weeks)	Clinician blinded Y/N	Cervical length cut-off (mm)	Incidence of SPB (%)	Definition of SPB (weeks)	Sensitivity	Specificity	PPV	NPV
Berghella et al. (1997)	102	14–30 (serial testing)	Y	<25	18	<35	59	85	45	91
Owen et al. (2001)	183	16–19 (single test)	Y	<25	26	<35	19	98	75	
Guzman et al. (2001)	469	15–24 (serial testing)	N	<=25	6	<32	83	67	15	98

Table 5.4. Cervical length and spontaneous preterm birth (SPB) in women in threatened preterm labour

Study	Number of cases	Mean (and range) of gestational age at testing	Singleton only Y/N	Cervical length cut-off (mm)	Definition SPB (weeks)	Incidence SPB (%)	Sensitivity (%)	Specificity (%)	PPV (%)	NPV (%)
Iams et al. (1994)	60	31(24–35)	N	<30	<36	40	100	44	55	100
Gomez et al. (1994)	59	30 (20–35)	Y	<18	<36	37	73	78	67	83
Timor-Tritsch et al. (1996)	70	29 (20–35)	Y	Funnelling	<37	27	100	74	60	100
Crane et al. (1997)	162	29 (23–33)	N	<30	<34	10	88	56	19	97
					<37	33	79	61	50	86
Rozenberg et al. (1997)	76	31	Y	<=26	<37	26	75	73	50	89
Rizzo et al. (1996)	108	30	Y	<=20	<37	43	68	79	71	76
Hincz et al. (2002)	82	30.5	Y	<=20	Within 28 days	17	57	93	62	91

Table 5.5. Cervical length and spontaneous preterm birth (SPB) in women with multiple pregnancies

Study	Number of cases	gestational age at testing (wks)	Clinician blinded Y/N	Twins or triplets	Cervical length cut-off (mm)	Outcome definition (weeks)	Incidence SPB (%)	Sensitivity (%)	Specificity (%)	PPV (%)	NPV (%)
Skentou et al. (2001)	434	23	N	Twins	<=20	<33	7.8	26.5*	97	41	94
Guzman et al. (2000a)	131	21–24	N	Twins	<=20	<32	9.2	42	85	22	94
To et al. (2000a)	38	23	N	Triplets	<=25	<33	16	50	91	50	91
Maymon et al. (2001)	34	26	Y	Triplets	<=25	<=33	50	59	94	91	70
Guzman et al. (2000b)	51	21–24	N	Triplets	<=25	<32	32	60	84	64	82

*pts without cerclage only

In unselected populations, the studies indicate that the measurement of cervical length will identify between 7% and 58% of cases delivering preterm and of those cases with a short cervix between 15% and 52% will actually deliver preterm. Similarly, amongst pregnancies at increased risk of delivering preterm between 19% and 83% of cases delivering preterm will be identified and of those cases with a short cervix between 15% and 75% will actually deliver preterm (Tables 5.2 and 5.3).

It is clear that there is considerable variation in the results of testing, which is partly due to differences in study design. Whilst cervical length measurement represents an improvement upon clinical risk scoring (Goldenberg *et al.* 1998), it is unlikely that cervical ultrasound alone will become a clinically useful predictor of spontaneous preterm birth (SPB) in asymptomatic women.

Amongst symptomatic (contracting) women, in common with fFn testing, a high NPV (Table 5.4) can be expected to be useful since this would indicate a low risk of preterm birth and permit observation or discharge rather than intervention. Unfortunately, most published studies do not provide data for the most clinically relevant outcomes such as delivery within one week. The accurate differentiation of women destined to deliver within a few days of presentation from those who will not is most clinically relevant since it will enhance the appropriate use of tocolysis, corticosteroids for the enhancement of fetal pulmonary maturity and possibly in utero transfer.

Endocrine factors

Investigation of the pathophysiological mechanisms underlying spontaneous pre-term labour and delivery has generated interest in the identification and evaluation of biological markers as predictors of spontaneous preterm birth. Several endocrine and inflammatory markers have been investigated and their capacity to predict SPB is described here.

Oestriol

Oestriol (E3) is first detectable in maternal blood at nine weeks' gestation and plasma concentrations increase throughout pregnancy. A rapid surge in levels precedes the onset of labour by three to five weeks (Darne *et al.* 1987). Oestriol binds to myometrial oestrogen receptors, promotes a uterotrophic response when administered continuously and stimulates prostaglandin production in endometrial cells.

Salivary levels of E3 reflect the concentration of free, unconjugated E3 in the plasma (Lachelin and McGarigle 1984). The advantages of measurement in saliva rather than serum include ease of use, non-invasive collection and stability during transport. Oestriol production is suppressed by the administration of maternal corticosteroids which might limit its applicability.

McGregor *et al.* (1995) evaluated salivary E3 levels obtained weekly from 22 weeks' gestation until birth in 241 women with singleton pregnancies. They reported a progressive increase in levels as pregnancy advanced, with a surge 3 weeks prior to delivery. At a threshold of 2.3 ng/ml, measurement of salivary E3 demonstrated a sensitivity of 71% and a false positive rate of 23% for delivery before 37 weeks.

In a larger study of 956 women with singleton pregnancies weekly samples of saliva were collected and preterm delivery was defined as occurring prior to 36 completed weeks. Elevated salivary E3 was again associated with an increased risk of SPB, and the presence of more than one positive test increased the risk still further (Heine *et al.* 2000). However, even amongst women considered at high risk from prior clinical risk scoring and with two positive salivary E3 tests the sensitivity and PPV for SPB were only 39% and 26% respectively. Measurement of salivary E3 appears to be more accurate than clinical risk scoring (Heine *et al.* 1999) but is unlikely to be sufficiently accurate for use in clinical practice.

Corticotrophin-releasing hormone

Corticotrophin-releasing hormone (CRH) is produced by the placenta and fetal membranes. Levels of CRH in maternal blood rise exponentially during the second and third trimesters and are further elevated in women with preterm labour (Warren *et al.* 1992). Elevated concentrations of CRH can be observed several months prior to preterm delivery and low second trimester CRH levels are seen in women whose pregnancies continue beyond term (McLean *et al.* 1995). The biological relationship of CRH to the onset of delivery is discussed in Chapter 2.

The association of a raised level of CRH with SPB has resulted in its evaluation as a predictor of premature delivery. Amongst 1047 low-risk pregnant women sampled between 15–20 weeks' of gestation, those delivering spontaneously before 34 weeks had significantly higher mid-trimester CRH levels (Leung *et al.* 1999). For a test cut-off of 1.9 mutiples of the median (MoM), the sensitivity and positive predictive values were 72.7% and 3.6% respectively, indicating poor test performance. Sampling later in gestation might improve test performance (Moawad *et al.* 2002) but even when testing is delayed to 26 weeks, approximately half preterm deliveries will not be predicted and of those predicted only half will actually deliver preterm (Inder *et al.* 2001).

Relaxin

Relaxin is a 6000 d polypeptide that is produced by the corpus luteum, placenta and decidua and is believed to play a role in the maturation of the cervix and fetal membranes.

In humans, both the cervix and the fetal membranes have relaxin receptors; relaxin stimulates collagenases in both these sites and weakens fetal membranes in vitro (Vogel *et al.* 2002). An association between elevated serum relaxin levels and preterm birth has been reported (Petersen *et al.* 1992).

Vogel *et al.* (2001) evaluated a possible association between serum relaxin levels during the 18th week of pregnancy and delivery prior to 34 weeks in a group of unselected primiparous women. High relaxin levels were associated with an increased risk of preterm delivery (odds ratio (OR) 11.3, 95% confidence interval (CI) 1.3–59.1) and spontaneous preterm delivery (OR 5.5, 95% CI 1.3–23). The sensitivity and specificity for predicting delivery before 34 weeks were 27% and 96% respectively.

Amongst women with preterm uterine activity, serum levels of relaxin are higher amongst those delivering before 34 weeks' gestation (Vogel *et al.* 2002). A raised serum relaxin ($> = 300$ pg/ml) had a sensitivity, specificity, PPV and NPV of 58%, 78%, 72% and 65% respectively in these symptomatic women.

Serum relaxin is unlikely to be a useful marker for preterm delivery amongst asymptomatic women; amongst symptomatic women its clinical utility is limited by its performance and current lack of availability of a readily available assay.

Inflammatory cytokines

The relationship between early spontaneous preterm birth and upper genital tract infection is well recognised (see Chapter 2), but obtaining appropriate samples for culture is impractical in other than a research setting.

Infection-related SPB is strongly associated with elevated amniotic fluid concentrations of the proinflammatory cytokines such as interleukin-6 (IL-6), both in symptomatic women (Romero *et al.* 1990; Yoon *et al.* 2001) and asymptomatic women (Ghidini *et al.* 1997; Wenstrom *et al.* 1998). The invasive nature of amniocentesis severely limits the clinical application of amniotic fluid IL-6 measurement, and whilst IL-6 is found in higher concentration in the cervices of women subsequently delivering preterm, cervical IL-6 levels are not independently associated with SPB (Goepfert *et al.* 2001).

Elevated maternal serum IL-6 concentrations have been reported in women with preterm premature rupture of membranes (pPROM) and clinical and/or histologic evidence of chorioamnionitis (Murtha *et al.* 1996). An IL-6 level greater than 8 pg/ml is not seen amongst asymptomatic controls whilst women with preterm contractions or pPROM with levels greater than this have a shorter interval to delivery time compared to similar cases with levels < 8 pg/ml (Murtha *et al.* 1998).

To determine whether cytokines measured in the serum of asymptomatic pregnant women can predict SPB, the Preterm Prediction Study evaluated plasma levels of granulocyte colony-stimulating factor (GCSF) at 24 and 28 weeks' gestation in women undergoing routine antenatal care (Goldenberg *et al.* 2000). Granulocyte colony-stimulating factor is a cytokine produced by monocytes, which attracts circulating leukocytes into tissue. Women delivering before 32 weeks' gestation had elevated serum levels of GCSF at both 24 and 28 weeks' gestation; plasma GCSF was not associated with SPB after 32 weeks' gestation. At 24 weeks' gestation the sensitivity of an elevated plasma GCSF for predicting spontaneous preterm birth at 24 to 28 weeks' gestation was 54%, with a specificity of 79%. The PPV and NPV were 2.2% and 99% respectively. At 28 weeks' gestation an elevated GCSF value had a sensitivity of 37% and a positive predictive value of only 7% for subsequent SPB at 28–31 weeks' gestation (Goldenberg *et al.* 2000). The measurement of inflammatory cytokines in the mother's serum is not sufficiently accurate to justify its use as a predictor of SPB in the general antenatal population.

Matrix metalloproteinase 9 (MMP-9)

Matrix metalloproteinases are a family of endopeptidases involved in the remodelling and degradation of extracellular matrix associated with trophoblast invasion during pregnancy and the onset of labour. Elevated MMP-9 levels have been identified in amniotic fluid in association with labour and premature rupture of membranes (Vadillo-Ortego *et al.* 1996).

Plasma MMP-9 levels have been assessed longitudinally in pregnancy (Tu *et al.* 1998). Prenatal values did not change significantly with advancing gestation, regardless of whether the woman delivered preterm or not. There was, however, a threefold increase once the woman was in spontaneous labour.

Agrez *et al.* (1999) reported a small study examining the utility of urine testing for the presence of MMP-9 to differentiate women for whom threatened preterm labour resolves from those in whom it leads to premature delivery. Using a cut-off for urinary MMP-9 levels of greater than or equal to 5 ng/ml, the sensitivity was 67% and the PPV 80% for delivery within 7 days. Further studies are required to determine whether MMP-9 measurement will become a clinically useful tool in the prediction of SPB.

Other circulating factors

Alpha-fetoprotein (AFP)

The use of maternal serum AFP (MSAFP) in screening for fetal structural anomalies is well established but, in addition, several studies have described an increased risk of adverse perinatal outcomes associated with a high level of MSAFP, including an increased risk of SPB (Davis *et al.* 1992). There is no single explanation for this association although it is generally believed that an abnormality in placentation is common to both a raised MSAFP and some cases of SPB.

Amongst 51 008 women undergoing AFP screening between 15–19 weeks' gestation there was a strong gradient of increasing risk of preterm birth with increasing levels of serum AFP (Waller *et al.* 1996). An MSAFP level exceeding 2.5 MoM was associated with high risk of preterm birth compared to those women in the lowest quartile (OR 8.7, 95% CI 7.1–10.7) but in this study there was no differentiation between SPB and iatrogenic prematurity. When MSAFP is measured at 24 weeks' gestation, a value greater than the 90th centile has an OR of 3.9 (95% CI 1.8–8.9) for SPB before 35 weeks' gestation but the sensitivity is only 35% (Moawad *et al.* 2002).

An unexplained raised MSAFP discovered at the time of prenatal screening is an indication for increased fetal surveillance but MSAFP measurement alone is insufficiently accurate to be a predictor of SPB.

Combining markers to estimate risk of preterm delivery

There is no currently available single test that can reliably identify those women who will and those who will not deliver prematurely. The more recently described tests involving the detection of cervico-vaginal fFn and the ultrasonographic measurement of cervical length appear to perform better than more traditional risk-factors based upon maternal characteristics and obstetric history (Goldenberg *et al.* 1998).

When the performances of fFn testing and cervical length measurement are compared in asymptomatic populations there are conflicting reports regarding which test most usefully predicts subsequent SPB (Heath *et al.* 2000; Iams *et al.* 2001). The presence of fFn, a short cervix (less than or equal to 25 mm) and a history of a previous SPB are the three strongest predictors for delivery before 32 weeks' gestation; the rate of SPB progressively rises from 0.5% for women with none of these factors to 50% if all three risk-factors are present at 22–24 weeks' gestation (Goldenberg *et al.* 1998).

Combining such markers in an effort to improve the prediction of SPB might be useful if the individual risk-factors assessed provide additional predictive capacity independently of each other. There appears to be little overlap of the most promising biological markers for SPB (cervical length, fFn and serum markers of the inflammatory response) suggesting that there are several pathways that lead to SPB and also suggesting that the combination of these markers might be a valid and fruitful way of improving the prediction of SPB (Goldenberg *et al.* 2001). Further prospective studies are required to elucidate the selection and timing of the biological markers that might be combined to maximise our ability to accurately predict SPB in asymptomatic women.

Amongst women experiencing preterm uterine activity, the presence of fFn performs better or at least as well as ultrasound measurement of the cervix in differentiating true from false preterm labour (Rizzo *et al.* 1996; Rozenberg *et al.* 1997). The resources required for cervico-vaginal fibronectin testing are less than those required for cervical assessment since bedside testing is uncomplicated (Senden and Owen 1996) and does not require expensive equipment or personnel trained in cervical length measurement.

The selective addition of fFn testing to women with these cervical length measurements has been proposed as a rational use of both tests. Amongst symptomatic women with cervical dilatation < 3 cm and intact membranes, below and above cervical lengths of 21 and 31 mm, fFn testing does not improve the ability to predict subsequent delivery within 28 days. However, fFn testing is independent of cervical length measurement between 21 and 31 mm and the selective application of fFn testing results in a two-step test with performance of 86%, 90%, 63% and 97% for sensitivity, specificity, positive and negative prediction respectively, which is an improvement upon the performance of either cervical length or fFn testing alone (Hincz *et al.* 2002). Further evaluation of this promising two-step test using a shorter, more clinically relevant interval from presentation to delivery is required.

Conclusions

A greater understanding of the biological mechanisms underlying the onset and maintenance of spontaneous preterm birth has permitted the evaluation of a number of novel markers as predictors of SPB. The multifactorial nature of SPB makes it unlikely that a single test can be a reliable and accurate predictor of SPB.

Amongst women at highest risk of SPB, presenting with preterm uterine activity, both fFn testing and ultrasonographic measurement of cervical length have clinical utility but neither test has been evaluated in a randomised controlled trial. Amongst asymptomatic women, there is currently no biological marker that can be recommended as a universal test for the prediction of SPB; developing a multi-marker test by combining a number of biological markers appears to be a promising avenue for future research.

REFERENCES

Agrez, M., Gu, X. and Giles, W. (1999) Matrix metalloproteinase 9 in urine of patients at risk for premature delivery. *Am. J. Obstet. Gynecol.* **181**, 387–8.

Andersen, H. F. (1991) Transvaginal and transabdominal ultrasonography of the uterine cervix during pregnancy. *J. Clin. Ultrasound* **19**, 77–83.

Bega, G., Lev-Toaff, A., Kuhlman, K. *et al.* (2000) Three-dimensional multiplanar transvaginal ultrasound of the cervix in pregnancy. *Ultrasound Obstet. Gynecol.* **16**, 351–8.

Berghella, V., Tolosa, J. E., Kuhlman, K. *et al.* (1997) Cervical ultrasonography compared with manual examination as a predictor of preterm delivery. *Am. J. Obstet. Gynecol.* **177**, 723–30.

Chien, P. F. W., Khan, K. S., Ogston, S. and Owen, P. (1997) The diagnostic accuracy of cervico-vaginal fetal fibronectin in predicting preterm delivery: an overview. *BJOG* **104**, 436–44.

Crane, J. M. G., Van Den Hof, M., Armson, B. A. and Liston, R. (1997) Transvaginal ultrasound in the prediction of preterm delivery: singleton and twin gestations. *Obstet. Gynecol.* **90**, 357–63.

Creasy, R. K., Gummer, B. A. and Liggins, G. C. (1980) System for predicting spontaneous preterm birth. *Obstet. Gynecol.* **55**, 692–5.

Darne, J., McGarrigle, H. H. G. and Lachelin, G. L. C. (1987) Saliva oestriol, oestradiol, oestrone and progesterone levels in pregnancy: Spontaneous labour at term is preceded by a rise in the saliva oestriol: progesterone ratio. *BJOG* **94**, 227–35.

Davis, R. O., Goldenberg, R. L., Boots, L. *et al.* (1992) Elevated levels of maternal serum alpha-fetoprotein are associated with preterm delivery but not with fetal growth retardation. *Am. J. Obstet. Gynecol.* **167**, 596–601.

Fujita, M. M., Brizot, M. L., Liao, A. W. *et al.* (2002) Reference ranges for cervical length in twin pregnancies. *Acta Obstet. Gynecol. Scand.* **81**(9), 856–9.

Ghidini, A, Jenkins, C. B., Spong, C. Y. *et al.* (1997) Elevated amniotic fluid interleukin-6 levels during the early second trimester are associated with greater risk of subsequent preterm delivery. *Am. J. Reprod. Immunol.* **37**, 227–31.

Gibson, J. L., Macara, L., Owen, P., *et al.* (2004) Prediction of preterm delivery in twin pregnancy: a prospective, observational study of cervical length and fetal fibronectin testing. *Ultrasound Obstet. Gynecol.* **23**, 561–6.

Goepfert, A. R., Goldenberg, R. L., Andrews, W. W. *et al*; National Institute of Child Health and Human Development Maternal-Fetal Medicine Units Network (2001) The Preterm Prediction Study: Association between cervical interleukin 6 concentration and spontaneous preterm birth. National Institute of Child Health and Human Development Maternal-Fetal Medicine Units Network. *Am. J. Obstet. Gynecol.* **184**, 483–8.

Goldenberg, R. L., Iams, J. D., Miodovnik, M. *et al.* (1996) The preterm prediction study: risk factors in twin gestations. National Institute of Child Health and Human Development Maternal-Fetal Medicine Units Network. *Am. J. Obstet. Gynecol.* **175**, 1047–53.

Goldenberg, R. L., Iams, J. D., Mercer, B. M. *et al.* (1998) The preterm prediction study: The value of new vs standard risk factors in predicting early and all spontaneous preterm births. NICHD MFMU Network. *Am. J. Obstet. Gynecol.* **88**, 233–8.

Goldenberg, R. L., Andrews, W., Mercer, B. *et al.* (2000) The preterm prediction study: Granulocyte colony-stimulating factor and spontaneous preterm birth. *Am. J. Obstet. Gynecol.* **182**, 625–30.

Goldenberg, R. L., Iams, J. D., Mercer, B. M. *et al.* Maternal-Fetal Medicine Units Network. (2001) The Preterm Prediction Study: Toward a multiple-marker test for spontaneous preterm birth. *Am. J. Obstet. Gynecol.* **185**, 643–51.

Gomez, R., Galasso, M., Romero, R. *et al.* (1994) Ultrasonographic examination of the uterine cervix is better than cervical digital examination as a predictor of the likelihood of premature delivery in patients with preterm labor and intact membranes. *Am. J. Obstet. Gynecol.* **171**, 956–64.

Guzman, E. R., Walters, C., O'Reilly-Green, C. *et al.* (2000a) Use of cervical ultrasonography in prediction of spontaneous preterm birth in twin gestations. *Am. J. Obstet. Gynecol.* **183**, 1103–7.

Guzman, E. R., Walters, C., O'Reilly-Green, C. *et al.* (2000b) Use of cervical ultrasonography in prediction of spontaneous preterm birth in triplet gestations. *Am. J. Obstet. Gynecol.* **183**, 1108–13.

Guzman, E. R., Walters, C., Ananth, C. V. *et al.* (2001) A comparison of sonographic cervical parameters in predicting spontaneous preterm birth in high-risk singleton pregnancies. *Ultrasound Obstet. Gynecol.* **18**, 204–10.

Hassan, S. S., Romero, R., Berry, S. *et al.* (2000) Patients with an ultrasonographic cervical length $< = 15\,mm$ have nearly a 50% risk of early spontaneous preterm delivery. *Am. J. Obstet. Gynecol.* **182**, 1458–67.

Heath, V. C., Southall, T. R., Souka, A. P., Elisseou, A. and Nicolaides, K. H. (1998) Cervical length at 23 weeks of gestation: prediction of spontaneous preterm delivery. *Ultrasound Obstet. Gynecol.* **12**, 312–17.

Heath, V. C., Daskalalis, G., Zagaliki, A., Carvalho, M. and Nicolaides, K. H. (2000) Cervicovaginal fibronectin and cervical length at 23 weeks of gestation: relative risk of early preterm delivery. *BJOG* **107**, 1276–81.

Heine, R. P., McGregor, J. A. and Dullien, V. K (1999) Accuracy of salivary estriol testing compared to traditional risk factor assessment in predicting preterm birth. *Am. J. Obstet. Gynecol.* **180**, S214–18.

Heine, R. P., McGregor, J. A., Goodwin, T. M. *et al.* (2000) Serial salivary estriol to detect an increased risk of preterm birth. *Obstet. Gynecol.* **96**, 490–7.

Hincz, P., Wilczynski, J., Kozarzewski, M. and Szaflik, K. (2002) Two-step test: the combined use of fetal fibronectin and sonographic examination of the uterine cervix for prediction of preterm delivery in symptomatic patients. *Acta Obstet. Gynecol. Scand.* **81**, 58–63.

Holbrook, R. H., Laros, R. K. and Creasy, R. K. (1989) Evaluation of a risk-scoring system for prediction of preterm labor. *Am. J. Perinatol.* **6**, 62–8.

Honest, H., Bachmann, L. M., Gupta, J. K., Kleijnen, J. and Khan, K. S. (2002) Accuracy of cervicovaginal fetal fibronectin test in predicting risk of spontaneous preterm birth: systematic review. *BMJ* **325**, 301–4.

Iams, J. D., Paraskos, J., Landon, M. B., Teteris, J. N. and Johnson, F. F. (1994) Cervical sonography in preterm labor. *Obstet. Gynecol.* **84**, 40–6.

Iams, J. D., Goldenberg, R. L., Meis, P. J. *et al.* (1996) The length of the cervix and the risk of spontaneous preterm delivery. *N. Engl. J. Med.* **334**, 567–72.

Iams, J. D., Goldenberg, R. L., Mercer, B. M. *et al.*; National Institute of Child Health and Human Development Maternal-Fetal Medicine Units Network. (2001) The Preterm Prediction Study: Can low-risk women destined for spontaneous preterm birth be identified? *Am. J. Obstet. Gynecol.* **184**, 652–5.

Iams, J. D., Newman, R. B., Thom, E. A. *et al.*; National Institute of Child Health and Human Development Network of Maternal-Fetal Medicine Units (2002) Frequency of uterine contractions and the risk of spontaneous preterm delivery. *N. Engl. J. Med.* **346**, 250–5.

Inder, W. J., Prickett, T., Ellis, J. *et al.* (2001) The utility of plasma CRH as a predictor of preterm delivery. *J. Clin. Endocrinol. Metab.* **86**, 5706–10.

Joffe, G. M., Jacques, D., Bemis-Heyes, R. *et al.* (1999) Impact of the fetal fibronectin assay on admissions for preterm labor. *Am. J. Obstet. Gynecol.* **180**, 581–6.

Keirse, M. J. N. C. (1989) An evaluation of formal risk scoring for preterm birth. *Am. J. Perinatol.* **6**, 226–33.

Keirse, M. J. N. C. (1992) Home uterine activity monitoring for preventing preterm delivery. In Pregnancy and Childbirth Module (eds. M. W. Enkin, M. J. N. C. Keirse, M. J. Renfrew, and J. P. Neilson) '*Cochrane Database Syst. Rev.*, Review No. 06656.

Lachelin, G. C. and McGarrigle, H. H. (1984) A comparison of saliva, plasma unconjugated, and plasma total oestriol throughout normal pregnancy. *BJOG* **91**, 1203–9.

Leitich, H., Brunbauer, M., Kaider, A., Egarter, C. and Husslein, P. (1999) Cervical length and dilatation of the internal cervical os detected by vaginal ultrasonography as markers for preterm delivery: A systematic review. *Am. J. Obstet. Gynecol.* **181**, 1465–72.

Leung, T. N., Chung, T. K., Madsen, G. *et al.* (1999) Elevated mid-trimester maternal corticotrophin-releasing hormone levels in pregnancies that delivered before 34 weeks. *BJOG* **106**, 1041–6.

Lockwood, C. J., Seneyi, A. E., Dische, R. *et al.* (1991) Fetal fibronectin in cervical and vaginal secretions as a predictor of preterm delivery. *N. Engl. J. Med.* **325**, 669–74.

Lumley, J. (1993) The epidemiology of preterm birth. *Baillieres Clin. Obst. Gynaecol.* **7**, 447–98.

Macdonald, R., Smith, P. and Vyas, S. (2001) Cervical incompetence: the use of transvaginal sonography to provide an objective diagnosis. *Ultrasound Obstet. Gynecol.* **18**, 211–16.

McGregor, J. A., Jackson, G. M., Lachelin, G. C. L. *et al.* (1995) Salivary estriol as risk assessment for preterm labor: a prospective trial. *Am. J. Obstet. Gynecol.* **173**, 1337–42.

McKenna, D. S., Chung, K. and Iams, J. D. (1999) Effect of digital cervical examination on the expression of fetal fibronectin. *J. Reprod. Med.* **44**, 796–800.

McLean, M., Bisits, A., Davies, J. *et al.* (1995) A placental clock controlling the length of human pregnancy. *Nat. Med.* **1**, 460–3.

Maymon, R., Herman, A., Jauniaux, E. *et al.* (2001) Transvaginal sonographic assessment of cervical length changes during triplet gestation. *Hum. Reprod.* **16**, 956–60.

Mercer, B. M., Goldenberg, R. L., Das, A. *et al.* (1996) The preterm prediction study: A clinical risk assessment system. *Am. J. Obstet. Gynecol.* **174**, 1885–95.

Moawad, A., Goldenberg R. L., Mercer, B. *et al.*; NICHD MFMU Network. (2002) The Preterm Prediction Study: The value of serum alkaline phosphatase, alpha-fetoprotein, plasma corticotrophin-releasing hormone, and other serum markers for the prediction of spontaneous preterm birth. *Am. J. Obstet. Gynecol.* **186**, 990–6.

Murtha, A. P., Greig, P. C., Jimmerson, C. E. *et al.* (1996) Maternal serum interleukin-6 concentrations in patients with preterm rupture of membranes and evidence of infection. *Am. J. Obstet. Gynecol.* **175**, 966–9.

Murtha, A. P., Greig, P. C., Jimmerson, C. E. and Herbert, W. N. (1998) Maternal serum interleukin-6 concentration as a marker for impending preterm delivery. *Obstet. Gynecol.* **91**, 161–4.

Newman, R. B., Campbell, B. A. and Stramm, S. L. (1990) Objective tocodynamometry identifies labor onset earlier than subjective maternal perception. *Obstet. Gynecol.* **76**, 1089–92.

Owen, J., Yost, N., Berghella, V. *et al.*; National Institute of Child Health and Human Development, Maternal-Fetal Medicine Units Network. (2001) Mid-trimester endovaginal sonography in women at high risk for spontaneous preterm birth. *JAMA* **286**, 1340–8.

Petersen, L. K., Skajaa, K. and Uldbjerg, N. (1992) Serum relaxin as a potential marker for preterm labour. *BJOG* **99**, 292–5.

Rizzo, G., Capponi, A., Arduini, D., Lorido, C. and Romanini, C. (1996) The value of fetal fibronectin in cervical and vaginal secretions and of ultrasonographic examination of the uterine cervix in predicting premature delivery for patients with preterm labor and intact membranes. *Am. J. Obstet. Gynecol.* **175**, 1146–51.

Romero, R., Avila, C., Santhanam, U. and Sehgal, P. B. (1990) Amniotic fluid interleukin-6 in preterm labor. *J. Clin. Invest.* **85**, 1392–400.

Rozenberg, P., Goffinet, F., Malagrida, L. *et al.* (1997) Evaluating the risk of preterm delivery: a comparison of fetal fibronectin and transvaginal ultrasonographic measurement of cervical length. *Am. J. Obstet. Gynecol.* **176**, 196–9.

Senden, I. P. and Owen, P. (1996) Comparison of cervical assessment, fetal fibronectin and fetal breathing in the diagnosis of preterm labour. *Clin. Exp. Obstet. Gynecol.* **23**, 5–9.

Skentou, C., Souka, A. P., To, M. S., Liao, A. W. and Nicolaides, K. H. (2001) Prediction of preterm delivery in twins by cervical assessment at 23 weeks. *Ultrasound Obstet. Gynecol.* **17**, 7–10.

Souka, A. P., Heath, V., Flint, S., Sevastopoulou, I. and Nicolaides, K. H. (1999) Cervical length at 23 weeks in twins in predicting spontaneous preterm birth. *Obstet. Gynecol.* **94**, 450–4.

Taipale, P. and Hiilesmaa, V. (1998) Sonographic measurement of uterine cervix at 18–22 weeks' gestation and the risk of preterm delivery. *Obstet. Gynecol.* **92**, 902–7.

Timor-Tritsch, I. E., Boozarjomehri, F., Masakowski, Y., Monteagudo, A. and Chao, C. R. (1996) Can a "snapshot" sagital view of the cervix by transvaginal ultrasonography predict active preterm labor? *Am. J. Obstet. Gynecol.* **174**, 990–5.

To, M. S., Skentou, C., Cicero, S., Liao, A. W. and Nicolaides, K. H. (2000) Cervical length at 23 weeks in triplets: prediction of spontaneous preterm delivery. *Ultrasound Obstet. Gynecol.* **16**, 515–8.

To, M. S., Skentou, C., Cicero, S. and Nicolaides, K. H. (2000) Cervical assessment at the routine 23–weeks' scan: problems with transabdominal sonography. *Ultrasound Obstet. Gynecol.* **15**, 292–6.

To, M. S., Skentou, C., Liao, A. W., Cacho, A. and Nicolaides, K. H. (2001) Cervical length and funnelling at 23 weeks of gestation in the prediction of spontaneous early preterm birth. *Ultrasound Obstet. Gynecol.* **18**, 200–3.

Tu, F. F., Goldenberg, R. L., Tamura, T. *et al.* (1998) Prenatal plasma matrix metalloproteinase-9 levels to predict spontaneous preterm birth. *Obstet. Gynecol.* **92**, 446–9.

United States Preventive Services Task Force (1993) Home uterine activity monitoring for preterm labor Policy Statement. *JAMA* **270**, 369–70.

Vadillo-Ortega, F., Hernandez, A., Gonzales-Avila, G. *et al.* (1996) Increased matrix metalloproteinase activity and reduced tissue inhibitor of metalloproteinases-1 levels in amniotic fluids from pregnancies complicated by premature rupture of membranes. *Am. J. Obstet. Gynecol.* **174**, 1371–6.

Vogel, I., Salvig, J., Secher, N. J. and Uldbjerg, N. (2001) Association between raised serum relaxin levels during the eighteenth gestational week and very preterm delivery. *Am. J. Obstet. Gynecol.* **184**, 390–3.

Vogel, I., Glavind-Kristensen, M., Thorsen, P., Armbruster, F. P. and Uldbjerg, N. (2002) S-relaxin as a predictor of preterm delivery in women with symptoms of preterm labour. *BJOG* **109**, 977–82.

Waller, D. K., Lustig, L. S., Cunningham, G. C., Feuchtbaum, L. B. and Hook, E. B. (1996) The association between maternal serum alpha-fetoprotein and preterm birth, small for gestational age infants, pre-eclampsia and placental complications. *Obstet. Gynecol.* **88**, 816–22.

Warren, W. B., Patrick, S. L. and Goland, R. S. (1992) Elevated maternal plasma corticotrophin-releasing hormone levels in pregnancies complicated by preterm labor. *Am. J. Obstet. Gynecol.* **166**, 1198–204.

Wenstrom, K. D., Andrews, W. W., Hauth, J. C. *et al.* (1998) Elevated second-trimester amniotic fluid interleukin-6 levels predict preterm delivery. *Am. J. Obstet. Gynecol.* **178**, 546–50.

Yoon, B. H., Romero, R., Moon, J. B. *et al.* (2001) Clinical significance of intra-amniotic inflammation in patients with preterm labor and intact membranes. *Am. J. Obstet. Gynecol.* **185**, 1130–6.

6

Prevention of preterm labour

John Morrison and Nandini Ravikumar

National University of Ireland

Introduction

The delivery of infants at preterm periods of gestation is a major factor contributing to perinatal morbidity and mortality in current obstetric practice in developed countries (ACOG Practice Bulletin 2001). It is associated with short- and long-term sequelae and constitutes a significant problem in terms of mortality, disability and cost to healthcare resources and society. Research efforts to address this problem have increased substantially over the last ten years but have failed in their attempts to improve prediction and prevention of preterm delivery.

Preterm delivery results from a series of disorders implicating maternal and fetal disease, some of which are explained and interrelated while many are of unknown aetiology (Iannucci et al. 1996; Burke and Morrison 2000). Epidemiological risk factors for preterm delivery, which are well established (Olsen et al. 1995; Mercer et al. 1996; Kramer et al. 2001), exert a huge influence on its incidence and outcome. In addition, the overall incidence of preterm delivery appears to be increasing in recent years (Goldenberg and Rouse 1998). The reasons for this increase are complex and have been the source of much debate. It has been speculated that there might have been a recent increased tendency to register live birth at very early gestational ages (i.e. 20–22 weeks) in some countries (Joseph et al. 1998). Increased obstetric intervention has also been suggested as a cause for recent increased preterm delivery rates (Joseph et al. 1998), as have other factors such as assisted reproduction techniques (Joseph et al. 1998), a higher number of multiple births (Sawdy and Bennett 1999), increased prevalence of substance abuse in urban areas (Olsen et al. 1995) and an increase in idiopathic preterm delivery rates heavily weighted by adverse socioeconomic factors (Olsen et al. 1995; Mercer et al. 1996; Kramer et al. 2001). While the overall preterm delivery rate within a population is an important statistic in public health terms, the main focus of attention must be on outcome measures in terms of morbidity and mortality. In most countries the preterm delivery statistics are calculated such that a delivery at

Preterm Labour Managing Risk in Clinical Practice, eds. Jane Norman and Ian Greer. Published by Cambridge University Press. © Cambridge University Press 2005.

34 weeks' gestation and a delivery at 27 weeks' gestation are given equal weight in the statistics. In terms of morbidity and mortality they are of course vastly different. For this reason, and because neonatal survival is effectively 100% after 32 weeks' gestation, there has been a recent trend towards evaluating and reporting outcome for the 1%–2% of births that occur before 32 weeks' gestation, separately from those occurring after this time (Morrison and Rennie 1997; El-Metwally *et al.* 2000; Burke and Morrison 2000; Wood *et al.* 2000).

Of all the epidemiological risk factors, parental Socioeconomic status, and the various socioeconomic and psychosocial variables that apply during pregnancy, each appear to play a huge role in terms of incidence and outcome for preterm delivery (Olsen *et al.* 1995; Mercer *et al.* 1996; Kramer *et al.* 2001; Slattery and Morrison 2002). The aim of this chapter is firstly to evaluate the role of these socioeconomic variables in relation to preterm delivery, and from a preventative view point, to assess benefits or otherwise of lifestyle modification in terms of reducing preterm delivery or improving its outcome. The second aim of this review is to consider management of maternal disease in pregnancy and its contribution to preterm delivery rates and the sequelae of preterm delivery. Thirdly, the role of prophylactic tocolysis for prevention of preterm delivery will be discussed. The fourth section of this review will deal with assessment of cervical status during pregnancy as a risk factor for preterm delivery, and specifically the role of cervical therapy for prevention of same. The final section of this chapter will deal with the role of antimicrobial therapy for prevention of preterm delivery. The problem of preterm delivery, and the various different predictive, preventative and therapeutic strategies that have been researched in recent years, is a very broad area in terms of clinical and scientific data. While the aims of this review are specific as outlined above, there will inevitably be overlap with topics covered in other chapters of this book.

Lifestyle modification

Socioeconomic factors

Whether defined by educational activity, income or occupation, social disadvantage is associated with a significantly increased risk of preterm birth (MacFarlane *et al.* 1988; Olsen *et al.* 1995; Morrison and Rennie 1997; Koupilova *et al.* 1998). It is frequently not clear why this should be the case but numerous explanations put forward include quality and quantity of antenatal care, increased prevalence of cigarette smoking, poorer nutritional status, greater use of recreational drugs such as cocaine, ecstasy or cannabis, higher incidence of fetal growth restriction, higher incidence of genital tract infection, higher levels of adverse physiological factors and occupations with a greater need for physically demanding work. Frequently, a combination of the above factors may pertain. It is hard to explain why greater financial income or education should have a direct effect on the duration of gestation (Kramer *et al.* 2001). It seems more likely that relative socioeconomic disadvantage as mediated by the different pathways outlined above, leading to unhealthy physical or psychological wellbeing in the mother, results in a greater incidence of spontaneous preterm delivery or the need for elective preterm delivery. The biological basis for the above outlined mechanisms is however rather weak.

Racial factors

While there is great racial variation in the incidence of preterm delivery, with the preterm birth rate for black women being almost twice that of white women of comparable age in the USA (Schieve and Handler 1996; Joseph *et al.* 1998; Ananth *et al.* 2001), this difference appears to exist irrespective of socioeconomic status (McGrady *et al.* 1992). In other words, after standardising for socioeconomic variables among black and white college graduates, the incidence of preterm birth was significantly higher among black participants (McGrady *et al.* 1992). It is not clear why this difference exists, but it appears that the preponderance of preterm deliveries in the black population occur in the idiopathic preterm labour group. For this reason it has been suggested that there is some intrinsic biological variation in the regulation of labour onset, and the length of gestation, in black women in comparison to white women. In global terms however the racial gap in preterm delivery rates has slightly diminished during the last ten years largely due to an increase in preterm delivery rates for white infants (Mattison *et al.* 2001).

Recreational drug abuse

In the last decade much research has focused on the issue of substance abuse during pregnancy and its link with preterm delivery. This has arisen because of the increasing problem of high preterm delivery rates in inner city deprived areas and the putative links with recreational drug abuse. What has always been controversial is the component of risk provided by the actual substance abuse and that which is related to other adverse socioeconomic factors. It is clear that preterm delivery occurs in approximately 25% of poly-drug using women (Boer *et al.* 1994). The reported findings for substance abuse in relation to preterm delivery vary significantly between reports, and between the actual substance used. There appears to be a clear association between cocaine use and increased preterm delivery rates (Cherukuri *et al.* 1988; Neerhof *et al.* 1989; Handler *et al.* 1991; Dinsmoor *et al.* 1994; Offidani *et al.* 1995); however, interpretation of findings from these studies can be rather difficult as highly selected populations are often studied, and it is difficult to control for potential confounding variables. In addition, various studies use different criteria as evidence of drug abuse, i.e. self-reporting, medical record documentation or urine assays. Interestingly, other studies have not demonstrated an increase in preterm birth rates with cocaine use during pregnancy (Shiono *et al.* 1995; Miller and Boudreaux 1999), and have suggested that numerous other lifestyle risk factors in cocaine users may account for adverse pregnancy outcomes.

In relation to cannabis or marijuana it appears that at least 5% of women use this substance during pregnancy and that this figure may in fact be an underestimate (Fergusson *et al.* 2002). The occasional use of cannabis during pregnancy is not apparently associated with increased risks of preterm delivery or increased perinatal morbidity mortality (Fried *et al.* 1984; Hatch and Bracken 1986; Shiono *et al.* 1995; Fergusson *et al.* 2002). However, a possible association between frequent and regular use of marijuana throughout pregnancy with small decrements in fetal birthweight has been suggested (Fergusson *et al.* 2002).

The principal biologically active component of marijuana, Δ^9 tetrahydrocannabinol (Δ^9 – THC), is a member of the cannabinoid family. The family of compounds are known to exert their effects via the cannabinoid receptor subtypes, CB_1 and CB_2 (Matsuda *et al.* 1990; Munro *et al.* 1993). In 1992, following discovery of the cannabinoid receptors, it was reported that arachidonoyl ethanolamine (AEA), also known as anandamide (ANAN), is an endogenous ligand for these receptors, i.e. is an endogenous cannabinoid or endocannabinoid (Devane *et al.* 1992). We have recently investigated the effects of endogenous and exogenous cannabinoids on human myometrial contractility during pregnancy in order to evaluate whether or not marijuana had a direct effect on the uterine smooth muscle (Dennedy *et al.* 2002). We have demonstrated that the exogenous cannabinoid Δ^9 – THC exerted a potent utero-relaxant effect on isolated human myometrial contrations in vitro. The effects of Δ^9 – THC (the active component of marijuana) on isolated human myometrial contractions in vitro are shown in Figure 6.1. A cumulatively progressive inhibitory effect is demonstrated. From a physiological point of view, our provisional results support the theory that cannabis use in itself, after standardising for other socioeconomic variables, may not be an independent risk factor for preterm delivery.

Cigarette smoking and high alcohol intake are more prevalent among the socially deprived, but these factors have not been shown to exert an independent adverse effect by increasing the risk of preterm delivery (Olsen *et al.* 1995; Kramer, 1996). Similarly, increased caffeine consumption does not appear to be associated with increased risk of preterm delivery (Golding 1995).

Psychological stress

Be it independent of Socioeconomic status, or related to social disadvantage, the question of whether or not physiological stress or stressful events during

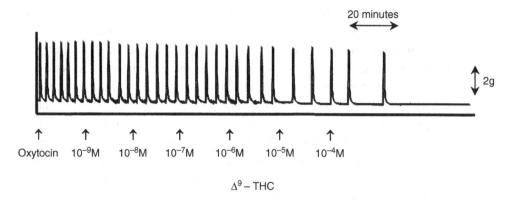

Oxytocin 10^{-9}M 10^{-8}M 10^{-7}M 10^{-6}M 10^{-5}M 10^{-4}M

$\Delta^9 - $THC

Figure 6.1   Representative recordings of the effects of $\Delta^9 - $THC on human pregnant myometrial contractility in vitro, demonstrating a cumulatively increasing relaxant effect.

pregnancy are linked to preterm delivery has interested clinicians and epidemiologists for many years. The pregnancy itself may be a source of stress for some women in terms of anxiety about fetal wellbeing or the wish to optimise pregnancy outcome. Within each culture there are set preconceived views about pregnancy and what a pregnant woman should pursue or actively avoid. Other life factors outside of the pregnancy may also be a source of stress to a woman during pregnancy. While some studies have demonstrated a positive association between psychosocial stress and pregnancies that end in preterm delivery (Gunter 1963; Lobel *et al.* 1992; Hedegaard *et al.* 1993; Pritchard and Teo 1994), many studies have not produced consistent results, and when a positive association has been present it has been small in size (Rutter and Quine 1990; Williams 1990; Lobel 1994; Hoffman and Hatch 1996). There is no sound biological basis to the mechanisms whereby psychological stress might increase the risk of preterm delivery. This is a difficult topic to study and individuals vary their biological responses to stress. Studies that have evaluated the role of elevated blood pressure, or alterations in levels of adrenocorticotrophic hormone or corticotrophin-releasing hormone, for example, have not been conclusive (Tambyrajia and Mongelli 2000; Hogue *et al.* 2001).

Enhanced social support

The central role of Socioeconomic parameters in the aetiology of preterm delivery has resulted in numerous studies evaluating the contribution of enhanced antenatal care, and increased social support during pregnancy, to the rate of preterm delivery. Similarly, the putative link between stress during pregnancy and the risk of preterm delivery, has prompted studies of enhanced social support for women deemed to be at high risk of psychological stress. The type of enhanced social support offered varies between different reports and generally includes an increase in the number of antenatal visits, bed rest programmes, home visits by midwives or social workers, the provision of psychological counselling sessions, nutritional education, counselling in relation to substance abuse or maternal cigarette smoking. Analysis of the results of 11 randomised controlled trials carried out in different countries (Europe, USA and Latin America), involving a number of women deemed to be at high risk because of socioeconomic or psychosocial stress reasons, found no significant difference in outcome between enhanced antenatal care versus the usual format of antenatal care in reducing preterm birth (Spencer *et al.* 1989; Klerman *et al.* 2001). There was no evidence, however, that enhanced antenatal care had any adverse effects, but it was associated with benefit. The lack of success in these trials may have been due to the heterogeneous nature of psychosocial deprivation, i.e. the trials may have been diluted by inclusion of women in the intervention group whose need for social report varied greatly. Some women may have been included who did not need social support. The design of trials to answer this particular question is undoubtedly difficult. In addition, there are many different levels of social support. However, the current level of evidence indicates that increased social intervention, or enhanced antenatal care or support, do not result in a reduced rate of preterm delivery or improved outcome.

Management of maternal disease

Medical disorders of pregnancy

Maternal disorders, either specific to pregnancy or generalised medical disorders, are associated with an increased risk of preterm delivery. Hypertensive disorders during pregnancy comprise the single largest category of disorders accounting for preterm delivery (Burke and Morrison 2000). Such disorders can cause up to 10% of all preterm deliveries by necessitating elective preterm delivery. Other important but less common causes, include diabetes mellitus, connective tissue disorders (particularly systematic lupus erythematosis (SLE)), renal disease and systemic diseases. Any systemic infection during pregnancy (e.g pyelonephritis (Fan *et al.* 1987) pneumonia (Madinger *et al.* 1989) or appendicitis (Anderson and Nielson 1999)), which occurs at a preterm period of gestation, may trigger labour onset. Other significant or common risk factors for preterm delivery include the presence of asymptomatic bacteriuria during pregnancy, urinary tract infection or pyelonephritis (How 1995).

Reproductive disorders

The risk of preterm delivery is substantially increased following conception with in vitro fertilisation (IVF) or gamete intrafallopian transfer (GIFT). This is particularly so for singleton pregnancies conceived by these methods in comparison to singleton pregnancies conceived naturally. Singleton pregnancies derived from such assisted reproduction technology methods have preterm delivery rates of the order of 20% (Lumley 1993; Fisch *et al.* 1997; Perri *et al.* 2001). These higher rates have been attributed to various factors such as cervical trauma, infection, uterine malformation, disturbed implantation and associated fertility factors. For mothers with ovarian failure, interestingly, no further increase in rates was observed with oocyte donation (Abdalla *et al.* 1998; Soderstrom-Anttila *et al.* 1998).

For twin pregnancies conceived following IVF or GIFT, there would not appear to be a statistically significant difference in the frequency of preterm delivery or mean gestational age at delivery, in comparison to twins conceived spontaneously (Bernasko *et al.* 1997). This may be linked to the fact that there is a reduced incidence of monozygotic twinning in an assisted reproduction technology group, in comparison to a naturally conceived group of twins.

Other maternal disorders specific to pregnancy which are linked to increased rates of preterm delivery include antepartum haemorrhage, persistent vaginal bleeding in pregnancy, intrauterine growth restriction and previous second trimester pregnancy loss (Goldenberg *et al.* 1993; Burke and Morrison 2000). The link with previous second trimester pregnancy loss may be due to cervical incompetence with dilatation at induced abortion or previous cone biopsy. Previous termination of pregnancy by itself appears to raise the risk of preterm delivery (Zhou *et al.* 1999). Finally, after adjusting for confounding variables, and stratifying by gravidity, the odds ratios of preterm singleton live births in women with one, two or more previously induced abortions were 1.89 (95% confidence interval (CI) 1.70–2.11), 2.66 (95% CI 2.09–3.37), and 2.03 (95% CI 1.29–3.19) respectively (Zhou *et al.* 1999).

In relation to maternal disorders, it is important that all sensible measures in terms of prophylactic medical care be taken prior to pregnancy onset and early during the pregnancy. For specific medical conditions such as diabetes mellitus, or SLE, it is desirable that pre-pregnancy counselling be arranged with the appropriate physician or with the specialist feto-maternal services. For pre-existing medical diseases the practice of joint review by the physician team, with feto-maternal expertise, as a joint clinic, is the most desirable practice. It is essential to aim for good control of metabolic diseases such as diabetes mellitus. Early and efficient control of hypertensive disorders is desirable. For women undergoing treatment for infertility, it is important that an awareness of the increased risk of preterm delivery and the use of potential screening tests such as transvaginal ultrasound scan of the cervix to be in place. While all these measures constitute standard medical care, the close link between these conditions and delivery at early periods of gestation should always be borne in mind. However, there is no clear indication from evidence based medicine that any of the above measures, albeit constituting sensible medical practice, lead to a reduction of the incidence of preterm delivery or benefits in terms of perinatal outcome.

Prophylactic tocolysis

The use of pharmacological agents to relax uterine smooth muscle therapeutically for prevention of preterm labour, or for inhibition of uterine contractions once preterm labour has already been initiated, has been part of standard clinical practice for more than 30 years now. Beta-2 adrenergic receptor agonists have been most widely used in clinical practice (The Canadian Preterm Labor Group 1992; Higby and Suiter 1999) and particularly ritodrine and terbutaline. Historically, because of the lack of efficacy with beta-2 adrenoreceptor agonists, and their high level of associated serious adverse effects, many other pharmacological compounds have been used in an attempt to relax the uterus prophylactically or during preterm labour. These agents include the prostaglandin synthetase inhibitors such as indomethacin, oxytocin antagonists such as atosiban, calcium channel blocking compounds such as nifedipine, nitric oxide donor compounds such as glyceryl trinitrate and magnesium sulphate (Hannah *et al.* 1995; Gyetvai *et al.* 1999; Higby and Suiter 1999; Lees *et al.* 1999; Abramov *et al.* 2000; Moutquin *et al.* 2000; Romero *et al.* 2000; Worldwide Atosiban versus Beta-agonists Study Group 2001; Tsatsaris *et al.* 2001). For women in preterm labour, it is apparent that beta-mimetics, atosiban, nifedipine and indomethacin all significantly delay delivery of the infant following preterm labour onset for 24–48 hours when compared with placebo or no treatment (Hannah *et al.* 1995; Gyetvai *et al.* 1999; Higby and Suiter 1999; Lees *et al.* 1999; Abramov *et al.* 2000; Moutquin *et al.* 2000; Romero *et al.* 2000; Worldwide Atosiban versus Beta-agonists Study Group 2001; Tsatsaris *et al.* 2001). However, when outcome measures in terms of perinatal death, respiratory distress syndrome, birthweight, necrotizing enterocolitis, patent ductus arteriosus, intraventricular haemorrhages, neonatal seizures, hypoglycaemia, and neonatal sepsis are examined, no significant difference in neonatal outcome for the infants of treated mothers was observed. The pharmacological treatment of preterm delivery offers no benefit to the neonate in comparison to placebo treatment. The use of tocolysis in any situation of preterm labour has therefore always been open to question.

Apart from the use of tocolytics for inhibiting preterm labour once initiated, as outlined above, much research has focused on the use of tocolytic compounds to prevent the onset of preterm labour (Wenstrom *et al.* 1997; Sanchez-Ramos *et al.* 1999; Crowther and Moore 2002). Such therapy could theoretically be used in women at high risk of preterm labour, or in those who have had one episode of threatened preterm labour in that pregnancy. The use of maintenance tocolytic therapy is not associated with a significant reduction in the rates of recurrent preterm labour or preterm labour (Wenstrom *et al.* 1997; Crowther and Moore 2002; Sanchez-Ramos *et al.* 1999). A more recent meta-analysis serves to confirm findings from earlier randomised clinical trials showing that maintenance therapy did not influence outcome in terms of incidence of preterm delivery (Macones *et al.* 1995).

Proper evidence based interpretation of the above clinical trials would indicate that tocolytic treatment does not have a place in either prevention or treatment of preterm labour. Despite this, tocolytic agents are used widely in clinical practice perhaps because primarily there is no other treatment regime, or secondarily, because the proven delay of 24–48 hours is deemed helpful for corticosteroid administration and parental preparation. However, it must be borne in mind that no significant perinatal benefit is conferred by tocolytic use. This should not, however, deter research efforts to develop more suitable and safer compounds that may have proven efficacy in the future. For example, there are limited clinical data in relation to the use of cyclooxygenase-2 (COX-2) inhibitors for preventing or treating preterm labour. The data that are available, mainly in terms of case reporting, have also highlighted the possibility of adverse neonatal effects (Peruzzi *et al.* 1999). Human chorionic gonadatrophin (hCG) appears to play a role in maintaining uterine quiescence in the third trimester (Peruzzi *et al.* 1999), and may be an endogenous tocolytic agent. Our research (Peruzzi *et al.* 1999) group has demonstrated that hCG exerts a potent myometrial relaxant effect in vitro in the third trimester and it also appears to inhibit preterm delivery in an animal model (Kurtzman *et al.* 1999).

Our understanding of the factors regulating smooth muscle contractility is continuously changing with elucidation of novel molecular and physiological pathways. In recent years, for example, it has become apparent that the process of calcium sensitisation, is a major pathway regulating the state of contractility of smooth muscle (Uehata *et al.* 1997) in addition to regulation of contractility by intracellular calcium concentration ($[Ca^{2+}]$) (Wray 1993; Iizuka *et al.* 1999). It is now known that a G protein, Rho A, is associated with inhibition of myosin light chain phosphatase (MLCP). Although the precise mechanism of action of Rho A has not been fully elucidated, two of its target proteins, Rho associated coil-forming protein kinase (ROCK I, also called p160ROCK) and its isoform ROCK II (also known as ROKα or Rho kinase) have been reported as having a key role in RhoA-mediated calcium sensitisation. These target proteins are collectively known as Rho kinases and when activated they enhance RhoA-mediated calcium sensitisation and smooth muscle contractility. We have identified expression of Rho A, ROCK I and ROCK II in mRNA in human pregnant myometrium (Moran *et al.* 2002). We have also recently investigated the effects of specific Rho kinase inhibitors on isolated uterine contractions in vitro (Moran *et al.* 2002) and we have

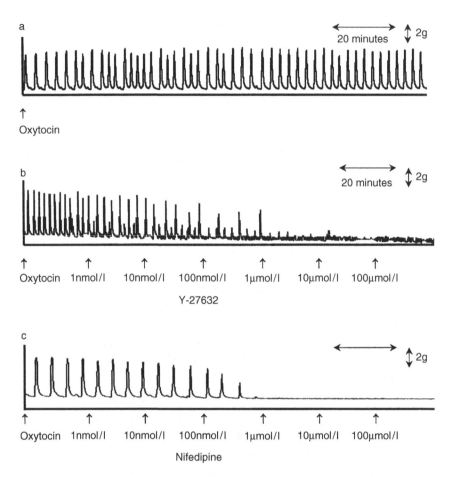

Figure 6.2   Representative recordings of oxytocin-stimulated (0.5nmol/l) contractions in pregnant human myometrium are shown. (a) Recording from a control strip and no further drug additions were made following incubation with oxytocin. (b and c) Effects of cumulative additions of Y-27632 and nifedipine respectively (1 nmol/l, 10nmol/l, 100nmol/l, 1μmol/l, 10μmol/l and 100μmol/l) at 20 min intervals. (Reproduced by permission of Oxford University Press/Human Reproduction (Moran *et al.* 2002)).

demonstrated that the specific Rho kinase inhibitor Y-27632, is a potent utero-relaxing agent, with similar potency to nifedipine. A representative recording from our in vitro data is shown in Figure 6.2 outlining a control recording and the cumulative effects of Y-27632 and nifedipine. These findings highlight the fact that inhibition of Rho kinase is a potential novel mechanism for pharmacological relaxation of uterine tissue. It is only by such scientific studies that novel therapeutic agents with the desired efficiency will be developed, to be later subjected to randomised clinical trials.

Cervical therapy

It is well established that a shortening of cervical canal length, less than the accepted normal of 40 mm, is associated with preterm delivery. With transvaginal ultrasound imaging it is possible to measure the cervical canal length very accurately from early periods of gestation. The role of cervical cerclage in women with short cervical length has been the topic of much research in recent years. In addition, the role of cervical cerclage in women with previous mid-trimester miscarriages, or preterm delivery, with or without short cervical length, has been controversial. While it is believed that insertion of a cervical suture may provide enhanced support for the cervix and hence help maintain cervical length, the evidence in terms of benefit from such practice, is conflicting.

The first randomised trial investigating cervical cerclage, and indeed the largest randomised trial, was conducted by the combined Medical Research Council/ Royal College of Obstetricians and Gynaecologists Working Party on Cervical Cerclage and was reported in 1993 (MRC/RCOG 1993). The results of this trial demonstrated that cervical cerclage had an important beneficial effect in only 1 in 25 cases in the trial (95% CI 1 in 12 to 1 in 300 sutures). There were fewer deliveries before 33 weeks in the cerclage group (13% with cerclage vs. 17% with no cerclage, $p = 0.03$). No significant risk reduction was observed between 33 and 36 weeks' gestation and the insertion of cervical surgical sutures was reported to double the risk of puerperal pyrexia. The trial suggested that, on balance, cervical cerclage should be offered to women at high risk, such as those with a history of three or more pregnancies ending before 37 weeks' gestation.

More recently published randomised controlled trials have failed to further clarify this issue. For women with preterm dilatation of the internal cervical os ultrasonographically between 16–24 weeks' gestation, it does not appear that treatment with McDonald cerclage confers any benefit in terms of perinatal outcome (Rust et al. 2000). In addition, for women with cervical shortening, membrane prolapse and internal os dilation, the use of cervical cerclage does not alter any perinatal outcome variable (Rust et al. 2001). However, the results of the cervical incompetence prevention randomised cerclage trial (CIPRACT) demonstrated that therapeutic cerclage with bed rest reduces preterm delivery before 34 weeks of gestation ($p = 0.002$) (Althuisius et al. 2001). In this study it also appeared that compound neonatal morbidity was reduced in the women in whom a cervical suture was inserted, in comparison to those who were managed with the bed rest alone.

Clinical practice in this area is therefore confusing. Other than the MRC/RCOG Working Party Trial, the other randomised trials included small numbers. There are in addition many observational and non-randomised studies, which have produced varying results. Many clinicians now reserve the use of cervical cerclage for women who have sonographically demonstrated reduction in cervical length and only recommend cerclage if the cervix shortens or if funnelling occurs. It is certainly reasonable to interpret from the evidence available that cerclage in such high-risk pregnancies may confer benefit.

Antimicrobial therapy

Because of the association between genital tract infection and preterm delivery much effort has been directed at evaluating the benefit of prophylactic antimicrobial therapy in the management of women at increased risk of preterm delivery. Meta-analyses of reports from randomised controlled trials on the efficacy of different combinations of antibiotics in the prevention and treatment of preterm labour are inconsistent (Kenyon *et al.* 2001a; Kenyon and Boulvain 2002; King and Flenady 2002). However, a recent large multicentre randomised controlled trials (including 6295 women in spontaneous preterm labour) has found no evidence supporting a role for routine antibiotic prophylaxis in the management of women presenting with spontaneous preterm labour (Kenyon *et al.* 2001a). This trial, because of its quality and size overrules the uncertainties of previous trials.

The beneficial effect of prophylactic antibiotic regimens in cases where the fetal membranes have ruptured prematurely (pPROM) is better defined. The ORACLE 1 study reported favourable outcomes including a significant prolongation of pregnancy, and improved neonatal outcome, in a large cohort of mothers treated with erythromycin for pPROM (Kenyon *et al.* 2001b). Speculative screening of asymptomatic mothers for microbes associated with an increased incidence of preterm birth, in particular those responsible for bacterial vaginosis (BV), (Kurkinen-Raty *et al.* 2000, Kekki *et al.* 2001) does not appear to be worthwhile (Guise *et al.* 2001). The treatment of established BV in early pregnancy decreases neither the incidence of preterm delivery nor the prevalence of peripartum infections (with the reported exception of mothers with a history of preterm labour) (McDonald *et al.* 2003). The empirical or blind treatment of all patients for BV in the first trimester may even be harmful, with recent reports suggesting that application of 2% clindamycin cream to pregnant women with normal vaginal flora stimulates the development of BV (Vermeulen *et al.* 2001).

Conclusion

In conclusion the epidemiological and clinical parameters associated with an increased risk of preterm delivery have been well defined in recent years. Extrapolation from this knowledge in order to design effective preventative strategies has been disappointing in its results. The social, clinical and pharmacological measures outlined above have not resulted in significant benefit by reducing the incidence of preterm birth, or improving outcome for infants delivered preterm in terms of mortality or morbidity. In addition, the preterm delivery rates appear to be rising slightly in recent years. Measures to redress these problems constitute a significant challenge to perinatal clinicians and scientists.

REFERENCES

Abdalla, H. I., Billett, A., Kan, A. K. *et al.* (1998) Obstetric outcome in 232 ovum donation pregnancies. *Br. J. Obstet. Gynaecol.* **105**, 332–7.

Abramov, Y., Nadjari, M., Weinstein, D. *et al.* (2000) Indomethacin for preterm labor: a randomised comparison of vaginal and rectal-oral routes. *Obstet. Gynecol.* **95**, 482–6.

Althuisius, S. M., Dekker, G. A., Hummel, P., Bekedam, D. J. and van Geijn, H. P. (2001) Final results of the Cervical Incompetence Prevention Randomized Prevention Trial (CIPRACT): therapeutic cerclage with bed rest versus bed rest alone. *Am. J. Obstet. Gynecol.* **185**, 1106–12.

American College of Obstetricians and Gynecologists (ACOG) Practice Bulletin (2001) Clinical Management Guidelines for Obstetrician-Gynecologists Number 31, October 2001. Assessment of risk factors for preterm birth. *Obstet. Gynecol.* **98**, 709–16.

Ananth, C. V., Misra, D. P., Demissie, K. and Smulian, J. C. (2001) Rates of preterm delivery among Black women and White women in the United States over two decades: an age-period-cohort analysis. *Am. J. Epidemiol.* **154**, 657–65.

Anderson, B. and Nielsen, T. F. (1999) Appendicitis in pregnancy: diagnosis, management and complications. *Acta Obstet. Gynecol. Scand.* **78**, 758–62.

Bernasko, J., Lynch, L., Lapinski, R. and Berkowitz, R. L. (1997) Twin pregnancies conceived by assisted reproductive techniques; maternal and neonatal outcomes. *Obstet. Gynecol.* **89**, 368–72.

Boer, K., Smit, B. J., van Huis, A. M. and Hogerzeil, H. V. (1994) Substance use in pregnancy: do we care? *Acta Paediatr. Suppl.* **404**, 65–71.

Burke, C. and Morrison, J. J. (2000) Perinatal factors and preterm delivery in an Irish obstetric population. *J. Perinat. Med.* **28**, 49–53.

Cherukuri, R., Minkoff, H., Feldman, J., Parekh, A. and Glass, L. (1988) A cohort study of alkaloidal cocaine ("crack") in pregnancy. *Obstet. Gynecol.* **72**, 147–51.

Crowther, C. A. and Moore, V. (2002) Magnesium for preventing preterm birth after threatened preterm labour (Cochrane Review). In *The Cochrane Library*, Issue 3. Oxford: Update Software

Dennedy, M. C., Friel, A. M., Houlihan, D. D., Smith, T. and Morrison, J. J. (2002) Cannabinoids and the human uterus during pregnancy. *J. Soc. Gynecol. Invest.* **9**, 52A.

Devane, W. A., Hanus, L., Breuer, A. *et al.* (1992) Isolation and structure of a brain constituent that binds to the cannabinoid receptor. *Science* **258**, 1946–9.

Dinsmoor, M. J., Irons, S. J. and Christmas, J. T. (1994) Premature rupture of the membranes associated with recent cocaine use. *Am. J. Obstet. Gynecol.* **171**, 305–8.

El-Metwally, D., Vohr, B. and Tucker, R. (2000) Survival and neonatal morbidity at the limits of viability in the mid 1990s: 22 to 25 weeks. *J. Pediatr.* **137**, 616–22.

Fan, Y. D., Pastorek, J. G., Miller, J. M. and Mulvey, J. (1987) Acute pyelonephritis in pregnancy. *Am. J. Perinatol.* **4**, 324–6.

Fergusson, D. M., Horwood, J. L. and Northstone, K. ALSPAC Study Team. Avon Longitudinal Study of Pregnancy and Childhood. (2002) Maternal use of cannabis and pregnancy outcome. *BJOG* **109**, 21–7

Fisch, B., Harel, L., Kaplan, B. *et al.* (1997) Neonatal assessment of babies conceived by in vitro fertilization. *J. Perinatol.* **17**, 473–98.

Fried, P. A., Watkinson, B. and Willan, A. (1984) Marijuana use during pregnancy and decreased length of gestation. *Am. J. Obstet. Gynecol.* **150**, 23–7.

Goldenberg, R. L. and Rouse, D. J. (1998) Prevention of premature birth. *N. Engl. J. Med.* **339**, 313–20.

Goldenberg, R. L., Mayberry, S. K., Copper, R. L., Dubard, M. B. and Hauth, J. C. (1993) Pregnancy outcome following a second-trimester loss. *Obstet. Gynecol.* **81**, 444–6.

Golding, J. (1995) Reproduction and caffeine consumption – a literature review. *Early Hum. Dev.* **43**, 1–14.

Guise, J. M., Mahon, S. M. Aickin, M. *et al.* (2001) Screening for bacterial vaginosis in pregnancy. *Am. J. Prev. Med.* **20**, S62–72.

Gunter, L. M. (1963) Psychopathology and stress in the life experience of mothers of premature infants. *Am. J. Obstet. Gynaecol.* **86**, 405–20.

Gyetvai, K., Hannah, M. E., Hodnett, E. D. and Ohlsson, A. (1999) Tocolytics for preterm labor: a systematic review. *Obstet. Gynecol.* **94**, 869–77.

Handler, A., Kistin, N., Davis, F. and Ferre, C. (1991) Cocaine use during pregnancy: perinatal outcomes. *Am. J. Epidemiol.* **133**, 818–21.

Hannah, M., Amankwah, K., Barret, J. *et al.* (1995) The Canadian consensus on the use of tocolytics for preterm labour. *J SOGC* **17**, 1089–115.

Hatch, E. E. and Bracken, M. B. (1986) Effect of marijuana use in pregnancy on fetal growth. *Am. J. Epidemiol.* **124**, 986–93.

Hedegaard, M., Brink Henriksen, T., Sabroe, S. and Secher, N. J. (1993) Psychological distress in pregnancy and preterm delivery. *Br. Med. J.* **307**, 234–9.

Higby, K. and Suiter, C. R. (1999) A risk-benefit assessment of therapies for premature labour. *Drug Saf.* **21**, 35–56.

Hoffman, S. and Hatch, M. C. (1996) Stress, social support and pregnancy outcome: a reassessment based on recent research. *Paediatr. Perinatal Epidemiol.* **10**, 380–405.

Hogue, C. J., Hofmann, S. and Hatch, M. C. (2001) Stress and preterm delivery: a conceptual framework. *Paediatr. Perinatal Epidemiol.* **15**, 30–40.

How, H. Y., Hughes, S. A., Vogel, R. L., Gall, S. A. and Spinnato, J. A (1995) Oral terbutaline in the out patient management of preterm labor. *Am. J. Obstet. Gynecol.* **173**, 1518–22.

Ianucci, T. A., Tomich, P. G. and Gianopoulos, J. G. (1996) Aetiology and outcome of extremely low-birth-weight infants. *Am. J. Obstet. Gynecol.* **174**, 1896–902.

Iizuka, K., Yoshii, A., Samizo, K. *et al.* (1999) A major role for the Rho-associated coiled coil forming protein kinase in G-protein-mediated Ca^{2+} sensitisation through inhibition of myosin phosphatase in rabbit trachea. *Br. J. Pharmacol.* **128**, 925–33.

Joseph, K. S., Kramer, M. S., Maecoux, S. *et al.* (1998) Determinants of preterm birth rates in Canada from 1981 through 1983 and from 1992 through 1994. *N. Engl. J. Med.* **339**, 1434–9.

Kekki, M., Kurki, T., Pelkonen, J., Kurkinen-Raty, M. and Cacciatore, B. J. (2001) Vaginal clindamycin in preventing preterm birth and peripartal infections in asymptomatic women with bacterial vaginosis: a randomised controlled trial. *Obstet. Gynecol.* **97**, 643–8.

Kenyon, S. and Boulvain, M. (2002) Antibiotics for preterm premature rupture of the membranes. In: Cochrane Library, issue 3.

Kenyon, S. L., Taylor, D. J. and Tarnow-Mordi, W.; ORACLE Collaborative Group. (2001a) Broad-spectrum antibiotics for spontaneous preterm labour: the ORACLE II randomised trial. *Lancet* **357**, 989–94.

Kenyon, S. L., Taylor, D. J. and Tarno-Mordi, W.; ORACLE Collaborative Group. (2001b) Broad-spectrum antibiotics for preterm, prelabour rupture of fetal membranes: the ORACLE I randomised trial. *Lancet* **357**, 979–88.

King, J. and Flenady, V. (2002) Antibiotics for preterm labour with intact membranes. In *The Cochrane Library*, Issue 3. Oxford: Update Software.

Klerman, L. V., Ramsey, S. L., Goldenberg, R. L. *et al.* (2001) A randomized controlled trial of augmented prenatal care for multiple-risk Medicaid eligible African American women. *Am. J. Public Health* **91**, 105–11.

Koupilova, I., Vagero, D., Leon, D. A. *et al.* (1998) Social variation in size at birth and preterm delivery in the Czech Republic and Sweden, 1981–1991. *Paediatr. Perinatal Epidemiol.* **12**, 7–24.

Kramer, M. S. (1996) Attributable causes of low birthweight. In F. Battaglia, F. Falkner, and C. Garza *et al.*, eds. *Maternal and Extra-uterine Nutritional Factors: their Influence on Fetal and Infant Growth.* Madrid: Ediciones Ergon, pp. 349–57.

Kramer, M. S., Goulet, L., Lydon, J. *et al.* (2001) socioeconomic disparities in preterm birth: casual pathways and mechanisms. *Paediatr. Perinatal Epidemiol.* **15**, 104–23.

Kurkinen-Raty, M., Vuopala, S., Koskela, M. *et al.* (2000) A randomised controlled trial of vaginal clindamycin for early pregnancy bacterial vaginosis. *BJOG* **107**, 1427–32.

Kurtzman, J. T., Spinnato, J. A., Goldsmith, L. J. *et al.* (1999) Human chorionic gonadotrophin exhibits potent inhibition of preterm delivery in a small animal model. *Am. J. Obstet. Gynecol.* **181**, 853–7.

Lees, C. C., Lojacono, A., Thompson, C. *et al.* (1999) Glyceryl trinitrate and ritodrine in tocolysis: an international multicenter randomized study. GTN Preterm Labour Investigation Group. *Obstet. Gynecol.* **94**, 403–8.

Lobel, M. (1994) Conceptualizations, measurement, and effects of prenatal maternal stress on birth outcomes. *J. Behav. Med.* **17**, 225–72.

Lobel, M., Dunkel-Schetter, C. and Scrimshaw, S. C. M. (1992) Prenatal maternal stress and prematurity: a prospective study of socioeconomically disadvantaged women. *Health Psychol.* **11**, 32–40.

Lumley, J. (1993) The epidemiology of preterm birth. *Baillieres Clin. Obstet. Gynaecol.* **7**, 477–98.

McDonald, H., Brocklehurst, P., Parsons, J. and Vigneswaran, R. (2003) Antibiotics for treating bacterial vaginosis in pregnancy. In *The Cochrane Library*, Issue 4. Oxford: Update Software.

MacFarlane, A., Cole, S., Johnson, A. and Botting, B. (1988) Epidemiology of birth before 28 weeks of gestation. *Br. Med. Bull.* **44**, 861–91.

McGrady, G. A., Sung, J. F., Rowley, D. L. and Hogue, C. J. (1992) Preterm delivery and low birthweight among first-born infants of black and white college graduates. *Am. J. Epidemiol.* **136**, 266–76.

Macones, G. A., Berlin, M. and Berlin, J. A. (1995) Efficacy of oral beta-agonist maintenance therapy in preterm labour: a meta-analysis. *Obstet. Gynecol.* **85**, 313–17.

Madinger, N. E., Greenspoon, J. S. and Ellrodt, A. G. (1989) Pneumonia during pregnancy: has modern technology improved maternal and fetal outcome? *Am. J. Obstet. Gynecol.* **161**, 657–62.

Matsuda, L. A., Lolait, S. J., Brownstein, M. J., Toung, A. C. and Bonner, T. I. (1990) Structure of a cannabinoid receptor and functional experssion of the cloned cDNA. *Nature* **346**, 561–4.

Mattison, D. R., Damus, K., Fiore, E., Petrini, J. and Alter, C. (2001) Preterm delivery: a public health perspective. *Paediatr. Perinatal Epidemiol.* **15**, 7–16.

Medical Research Council/Royal College of Obstetricians and Gynaecologists (MRC/RCOG) Working Party on Cervical Cerclage. (1993) Final report of the Medical Research Council/ Royal College of Obstetricians and Gynaecologists Multicentre Randomized Trial of Cervical Cerclage. *BJOG* **100**, 516–23.

Mercer, B. M., Goldenberg, R. L., Das, A. *et al.* (1996) The preterm prediction study: A clinical risk assessment system. *Am. J. Obstet. Gynecol.* **174**, 1885–95.

Miller, J. M. and Boudreaux, M. C. (1999) A study of antenatal cocaine use – chaos in action. *Am. J. Obstet. Gynecol.* **180**, 1427–31.

Moran, C. J, Friel, A. M., Smith, T. J., Cairns, M. and Morrison, J. J. (2002) Expression and modulation of Rho kinase in human pregnant myometrium. *Mol. Hum. Rep.* **8**, 196–200.

Morrison, J. J. and Rennie, J. M. (1997) Clinical, scientific and ethical aspects of fetal and neonatal care at extreme preterm periods of gestation. *BJOG* **104**, 1341–50.

Moutquin, J. M., Sherman, D., Cohen, H. (2000) Double blind, randomized, controlled trial of atosiban and ritodrine in the treatment of preterm labor: a multicenter effectiveness and safety study. *Am. J. Obstet. Gynecol.* **182**, 1191–9.

Munro, S., Thomas, K. L. and Abu Shaar, M. (1993) Molecular characterization of a peripheral receptor for cannabinoids. *Nature* **365**, 61–5.

Neerhof, M. G., MacGregor, S. N., Retzky, S. S. and Sullivan, T. P. (1989) Cocaine abuse during pregnancy: peripartum prevalence and perinatal outcome. *Am. J. Obstet. Gynecol.* **161**, 633–8.

Offidani, C., Pomini, F., Caruso, A. *et al.* (1995) Cocaine during pregnancy: a critical review of the literature. *Minerva Ginecol.* **47**, 381–90.

Olsen, P., Laara, E., Rantakillio, P. *et al.* (1995) Epidemiology of preterm delivery in two birth cohorts with an interval of 20 years. *Am. J. Epidemiol.* **142**, 1184–93.

Perri, T., Chen, R., Yoeli, R. *et al.* (2001) Are singleton assisted reproductive technology pregnancies at risk of prematurity. *J. Assist. Reprod. Genet.* **18**, 245–9.

Peruzzi, L., Gianoglio, B., Porcellini, M. G. and Coppo, R. (1999) Neonatal end-stage renal failure associated with maternal ingestion of cyclo-oxygenase-type-1 selective inhibitor nimesulide as tocolytic. *Lancet* **354**, 1615.

Pritchard, C. W. and Teo, P. Y. (1994) Preterm birth, low birthweight and stressfulness of the household role for the pregnant woman. *Soc. Sci. Med.* **38**, 89–96.

Romero, R., Sibai, B. M., Sanchez-Ramos, L. *et al.* (2000) An oxytocin receptor antagonist (atosiban) in the treatment of preterm labor: a radomized, double blind, placebo-controlled trial with tocolytic rescue. *Am. J. Obstet. Gynecol.* **182**, 1173–83.

Rust, O. A., Atlas, R. O., Jones, K. J., Benham, B. N. and Balducci, J. (2000) A randomised trial of cerclage versus no cerclage among patients with ultrasonographically detected second trimester prefers dilation of the internal os. *Am. J. Obstet. Gynecol.* **183**, 830–5.

Rust, O. A., Atlas, R. O., Reed, J., van Gaalen, J. and Balducci, J. (2001) Revisiting the short cervix detected by transvaginal ultrasound in the second trimester: why cerclage therapy may not help. *Am. J. Obstet. Gynecol.* **185**, 1098–105.

Rutter, D. R. and Quine, L. (1990) Inequalities in pregnancy outcome: review of psychosocial and behavioural mediators. *Soc. Sci. Med.* **30**, 553–68.

Sanchez-Ramos, L., Kaunitz, A. M., Gaudier, F. L. and Delke, I. (1999) Efficacy of maintenance therapy after acute tocolysis: A meta-analysis. *Am. J. Obstet. Gynecol.* **181**, 484–90.

Sawdy, R. J. and Bennett, P. R. (1999) Recent advances in the therapeutic management of preterm labour. *Curr. Opin. Obstet. Gynecol.* **11**, 131–9.

Schieve, L. A. and Handler, A. (1996) Preterm delivery and perinatal death among black and white infants in a Chicago-area perinatal registry. *Obstet. Gynecol.* **88**, 356–63.

Shiono, P. H., Klebanoff, M. A., Nugent, R. P. *et al.* (1995) The impact of cocaine and marijuana use on low birthweight and preterm birth: a multicenter study. *Am. J. Obstet. Gynecol.* **172**, 19–27.

Slattery, M. M. and Morrison, J. J. (2002) Preterm Delivery. *Lancet* **360**, 1485–97.

Soderstrom-Anttila, V., Sajaniemi, N., Tiitinen, A. and Hovatta, O. (1998) Health and development of children born after oocyte donation compared with that of those born after in vitro fertilization, and parents' attitudes regarding secrecy. *Hum. Reprod.* **13**, 2009–15.

Spencer, B., Thomas, H. and Morris, J. (1989) A randomized controlled trial of the provision of a social support service during pregnancy; the South Manchester Family Worker project. *BJOG* **96**, 281–8.

Tambyrajia, R. L. and Mongelli, M. (2000) Sociobiological variables and pregnancy outcome. *Int. J. Gynaecol. Obstet.* **70**, 105–12.

The Canadian Preterm Labor Investigators Group. (1992) Treatment of preterm labor with the beta adrenergic agonist ritodrine. The Canadian Preterm Labor Investigators Group. *N. Engl. J. Med.* **327**, 308–12.

Tsatsaris, V., Papatsonis, D., Goffinet, F., Dekker, G. and Carbonne, B. (2001) Tocolysis with nifedipine or beta-adrenergic agonists: a meta-analysis. *Obstet. Gynecol.* **97**, 840–7.

Uehata, M., Ishizaki, T., Satoh, H. *et al.* (1997) Calcium sensitisation of smooth muscle mediated by a Rho-associated protein kinase in hypertension. *Nature* **389**, 990–4.

Vermeulen, G. M., van Zwet, A. A. and Bruinse, H. W. (2001) Changes in the vaginal flora after two percent clindamycin vaginal cream in women at high risk of spontaneous prefer birth. *BJOG* **108**, 697–700.

Wenstrom, K. D., Weiner, C. P., Merrill, D. and Niebyl, J. (1997) A placebo controlled randomized trial of the terbutaline pump for prevention of preterm delivery. *Am. J. Perinatal.* **14**, 87–91.

Williams, D. R. (1990) Socioeconomic differentials in health: a review and redirection. *Soc. Psychol. Quart.* **53**, 81–99.

Wood, N. S., Marlow, N., Costeloe, K., Gibson, A. T. and Wilkinson, A. R. EPICure study group (2000) Neurological and developmental disability after extremely preterm birth. *N. Engl. J. Med.* **343**, 378–84.

Worldwide Atosiban versus Beta-agonists Study Group. (2001) Effectiveness and safety of the oxytocin antagonist atosiban versus beta-adrenergic agonists in the treatment of preterm labour. The Worldwide Atosiban versus Beta-agonists Study Group. *BJOG* **108**, 133–42.

Wray, S. (1993) Uterine contraction and physiological mechanisms of modulation. *Am. J. Physiol.* **264**, C1–18.

Zhou, W., Sorensen, H. T. and Olsen, J. (1999) Induced abortion and subsequent pregnancy duration. *Obstet. Gynecol.* **94**, 948–53.

7

Management of preterm premature ruptured membranes

Donald Peebles

University College London

Introduction

It would be reasonable to question the need for a separate chapter dealing with the management of preterm, premature rupture of the fetal membranes (pPROM). After all, pPROM is present in up to 40% of cases of premature labour, almost always results in birth of a premature infant and has a common infectious aetiology with preterm labour. However, important data, such as those from the ORACLE 1 randomised trial which showed therapeutic benefit from maternal antibiotic treatment after pPROM but not preterm labour with intact membranes, suggest that in some respects these two clinical scenarios should be considered as separate, but related entities.

The increasing realisation that the fetal inflammatory response to materno-fetal infection can lead to bronchopulmonary dysplasia and long-term neurological disability is now a key factor in the management of pPROM. The high frequency of proven intra-amniotic infection (approximately 30%) with pPROM, potentially long delays between presentation and spontaneous onset of labour, and evidence that the rate of microbial invasion increases over time (up to 75% by the onset of labour), give rise to management issues unique to this pregnancy complication. These issues include: how is materno-fetal infection and its inflammatory consequences best detected, are there therapeutic interventions which can ameliorate the fetal inflammatory response and so reduce perinatal and long-term morbidity, and when is the optimal time to deliver the fetus? As will become clear, the data are not yet available to answer many of these questions.

Diagnosis

Diagnosis of membrane rupture

A history of a gush of fluid lost vaginally followed by continuous or intermittent watery loss is strongly suggestive of PROM, with the diagnosis confirmed in up to

Preterm Labour Managing Risk in Clinical Practice, eds. Jane Norman and Ian Greer. Published by Cambridge University Press. © Cambridge University Press 2005.

90% cases (Friedman and McElinin 1969). In the absence of uterine activity, visual inspection of the cervix using a speculum, introduced using an aseptic technique, will reveal a pool of watery fluid collecting in the posterior blade of the speculum. This should be Nitrazine test positive with a blue colour appearing at a pH above 6, and will display microscopic ferning if allowed to dry on a slide. Nitrazine testing for pPROM has a sensitivity of between 81% and 97%, although the false positive rate is high if taken from the cervix (specificity 57%), as opposed to the vagina (Kishida *et al.* 1996). As well as confirming the diagnosis of ruptured membranes, swabs should be taken from the vagina (to detect group B streptococcus, *Mycoplasma* spp, *Ureaplasma Urealyticum*) and cervix (*Neisseria gonorrhoea*, *Chlamydia trachomatis*). Only if there is evidence of cervical dilatation on visual inspection and/or regular uterine contractions should the cervix be assessed by digital examination. Although there is little evidence that digital examination increases the risk of neonatal infection (Seaward *et al.* 1998), it reduces the latent period between rupture of membranes and onset of labour (Lewis *et al.* 1992). Transvaginal or translabial ultrasonography can be a useful adjunct to digital examination, providing information about cervical length, dilatation, opening of the internal os and funnelling of membranes (Carlan *et al.* 1997). Ultrasonographic detection of oligohydramnios in combination with suggestive history and examination helps confirm the diagnosis of ruptured membranes, but should not be used in isolation as there are many causes of oligohydramnios, such as placental dysfunction or pathology of the fetal urinary tract.

Diagnosis of materno-fetal infection
Amniocentesis

An increasing recognition of the deleterious consequences of fetal exposure to infection in utero has highlighted the importance of early detection of bacterial colonisation of fetal membranes, amniotic fluid and fetal blood. Unfortunately, in normal clinical practice the accurate detection of infection remains an elusive goal. Amniotic fluid culture has been considered the "gold standard" for bacterial detection. The rate of positive amniotic fluid cultures increases from approximately 32% at presentation with pPROM to 75% by the time labour commences (Goncalves *et al.* 2002). It is possible that the incidence of bacterial infection is even higher than these figures suggest; bacteria specific 16S rRNA, detected by polymerase chain reaction (PCR), is present in 36% of culture negative amniotic fluid samples (Hitti *et al.* 1997). Using species-specific primers it is possible to detect 16S rRNA from bacteria normally found in the mouth, (e.g. *Fusobacterium nucleatum* and *Streptococcus* spp)in amniotic fluid (Bearfield *et al.* 2002). However, the need to perform an amniocentesis to obtain a suitable sample restricts the clinical use of amniotic fluid culture, PCR or cytokine assays. This is partly because retrieval of amniotic fluid can be technically difficult after pPROM, and partly due to concern that amniocentesis may trigger preterm labour. In addition, it is not yet clear how knowledge of amniotic fluid infection or inflammation changes management – e.g. should detection of an organism in the amniotic fluid (which may have been present from much earlier in pregnancy) of a woman with pPROM but no other clinical evidence of infection, prompt delivery? The data are not available to answer this important question.

Clinical signs of infection and C-reactive protein

Chorioamnionitis is often subclinical; clinical signs of infection, such as pyrexia, uterine tenderness and foul smelling liquor, are present in only 30% of cases with proven microbial invasion (Goncalves *et al.* 2002). Histological chorioamnionitis, with evidence of leucocyte recruitment within the fetal membranes is present in up to 70% cases of preterm labour, often in the absence of any clinical signs of infection (Pankuch *et al.* 1984; Hillier *et al.* 1993). In a group of women with pPROM, evidence of fetal bacteraemia and positive amniotic fluid cultures, only 16% were pyrexial and 33% had a raised C-reactive protein level (Carroll *et al.* 1995a). Yoon *et al.* (1996a) found that in women with pPROM, a raised C-reactive protein had a sensitivity of 56% and a positive predictive value of 83% to detect a positive amniotic fluid cultures. Positive genital tract swabs only predict 40% of positive fetal blood and 53% of positive amniotic fluid cultures and have a high false positive rate of 24% and 25% respectively (Carroll *et al.* 1996). Taken together these data suggest that without performing an amniocentesis subclinical chorioamnionitis cannot be excluded. On the other hand, a woman with pPROM and clinical signs of infection is very likely to have chorioamnionitis.

Cordocentesis

An even greater clinical challenge than detection of chorioamnionitis is fetal assessment for evidence of infection and/or an inflammatory response. This is important, as the association between infection/inflammation and poor neonatal outcome is much stronger with markers of fetal rather than placental membrane inflammation (Leviton *et al.* 1999). An additional drawback of amniocentesis is that it does not specifically identify the infected fetus, since fetal bacteraemia is present in only 33% of pregnancies with a positive amniotic fluid culture (Carroll *et al.* 1996). Cordocentesis can be used to obtain fetal blood which can be analysed for the presence of bacteria and a proinflammatory cytokine response; however, this is a technically demanding procedure and of uncertain clinical relevance.

Ultrasound

In view of the above, non-invasive, ultrasonographic methods have been used in fetal assessment in pPROM. Not surprisingly, a low biophysical score, which is likely to indicate severe fetal compromise, correlates with fetal infection after premature membrane rupture (Vintizilios *et al.* 1985). However, early signs of fetal infection are not particularly reliable; tachycardia, although observed in fetal sheep following endotoxin exposure and neonates with an inflammatory cytokinaemia, is a non-specific finding (Yanowitz *et al.* 2002; Dalitz *et al.* 2003). Doppler studies, which show no correlation between blood flow in the umbilical or middle cerebral arteries and fetal bacteraemia, are in agreement with animal data showing that cerebral blood flow does not significantly change following systemic administration of small doses of endotoxin (Carroll *et al.* 1995b; Dalitz *et al.* 2003). Better methods for detecting fetal inflammation are urgently required, but have to be well evaluated, as decisions concerning proactive delivery will be influenced by such information. It is possible that careful assessment of fetal cardiac function might show changes in cardiac output or ventricular contractility in those fetuses with a pro-inflammatory cytokine response (Yanowitz *et al.* 2002).

Materno-fetal complications of pPROM

There are three main causes of poor fetal outcome related to rupture of the membranes before 37 weeks' gestation and all of them are more likely the earlier in pregnancy the membranes rupture: premature delivery, oligohydramnios and chorioamnionitis, the latter either pre-existent and the cause of pPROM, or due to ascending infection after pPROM. In the absence of specific complications, pPROM itself does not appear to be a specific risk factor for adverse fetal outcome. The main sources of maternal morbidity are chorioamnionitis, endometritis (14%), placental abruption (3%) and postpartum haemorrhage (12%) (Mercer 2003).

Prematurity

Premature rupture of the membranes almost inevitably results in delivery of a premature infant. There is an inverse correlation between the length of the latent phase (the time between membrane rupture and labour) and gestation (Savitz *et al.* 1997); however, even at 25 weeks 50% will deliver within 1 week, and at 28 weeks 80% will deliver within 2 weeks. The neonatal complications of premature delivery, discussed in detail in Chapter 4, are the single largest source of perinatal mortality and morbidity. Survival increases exponentially from approximately 5% at 23 weeks to 95% at 31 weeks (Rutter 1995), although the figures will vary from unit to unit depending on experience, size and a proactive approach to resuscititation at the extremes of prematurity. Of a large cohort of babies born before 26 weeks' gestation 39% survived, with 17% of survivors having brain lesions, 14% receiving treatment for retinopathy of prematurity and 51% needing supplementary oxygen at the expected date of delivery (Costeloe *et al.* 2000). At 30 months of age 23% of these children had a severe form of disability (Wood *et al.* 2000). The major causes of death were pulmonary insufficiency, respiratory distress syndrome, infection and intraventricular haemorrhage. Interestingly, the presence of chorioamnionitis *improved* survival to a similar degree to the antenatal administration of steroids. Two other complications related to pPROM can exacerbate the pulmonary consequences of prematurity – oligohydramnios and infection.

Consequences of oligohydramnios

Oligohydramnios occurring during the canalicular stage of lung development (between 17 and 26 weeks' gestation) can lead to pulmonary hypoplasia. In general the lung morphology at delivery is similar to that at which pPROM and severe oligohydramnios occurred, although reaccumulation of fluid or only mild to moderate degrees of oligohydramnios can be associated with normal lung growth (Kilbride and Thibeault 2001). Overall the incidence of pulmonary hypoplasia with pPROM is approximately 16% (Kilbride and Thibeault 2001), but is higher with membrane rupture at earlier gestation and longer latent periods with oligohydramnios. Rotschild *et al.* (1990) estimated the incidence of pulmonary hypoplasia to be 50% at 19 weeks and 10% at 25 weeks. A combination of clinical (gestation < 20 weeks, duration of oligohydramnios > 8 weeks), ultrasound (deepest pool of liquor of < 1 cm), biometric (thoracic/abdominal circumference ratio < 5th centile) and Doppler (peak systolic velocity in proximal pulmonary artery < 5th centile) parameters best predicts lethal hypoplasia with a positive predictive value of 100% and sensitivity of 71% (Laudy *et al.* 2002).

Chorioamnionitis

Perinatal brain injury

A growing body of epidemiological data suggest that intrauterine infection is an important cause of brain injury in infants born before 32 weeks' gestation. Characteristically, damage is localised to the white matter, involving both a diffuse astrogliosis with subsequent loss of myelin-producing oligodendrocytes, as well as multifocal necroses resulting in cystic change (periventricular leukomalacia, PVL) (Volpe 2001). Such lesions lead to cerebral palsy in 60 to 90% of affected infants. Studies in a variety of animals show that exposure to bacteria or endotoxin at a critical stage in fetal development results in white matter damage (Yoon *et al.* 1997b, Peebles *et al.* 2003) (see Figure 7.1). Clinical antecedents linked with this type of injury include maternal pyrexia, prolonged preterm rupture of membranes and maternal leukocytosis. In a recent meta-analysis clinical chorioamnionitis was significantly associated with both PVL (Relative risk (RR), 3.0; 95% confidence interval (CI), 2.2–4.0) and cerebral palsy (RR, 1.9; 95% CI, 1.4–2.5) (Wu and Colford 2000). Histological evidence of chorioamnionitis, present in up to 50% of

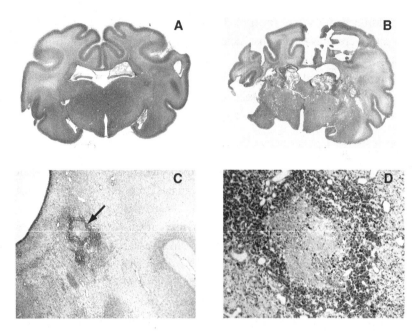

Figure 7.1   Sections from fetal ovine brains at circa 98–100 days' gestation, stained with haematoxylin and eosin, after iv saline (control, A) and 72 hours after 100 ng/kg lipopolysaccharide iv. (B). A focal area of necrosis in periventricular white matter (indicated by the arrow) is shown in C (x2 magnification). The same lesion is seen at higher magnification (x10) in D.

women who deliver preterm and often not associated with clinical signs, correlates significantly with PVL (RR, 2.1; 95% CI, 1.5–2.9) but has a weaker association with cerebral palsy (RR, 1.6; 95% CI, 0.9–2.7) (Wu and Colford 2000). It appears that the presence of a fetal inflammatory response, rather than maternal infection itself, is the most important aetiological factor. Fetal vasculitis, but not placental membrane inflammation, is associated with ultrasonographically detected echolucencies in white matter (Leviton *et al.* 1999), and the risk of neonatal complications is higher in infants with elevated pro-inflammatory cytokine levels (interleukin-6 (IL-6) > 11 pg/ml) in blood collected by cordocentesis (Gomez *et al.* 1998). The same authors have shown elevated levels of inflammatory cytokines in cord blood (IL-6) and amniotic fluid (IL-6, IL-1β and tumor necrosis factor-α) of infants with white matter damage and cerebral palsy (Yoon *et al.* 1996b, 1997a).

Lung injury

There is evidence that fetal exposure to inflammation may initiate events that lead to long-term lung injury (bronchopulmonary dysplasia, BPD) in the preterm infant (Matsuda *et al.* 1997, Yoon *et al.* 1997c). Preterm infants born within seven days of detection of elevated levels of the pro-inflammatory cytokines

IL-1β, -6 and -8 in amniotic fluid had a > tenfold increased risk of BPD, compared with those with normal cytokine levels (Yoon *et al.* 1997c). Watterberg *et al.* (1996) found a similar association between histologically detectable amnionitis and long-term lung injury, but also reported a *decreased* risk of acute respiratory distress syndrome. Similarly, Sims *et al.* (2002) found a correlation between pPROM and a *reduced* frequency of respiratory distress syndrome. This slightly paradoxical finding is in agreement with experimental data showing that exposure to a single bolus dose of endotoxin, injected intra-amniotically, improved postnatal lung compliance and surfactant production (Jobe *et al.* 2000). However, intra-amniotic endotoxin, whilst maturing the lungs, does not cause an intense inflammatory infiltrate; it is possible that a more chronic exposure to bacterial infection following pPROM leads to a greater fetal inflammatory response and worse lung injury. The worst outcome is associated with antenatal colonisation of the fetal lungs with bacteria, leading to congenital pneumonia and impaired postnatal lung function. Exposure to pro-inflammatory cytokines or stimulation of endogenous inflammatory processes by endotoxin may improve surfactant production in the short term but lead to tissue damage and BPD in the long term.

Placental abruption and fetal hypoxia

Preterm premature rupture of the fetal membranes is significantly related to the risk for placental abruption. Approximately 5% pregnancies with pPROM will end with an abruption and this is more likely if rupture of membranes is preceded by vaginal bleeding (Major *et al.* 1995). Oligohydramnios is also associated with an increased risk of umbilical cord compression, which may in turn lead to fetal hypoxia, particularly in the presence of uterine contractions.

Risk benefit analysis of immediate versus delayed delivery

The appropriate time to initate delivery after pPROM depends on the factor representing the greater risk to maternal and fetal health – prematurity or infection. As gestation advances, the relative risk of infectious morbidity becomes greater than that of prematurity and immediate delivery is favoured, whilst at earlier gestations conservative management to allow steroid administration and improved fetal maturity is associated with a better outcome. At any gestation, evidence of maternal or fetal sepsis would be an indication for delivery.

pPROM before fetal viability

Perinatal survival following pPROM before 25' weeks gestation is poor, with figures ranging from 22%–64% (Major and Kitzmiller 1990; Farooqi *et al.* 1998; Xiao *et al.* 2000; Winn *et al.* 2000). Factors associated with particularly high mortality and morbidity are the same as those for pulmonary hypoplasia i.e. severe oligohydramnios and early rupture of membranes. The live birth rate after PROM before 22 weeks is approximately 60% but the perinatal mortality rate is very high at 80–90% (Morales and Talley 1993, Dewan and Morris 2001). Hadi *et al.* (1994) related the neonatal outcome in pregnancies with PROM between 20 and 25 weeks' gestation to amniotic fluid volume; 40% of the group delivered before 25 weeks and only 5% of these survived. Pregnancies where the amniotic fluid volume was considered adequate were less likely to deliver before 25 weeks, less likely to have chorioamnionitis (24% vs. 69% with oligohydramnios) and had a better perinatal survival (2.1% vs. 69%). The major source of morbidity in survivors is pulmonary insufficiency and the risk is inversely related to gestation at membrane rupture. Survival without major impairment was observed in 75%, 80% and 100% of survivors when membranes ruptured at 14–19 weeks, 20–25 weeks and 26–28 weeks respectively (Farooqi *et al.* 1998). Others have reported a similar 20%–30% incidence of substantial impairment with ROM before 25 weeks (Kurkinen-Raty *et al.* 1998; Spitz *et al.* 1999).

These data suggest that if PROM occurs before 22 weeks' gestation, and there is persistent severe oligohydramnios the prognosis for neonatal survival without impairment is poor. In addition, there is a small, but important, risk of maternal sepsis (0.8%). The Confidential Enquiry into Maternal Death 1997–1999 includes a case of pPROM following insertion of cervical cerclage complicated by sepsis (Confidential Enquiries 1997–1999). Additionally, Moretti and Sibai (1988) reported one maternal death out of 731 cases of second trimester PROM. Counselling in this situation should therefore include the possibility of expediting delivery using either prostaglandins or oxytocin. The alternative is expectant management, hoping that delivery will not occur until at least 25 weeks' gestation.

pPROM between 25 and 31 weeks' gestation

Conservative management, aimed at prolonging pregnancy and reducing gestational-age dependent neonatal morbidity is widely considered to represent the best chance of good perinatal outcome in this group. Even with conservative management, many women will deliver within 7 days of membrane rupture; however, median latency periods of 10 days have been described with up to 30% women remaining undelivered at 20 days (Farooqi *et al.* 1998). Therapeutic interventions such as antenatal steroids and antibiotics (see below) can increase both the length of the latent period and neonatal outcome. The concern outlined previously was that increasing the latent period might decrease complications due to prematurity but increase infection related morbidity. This does not appear to be the case; Farooqi *et al.* (1998) had no fetal deaths and survival without impairment in 81% of infants born after ROM between 26 and 28 weeks. Others have found that increasing latency periods are associated with improved outcome (Winn *et al.* 2000). However, major advances in standards of neonatal care and improving survival rates at lower gestations mean that the threshold for expediting delivery because of concern either about fetal-wellbeing or infection, is gradually being lowered. This more proactive policy also includes the increasingly liberal use of caesarean section at the limits of viability (Bottoms *et al.* 1997).

pPROM at 32–36 weeks

At these gestations, latency periods are shorter and more similar to those at term (Savitz *et al.* 1997), which limits the potential benefit of expectant management. A gestation of 34 weeks could be considered as a break point after which fetal delivery will normally closely follow ROM (Neerhof *et al.* 1999). Neonatal morbidity after this gestation is low and steroids are not usually given; in addition, expectant management is associated with an increased risk of chorioamnionitis (Naef *et al.* 1998). Management of PROM at 32 weeks is slightly more controversial in that the risk of prematurity-related complications, such as respiratory distress syndrome, is still relatively high and delay of delivery for at least 48 hours to allow maximal benefit from steroids might have advantages. However, expectant management between 32 and 34 weeks is not associated with marked increases in latency period or improvements in neonatal outcome, whilst chorioamnionitis and evidence of fetal heart rate abnormalities are more common (Mercer *et al.* 1993; Cox and Leveno 1995).

Outpatient versus inpatient management

Although up to 50% of women presenting with pPROM will have delivered within one week, the latency period can be much longer. If management is expectant, women will be kept in hospital and monitored for evidence of infection; however, after initial treatment with steroids and antibiotics, they will receive no further therapeutic intervention. Is it safe for them to be discharged home and monitored as an outpatient? This question has not been adequately addressed in the literature. In one study only a small proportion of cases (18%) met the required criteria for outpatient management; these included a cephalic presentation, clear amniotic fluid, amniotic fluid index > 3 cm, normal maternal temperature, home not too distant from hospital and a suitable environment (Carlan *et al.* 1993). Two small studies concluded that, in appropriately selected women, outpatient management resulted in a decrease in the number of days spent in hospital with no worsening of neonatal outcome. Outpatient monitoring included six hourly measurement of pulse and temperature, fetal kick charts, twice weekly cardiotocographs and full blood counts and a weekly ultrasound scan (Carlan *et al.* 1993, Ayres 2002). A group of women who may be suitable for outpatient care are those where

ROM occurs before fetal viability; the emphasis here will be on early detection of infection. There are few absolute contraindications to outpatient care for women with pPROM; the main ones would be evidence of infection and inability to access hospital services easily.

Antimicrobials

Prophylactic antibiotic use and pPROM

Pre-existing infection leading to pPROM or ascending infection occurring after pPROM can lead to both premature labour and to activation of fetal inflammatory processes and long-term neurological and respiratory damage. Early treatment with antibiotics could therefore delay premature labour and reduce maternal and neonatal infectious morbidity. The most recent Cochrane review provides evidence that both assumptions may be true (Kenyon *et al.* 2002). There were 13 trials included in the review that randomised over 6000 women and their babies. The use of antibiotics following pPROM was associated with a statistically significant reduction in maternal infection after delivery prior to discharge from hospital (RR 0.85, 95% CI 0.76–0.96) and morbidity (RR 0.62, 95% CI 0.51, 0.75). The number of babies born within 48 hours (RR 0.77, 95% CI 0.72–0.83) and seven days (RR 0.88, 95% CI 0.84–0.92) was also significantly reduced. Neonatal infection (including pneumonia) (RR 0.67, 95% CI 0.52–0.85) and positive blood cultures (RR 0.75, 95% CI 0.60–0.93) were statistically significantly reduced in the babies whose mothers received antibiotics as was the numbers of babies requiring oxygen therapy overall (RR 0.88, 95% CI 0.81–0.96) and at 28 days of age or older (RR 0.81, 95% CI 0.68–0.97).

More precise information about the impact of broad-spectrum antibiotics on neonatal outcome is provided by the largest trial in the review – the ORACLE 1 study (Kenyon *et al.* 2001a). Four thousand, eight hundred and twenty six women with pPROM were randomised to receive either erythromycin, co-amoxiclav, both erythromycin and co-amoxiclav or placebo. The primary outcome measure was a composite of neonatal death, chronic lung disease, or major cerebral abnormality on ultrasonography before discharge from hospital. In singleton pregnancies there was a significant reduction in the number of neonates with the primary composite outcome with the use of erythromycin compared to placebo (125 of 1111 (11.2%) vs. 166 of 1149 (14.4%), $p = 0.02$). This effect was not seen with either co-amoxiclav alone or in combination with erythromycin. Erythromycin use was also associated with a prolongation of pregnancy, reductions in neonatal treatment with surfactant, decreases in oxygen dependence at 28 days and fewer major cerebral abnormalities on ultrasound. The findings are, in general, similar but less significant if multiple pregnancies are included in the analysis. The "dilution" of significance by inclusion of multiple pregnancies is biologically plausible as infection is less likely to be the cause of ROM in multiple pregnancies and so the rationale for antibiotic therapy is weakened. Importantly, these investigators have been funded to follow up the neonates from this study to see if the improvement in early neonatal outcome with antenatal erythromycin use is mirrored by a reduction in the risk of long-term handicap from bronchopulmonary dysplasia and cerebral palsy. Based on these results the use of erythromycin in women presenting with pPROM is justified. This is in contrast to the findings of ORACLE II, which followed a similar trial protocol as ORACLE 1, except that the study population was women in spontaneous preterm labour (Kenyon *et al.* 2001b); this failed to show any improvement in the primary outcome with any antibiotic, and concluded that antibiotics should not be prescribed for women in spontaneous preterm labour with no evidence of infection.

The ORACLE 1 study also demonstrates the possible dangers of antibiotic use. Co-amoxiclav, although associated with prolongation of pregnancy was also associated with a fourfold increase in proven necrotising enterocolitis, compared with placebo. This may be because co-amoxiclav changes the balance of microbial colonisation in the neonatal gut, leading to overgrowth of one or a few species. In the adult co-amoxiclav is known to select for *Clostridium difficile*, implicated in the development of pseudomembranous colitis. Another possible mechanism lies in the different modes of action of macrolide antibiotics such as erythromycin and clindamycin and the beta-lactams (penicillin and cephalosporin). It is known that the amount of endotoxin, a constituent of the outer membrane of the cell wall of gram-negative bacteria and a potent stimulant of pro-inflammatory cytokine release, found in blood varies depending on the type of antibiotic used (Prins *et al.* 1995). So, macrolide antibiotics, which reduce bacterial virulence, may have advantages over the beta-lactams that, by destroying bacteria, lead to higher endotoxin levels and a larger cytokine response. The significance of the association between co-amoxiclav and necrotising enterocolitis has been questioned by those who point out that no such effect was seen in ORACLE II, i.e. premature labour without ruptured membranes. This may be because of the higher burden of fetal/neonatal infection seen with pPROM, which, when combined with a bactericidal antibiotic, could lead to particularly high endotoxin/cytokine levels. The follow-up study will be important to show whether this differential antibiotic effect influences long-term outcome.

Treatment of chorioamnionitis

The antibiotic regime described above is appropriate for prophylaxis after pPROM. However, if there is strong evidence of chorioamnionitis treatment with intravenous broad-spectrum antibiotics is indicated; a combination of amoxicillin and gentamycin, co-amoxiclav, a cephalosporin, or clindamycin are all commonly used.

Tocolysis

It is clear that both antibiotics and steroids improve neonatal outcome if given prophylactically to mothers with pPROM; in particular, they can both prolong pregnancy. It remains unclear whether conventional tocolytics such as β–mimetics, oxytocin antagonists, indomethacin or magnesium sulphate, lead to further improvements in outcome. The well-reported ability of tocolytics to reduce the likelihood of delivery for a short period of time (up to seven days) in women with threatened preterm labour (Gyetvai et al. 1999), has also been described with pPROM (Fortunato et al. 1990; Matsuda et al. 1993). However, the use of antibiotics in these trials could be a confounding factor and the absence of any demonstrable improvement in neonatal outcome suggests that the additional benefit of a tocolytic may be small. In addition, the potential to do harm by delaying delivery of a fetus that may be exposed to damaging bacterial endotoxins and a cascade of inflammatory cytokines is greater at the early gestations at which delaying labour to maximise the therapeutic effects of steroids is also highest. Currently, in the face of pPROM and any evidence of materno-fetal infection tocolysis is probably not indicated. Interestingly, endotoxin exposure in sheep fetuses matured the lungs better than antenatal glucocorticoids (Jobe et al. 2000), another reason why tocolysis may be less necessary following ruptured membranes. Data from a large randomised trial are still needed to show whether tocolysis adds benefit to the use of antibiotics and steroids when infection has been excluded, possibly by the use of amniocentesis.

Other antenatal interventions to improve neonatal outcome

Steroids

The most recent Cochrane review (Crowley 2002) makes it clear that corticosteroids (2 doses of either 12 mg dexamethasone or betamethasone given 12 hours apart) given to the mother at risk of premature delivery substantially reduce the incidence of neonatal respiratory distress syndrome if delivery occurs within 7 days of steroid administration. Antenatal corticosteroid therapy also reduces neonatal mortality and the incidence of intraventricular haemorrhage. There do not appear to be any adverse effects of this treatment and in particular, fetal and neonatal infection was no more common, even after PROM. Maternal infection, however, although not increased overall, was more common following steroids if membranes had been ruptured for more than 24 hours. Significant improvements in outcome were only observed when 48 hours had elapsed between steroid treatment and delivery and if given after 24 weeks' gestation. However, there was a trend to better outcome with treatment at earlier gestations and shorter time intervals. The clinical implication is that all women with PROM, when delivery of a viable fetus is possible, should receive corticosteroids on admission.

The antenatal administration of glucocorticoids to the mother appears to reduce the risk of neonatal complications such as intraventricular haemorrhage. Because of their anti-inflammatory effects a similar protective role for steroids in prevention of white matter injury has been postulated. A large observational study suggests that this might be true for antenatal betamethasone, which was associated with a lower risk of cystic PVL than was either the absence of glucocorticoid therapy (odds ratio (OR), 0.5; 95% CI 0.2 to 0.9) or exposure to dexamethasone (OR, 0.3; 95% CI 0.1 to 0.7) (Baud *et al.* 1999). Betamethasone is therefore the steroid of choice to enhance lung maturation. However, currently there is no evidence to support the use of steroids or other anti-inflammatory therapies in the setting of maternal infection.

Amnioinfusion

The strong association between oligohydramnios and poor neonatal outcome has prompted some to try and restore liquor volume using amnioinfusion. Serial transabdominal amnioinfusions in women with pPROM and oligohydramnios before 26 weeks were considered successful if they resulted in an amniotic fluid pool of >2 cm for at least 48 hours; the outcome in this group was better than those where oligohydramnios persisted, but not so good as in pregnancies where liquor volume was maintained naturally (Locatelli *et al.* 2000). A similar amnioinfusion policy reduced the rate of pulmonary hypoplasia, compared with untreated controls, but did not affect age at delivery, latency or survival (Vergani *et al.* 1997). These studies are small and, although they suggest some benefit from a policy of amnioinfusion, need to be repeated in a randomised, controlled environment.

Endoscopic repair

The ability to visualise the membrane defect using an endoscope in women with spontaneous ROM has led to attempts to place an amniopatch consisting of a combination of cryoprecipitate and platelets, or a collagen graft, over the hole. In the one reported study to date, amniotic integrity was restored for a maximum of 72 hours in 4 women treated (Quintero *et al.* 1998). The author suggests that the technique may be suitable for women with no evidence of infection and where the defect is small and well-defined. However, the numbers of women treated are small and further research needs to be done.

Retention of cervical stitch

Cervical cerclage is a risk factor for PROM; rupture of membranes complicates 25% of pregnancies with a cervical stitch *in situ*. However, the management of women with pPROM and a cervical stitch *in situ* is controversial: should the stitch be removed as soon as possible because leaving it will increase the risk of materno-fetal infection, or will removing it precipitate delivery? There are no prospective data that address this question. Perinatal outcome was similar in pregnancies with pPROM when the suture was removed on admission and a control group that had pPROM and no cervical stitch (Yeast and Garite 1988). Another study found no evidence of difference in latency period, chorioamnionitis or neonatal outcome between pregnancies where the cervical suture was removed or retained (McElrath *et al.* 2000). However, a cautionary note is sounded by data showing that stitch retention prolonged pregnancy but at the cost of a higher perinatal mortality (70% vs. 10% in the immediate removal group) (Ludmir *et al.* 1994). Additionally, a maternal death has also been reported in this scenario (Confidential Enquiries into Maternal Deaths in the UK, 1997–1999). Until prospective data suggest otherwise, a reasonable approach might be to remove the stitch on admission, except in women where a short prolongation of pregnancy would be particularly advantageous, either to give steroids or to improve the risk of prematurity related neonatal complications.

Mode of delivery

In addition to triggering a sequence of inflammatory processes that can themselves damage developing white matter, there is some evidence that fetal infection might sensitise the brain to the effects of subsequent hypoxia-ischaemia. Administration of lipopolysaccharide (LPS) to the neonatal rat pup, four hours before unilateral hypoxia-ischaemia, leads to a much larger lesion than with either LPS or hypoxia alone (Eklind *et al.* 2001). In the adult, recent bacterial and viral infections are a risk factor for stroke (Grau *et al.* 1998), whilst in the term fetus, combined exposure to infection and intrapartum hypoxia-ischaemia dramatically increases the risk of spastic cerebral palsy (OR 78; 95%CI 4.8–406) compared with hypoxia alone (Nelson and Grether 1998). It seems plausible that pre-existing infection may lower the threshold at which hypoxia-ischaemia becomes neurotoxic, although whether this is by increasing fetal temperature or activating inflammatory pathways, or a combination of both, is not clear.

Currently, when faced with evidence of chorioamnionitis and pPROM most clinicians would try to avoid Caesarean section, and either wait for spontaneous onset of labour (itself often a manifestation of underlying infection), or would stimulate labour with syntocinon. Operative delivery may be associated with difficulty in delivering the very premature fetus and might carry an increased risk of maternal wound infection in the presence of chorioamnionitis. However, if fetal cerebral inflammation sensitises the brain to hypoxia-ischaemia a reasonable hypothesis would be that avoidance of labour, a period commonly associated with a degree of hypoxic fetal stress, would be neuroprotective. In the large Australian case-control study of newborn encephalopathy in term infants, *elective* Caesarean section was associated with a highly significant reduction in term neonatal encephalopathy (OR 0.17, 95% CI 0.05 to 0.56) whereas *emergency* Caesarean section was associated with an increased risk (Badawi *et al.* 1998). Baud *et al.* (1998) reported that in 110 preterm pregnancies complicated by chorioamnionitis, delivery by Caesarean section was associated with a dramatic decrease in the risk of periventricular leukomalacia (OR 0.15, 95% CI 0.04–0.57). However, this study has been criticised because of the high incidence of PVL (20%) and culture-proven neonatal sepsis (60%), which makes it unrepresentative of most preterm pregnancies with chorioamnionitis. Further large, well-conducted observational studies are required to address the relationship between fetal infection, its timing, mode of delivery and neurological outcome. At present there is insufficient data to support the choice of Caesarean section as the standard method of delivery in the presence of chorioamnionitis.

Conclusion

Because of its potentially serious consequences for mother and neonate, pPROM remains one of the most difficult obstetric conditions to manage. The problem is compounded by an incomplete understanding of the underlying mechanisms and the small number of randomised controlled trials available. Further developments in preventing pPROM and improving the management of pregnancies with pPROM will rely on an improved understanding of the relationship between inflammation, infection and neonatal outcome. Central to this research is better definition of maternal infection, particularly looking for evidence of an inflammatory response much earlier in the process, before there is obvious chorioamnionitis. Animal and clinical epidemiological studies will help determine the precise effects of inflammation on fetal/neonatal function. This information will guide development of interventions such as anti-inflammatory drugs or timing of delivery, which will then need to be tested in large randomised controlled trials.

REFERENCES

Ayres, Ar. W. (2002) Home management of preterm premature rupture of membranes. *Int. J. Obstet. Gynecol.* **78**, 153–5.

Badawi, N., Kurinczuk, J. J., Keogh, J. M. *et al.* (1998) Intrapartum risk factors for newborn encephalopathy: the Western Australian case-control study. *BMJ* **317**, 1554–8.

Baud, O., Ville, Y., Zupan, V. *et al.* (1998) Are neonatal brain lesions due to intrauterine infection related to mode of delivery? *BJOG* **105**, 121–4.

Baud, O., Foix-L'Helias, L., Kaminski, M. *et al.* (1999) Antenatal glucocorticoid treatment and cystic periventricular leukomalacia in very preterm infants. *N. Engl. J. Med.* **341**, 1190–6,

Bearfield, C., Davenport, E. S., Sivapathasundaram, V. and Allaker, R. P. (2002) Possible association between amniotic fluid micro-organism infection and microflora in the mouth *BJOG* **109**, 527–33.

Bottoms, S. F., Paul, R. H., Iams, J. D. *et al.* (1997) Obstetric determinants of neonatal survival: influence of willingness to perform Caesarean delivery on survival of extremely low-birth-weight infants. *Am. J. Obstet. Gynecol.* **176**, 960–6.

Carlan, S. J., O'Brien, W. F., Parsons, M. T. and Lense, J. J. (1993) Preterm premature rupture of membranes: a randomized study of home versus hospital management. *Obstet. Gynecol.* **81**, 61–4.

Carlan, S. J., Richmond, L. B and O'Brien, W. F. (1997) Randomized trial of endovaginal ultrasound in preterm premature rupture of membranes. *Obstet. Gynecol.* **89**, 458–61.

Carroll, S. G., Papaioannou, S., Davies, E. T. and Nicolaides, K. H. (1995a) Maternal assessment in the prediction of intrauterine infection in preterm prelabor amniorrhexis. *Fetal Diagn. Ther.* **10**, 290–6.

Carroll, S. G., Papaioannou, S. and Nicolaides, K. H. (1995b) Doppler studies of the placental and fetal circulation in pregnancies with preterm prelabor amniorrhexis. *Ultrasound Obstet. Gynecol.* **5**, 184–8.

Carroll, S. G., Papaioannou, S., Ntumazah, I. L., Philpott-Howard, J. and Nicolaides, K. H. (1996) Lower genital tract swabs in the prediction of intrauterine infection in preterm prelabour rupture of the membranes. *BJOG* **103**, 54–9.

Confidential Enquiries 1997–1999. *Why Mothers Die 1997–1999; Confidential Enquiries into maternal deaths in the United Kingdom.* RCOG Press 2001.

Costeloe, K., Hennessy, E., Gibson, A. T., Marlow, N. and Wilkinson, A. R. (2000) The EPICure study: outcomes to discharge from hospital for infants born at the threshold of viability. *Pediatrics* **106**, 659–71.

Cox, S. M. and Leveno, K. J. (1995) Intentional delivery versus expectant management with preterm premature ruptured membranes at 30–34 weeks' gestation. *Obstet. Gynecol.* **86**, 875–9.

Crowley, P. (2002) Prophylactic corticosteroids for preterm birth (Cochrane review). In *The Cochrane Library*, Issue 2, Oxford: Update Software.

Dalitz, P., Harding, R., Rees, S. M. and Cock, M. L. (2003) Prolonged reductions in placental blood flow and cerebral oxygen delivery in preterm fetal sheep exposed to endotoxin: possible factors in white matter injury after acute infection. *J. Soc. Gynecol. Investig.* **10**: 283–90.

Dewan, H. and Morris, J. M. (2001) A systematic review of pregnancy outcome following preterm premature rupture of membranes at a periviable gestation. *Aust. N. Z. J. Obstet. Gynaecol.* **41**, 389–94.

Eklind, S., Mallard, C., Leverin, A-L. *et al.* (2001) Bacterial endotoxin sensitizes the immature brain to hypoxic-ischemic injury. *Eur. J. Neurosci.* **13**, 1101–6.

Farooqi, A., Holmgren, P. A., Engberg, S. and Serenius, F. (1998) Survival and 2 year outcome with expectant mangement of second trimester rupture of membranes. *Obstet. Gynecol.* **92**, 895–901.

Fortunato, S. J., Welt, S. I., Eggleston, M. *et al.* (1990) Prolongation of the latency period in preterm premature rupture of membranes using prophylactic antibiotics and tocolysis. *J. Perinatol.* **10**, 252–6.

Friedman, M. L. and McElin, T. W. (1969) Diagnosis of ruptured fetal membranes: clinical study and review of the literature. *Am. J. Obstet. Gynecol.* **104**, 544–50.

Gomez, R., Romero, R., Ghezzi, F. *et al.* (1998) The fetal inflammatory response syndrome. *Am. J. Obstet. Gynecol.* **179**, 194–202.

Goncalves, L. F., Chaiworapongsa, T. and Romero, R. (2002) Intrauterine infection and prematurity. *Met. Retard. Dev. Disabil. Res. Rev.* **8**, 3–13.

Grau, A. J., Buggle, F., Becher, H. *et al.* (1998) Recent bacterial and viral infection is a risk factor for cerebrovascular ischaemia: clinical and biochemical studies. *Neurology* **50**, 196–203.

Gyetvai, K., Hannah, M. E., Hodnett, E. D. and Ohlsson, A. (1999) Tocolytics for preterm labor: a systematic review. *Obstet. Gynecol.* **94**, 869–77.

Hadi, H. A., Hodson, C. A. and Strickland, D. (1994) Premature rupture of the membranes between 20 and 25 weeks gestation: role of amniotic fluid volume in perinatal outcome. *Am. J. Obstet. Gynecol.* **170**, 1139–44.

Hillier, S. L., Witkin, S. S., Krohn, M. A. *et al.* (1993) The relationship of amniotic fluid cytokines and preterm delivery, amniotic fluid infection, histological chorioamnionitis and chorioamnion infection. *Obstet. Gynecol.* **81**, 941–8.

Hitti, J., Riley, D. E., Krohn, M. A. *et al.* (1997) Broad-spectrum bacterial rDNA polymerase chain reaction assay for detecting amniotic fluid infection among women in premature labor. *Clin. Infect. Dis.* **24**, 1228–32.

Jobe, A. H., Newham, J. P., Willett, K. E. *et al.* (2000) Effects of antenatal endotoxin and glucocorticoids on the lungs of preterm lambs. *Am. J. Obstet. Gynecol.* **182**, 401–8.

Kenyon, S. L., Taylor, D. J. and Tarnow-Mordi, W; ORACLE Collaborative Group. (2001a) Broad-spectrum antibiotics for preterm, prelabour rupture of fetal membranes: the ORACLE I randomised trial. *Lancet* **357**, 979–88.

Kenyon, S. L., Taylor, D. J. and Tarnow-Mordi, W.; ORACLE Collaborative Group. (2001b) Broad-spectrum antibiotics for spontaneous preterm labour: the ORACLE II randomised trial. *Lancet* **357**, 989–94.

Kenyon, S. L., Boulvain, M. and Neilson, J. (2002) Antibiotics for preterm premature rupture of membranes (Cochrane review). In *The Cochrane Library,* Issue 2, Oxford: Update software

Kilbride, H. W. and Thibeault, D. W. (2001) Neonatal complications of preterm premature rupture of membranes. Pathophysiology and management. *Clin. Perinatol.* **28**, 761–5.

Kishida, T., Yamada, H., Negishi, H. *et al.* (1996) Diagnosis of premature rupture of the membranes in preterm patients, using an improved AFP kit: comparison with ROM-check and/or nitrazine test. *Eur. J. Obstet. Gynecol. Reprod. Biol.* **69**, 77–82.

Kurkinen-Raty, M., Koivisto, M. and Jouppila, P. (1998) Perinatal and neonatal outcome and late pulmonary sequelae in infants born after preterm premature rupture of membranes. *Obstet. Gynecol.* **92**, 408–15.

Laudy, J. A., Tibboel, D., Robben, S. G. *et al.* (2002) Prenatal prediction of pulmonary hypoplasia: clinical, biometric, and Doppler velocity correlates. *Pediatrics* **109**, 250–8.

Leviton, A., Paneth, N., Reuss, M. L. *et al.* (1999) Maternal infection, fetal inflammatory response, and brain damage in very low birth weight infants. Developmental Epidemiology Network Investigators. *Pediatr. Res.* **46**, 566–75.

Lewis, D. F., Major, C. A., Towers, C. V. *et al.* (1992) Effects of digital examinations on latency period in preterm premature rupture of membranes. *Obstet. Gynecol.* **80**, 630–4.

Locatelli, A., Vergani, P., Di Pirro, G. *et al.* (2000) Role of amnioinfusion in the mangement of premature rupture of the membranes at < 26 weeks' gestation. *Am. J. Obstet. Gynecol.* **183**, 878–82.

Ludmir, J., Bader, T., Chen, L., Lindenbaum, E. S. and Wong, G. (1994) Poor perinatal outcome associated with retained cerclage in patients with premature rupture of membranes. *Obstet. Gynecol.* **84**, 823–6.

Major, C. A. and Kitzmiller, J. L. (1990) Perinatal survival with expectant management of midtrimester rupture of membranes. *Am. J. Obstet. Gynecol.* **163**, 838–44.

Major, C. A., de Veciana, M., Lewis, D. F. and Morgan, M. A. (1995) Preterm premature rupture of membranes and abruptio placentae: is there an association between these pregnancy complications? *Am. J. Obstet. Gynecol.* **172**, 672–6.

Matsuda, T., Nakajima, T., Hattori, S. *et al.* (1997) Necrotising funisitis: clinical significance and association with chronic lung disease in premature infants. *Am. J. Obstet. Gynecol.* **177**, 1402–7.

Matsuda, Y., Ikenoue, T. and Hokanishi, H. (1993) Premature rupture of the membranesaggressive versus conservative approach: effect of tocolytic and antibiotic therapy. *Gynecol. Obstet. Invest.* **36**, 102–7.

McElrath, T. F., Norwitz, E. R., Lieberman, E. S. and Heffner, L. J. (2000) Management of cervical cerclage and preterm premature rupture of the membranes: should the stitch be removed? *Am. J. Obstet. Gynecol.* **183**, 840–6.

Mercer, B. M. (2003) Preterm premature rupture of the membranes. *Obstet. Gynecol.* **101**, 178–93.

Mercer, B. M., Crocker, L. G., Boe, N. M. and Sibai, B. M. (1993) Induction versus expectant management in premature rupture of the membranes with mature amniotic fluid at 32 to 36 weeks: a randomized trial. *Am. J. Obstet. Gynecol.* **169**, 775–82.

Morales, W. J. and Talley, T. (1993) Premature rupture of membranes at <25 weeks: a management dilemma. *Am. J. Obstet. Gynecol.* **168**, 503–7.

Moretti, M. and Sibai, B. (1988) Maternal and perinatal outcome of expectant management of premature rupture of the membranes in the midtrimester. *Am. J. Obstet. Gynecol.* **159**, 390–6.

Naef, R. W., Allbert, J. R., Ross, E. L. *et al.* (1998) Premature rupture of membranes at 34 weeks to 37 weeks' gestation: aggressive versus conservative management. *Am. J. Obstet. Gynecol.* **178**, 126–30.

Neerhof, M. G., Cravello, C., Haney, E. I. and Silver, R. K. (1999) Timing of labor induction between 32 and 36 weeks' gestation. *Am. J. Obstet. Gynecol.* **180**, 349–52.

Nelson, K. B. and Grether, J. K. (1998) Potentially asphyxiating conditions and spastic cerebral palsy in infants of normal birth weight. *Am. J. Obstet. Gynecol.* **179**, 507–13.

Pankuch, G. A., Appelbaum, P. C., Lorenz, R. P. (1984) Placental microbiology and histology and the pathogenesis of chorioamnionitis. *Obstet. Gynecol.* **64**, 802–6.

Peebles, D. M., Miller, S. L., Newman, J. P., Scott, R. and Hanson, M. A. (2003)The effect of systemic administration of lipopolysaccharide on cerebral haemodynamics and oxygenation in the 0.65 gestation ovine fetus in utero. *BJOG* **110**, 735–43

Prins, J. M., Kuiper, E. J., Mevissen, M. L. C. M., Speelman, P. and van Deventer, S. J. H. (1995) Release of tumor necrosis factor alpha and interleukin 6 during antibiotic killing of Escherichia coli in whole blood: influence of antibiotic class, antibiotic concentration, and presence of septic serum. *Infect. Immun.* **63**, 2236–42.

Quintero, R. A., Morales, W. J., Kalter, C. S. *et al.* (1998) Transabdominal intra-amniotic endoscopic assessment of previable premature rupture of membranes. *Am. J. Obstet. Gynecol.* **179**, 71–6.

Rotschild, A., Ling, E. W., Puterman, M. L. and Farquharson. D. (1990) Neonatal outcome after prolonged rupture of the membranes. *Am. J. Obstet. Gynecol.* **162**, 46–52.

Rutter, N. (1995) The extremely preterm infant. *BJOG* **102**, 682–7.

Savitz, D. A., Ananth, C. V., Luther, E. R. and Thorp, J. M. Jr. (1997) Influence of gestational age on the time from spontaneous rupture of the chorioamniotic membranes to the onset of labor. *Am. J. Perinatol.* **14**, 129–33.

Seaward, P. G., Hannah, M. E., Myhr, T. L. *et al.* (1998) International multicenter PROM study: evaluation of predictors of neonatal infection in infants born to patients with premature rupture of membranes at term. *Am. J. Obstet. Gynecol.* **179**, 635–9

Sims, E. J., Vermilion, S. T. and Soper, D. E. (2002) Preterm premature rupture of the membranes is associated with a reduction in neonatal respiratory distress syndrome. *Am. J. Obstet. Gynecol.* **187**, 268–72.

Spitz, B., Vossen, C., Devlieger, R. and Van Assche, F. A. (1999) Rupture of membranes before 26 weeks of gestation: outcome of 148 consecutive cases. *J. Perinat. Med.* **27**, 451–7.

Vergani, P., Locatelli, A., Strobelt, N. *et al.* (1997) Amnioinfusion for prevention of pulmonary hypoplasia in second trimester rupture of membranes. *Am. J. Perinatol.* **14**, 325–9.

Vintizileos, A. M., Campbell, W. A., Nochimson, D. J. *et al.* (1985) The fetal biophysical profile in patients with premature rupture of the membranes – an early predictor of fetal infection. *Am. J. Obstet. Gynecol.* **152**, 510–6.

Volpe, J. J. (2001) Neurobiology of periventricular leukomalacia in the premature infant. *Pediatr. Res.* **50**, 553–62.

Watterberg, K. L., Demers, L. M., Scott, S. M. and Murphy, S. (1996) Chorioamnionitis and early lung inflammation in infants in whom bronchopulmonary dysplasia develops. *Pediatrics* **97**, 210–5.

Winn, H. N., Chen, M., Amon, E. *et al.* (2000) Neonatal pulmonary hypoplasia and perinatal mortality in patients with mid trimester rupture of amniotic membranes: a critical analysis. *Am. J. Obstet. Gynecol.* **182**, 1638–44.

Wood, N. S., Marlow, N., Costeloe, K., Gibson, A. T. and Wilkinson, A. R. (2000) Neurologic and developmental disability after extremely preterm birth. EPICure study group. *N. Engl. J. Med.* **343**, 378–84.

Wu, Y. W. and Colford, J. M. Jr. (2000) Chorioamnionitis as a risk factor for cerebral palsy: A meta-analysis. *JAMA* **284**, 1417–24.

Xiao, Z. H., Andre, P., Lacaze-Masmonteil, T. *et al.* (2000) Outcome of premature infants delivered after prolonged premature rupture of membranes before 25 weeks of gestation. *Eur. J. Obstet. Gynecol. Reprod. Biol.* **90**, 67–71.

Yanowitz, T. D., Jordan, J. A., Gilmour, C. H. *et al.* (2002) Hemodynamic disturbances in premature infants born after chorioamnionitis: association with cord blood cytokine concentrations. *Pediatr. Res.* **51**, 310–16.

Yeast, J. D. and Garite, T. R. (1988) The role of cerclage in the management of preterm premature rupture of membranes. *Am. J. Obstet. Gynecol.* **158**, 106–10.

Yoon, B. H., Jun, J. K., Park, K. H. *et al.* (1996a) Serum C-reactive protein, white blood cell count, and amniotic fluid white blood cell count in women with premature rupture of membranes. *Obstet. Gynecol.* **88**, 1034–40.

Yoon, B. H., Romero, R., Yang, S. H. *et al.* (1996b) Interleukin-6 concentrations in umbilical cord plasma are elevated in neonates with white matter lesions associated with periventricular leukomalacia. *Am. J. Obstet. Gynecol.* **174**, 1433–40.

Yoon, B. H., Jun, J. K., Romero, R. *et al.* (1997a) Amniotic fluid inflammatory cytokines (interleukin-6, interleukin -1β and tumor necrosis factor-alpha). Neonatal brain white matter lesions, and cerebral palsy. *Am. J. Obstet. Gynecol.* **177**, 19–26.

Yoon, B. H., Kim, C. J., Romero, R. *et al.* (1997b) Experimentally induced intrauterine infection causes fetal brain white matter lesions in rabbits. *Am. J. Obstet. Gynecol.* **177**, 797–802

Yoon, B. H., Romero, R., Jun, J. K. *et al.* (1997c) Amniotic fluid cytokines (interleukin-6, tumor necrosis factor-alpha, interleukin-1beta and interleukin-8) and the risk for the development of bronchopulmonary dysplasia. *Am. J. Obstet. Gynecol.* **177**, 825–30.

8

Management of threatened preterm labour

Manu Vatish[1], Katie Groom[2], Phillip Bennett[2] and Steven Thornton[1]

[1]Warwick Medical School
[2]Imperial College School of Medicine

Diagnosis

Preterm labour (PTL) is the onset of labour (regular uterine contractions and cervical effacement and dilatation) between the limit of viability and term. In practice, it is defined as labour between 20 and 37 completed weeks of gestation.

Clinical assessment

The history is notoriously unreliable in the diagnosis of PTL, as the only symptom (maternal perception of contraction frequency or strength) is a poor guide to the outcome. Approximately 50% of patients presenting with threatened PTL will deliver at term even without treatment (Lockwood et al. 1991). However, in a proportion of patients, temporal changes in symptoms within an individual are helpful in guiding management. Clinical examination, particularly palpation of the uterus is often unreliable in assessing contraction strength. Vaginal speculum examination is useful however, to determine cervical effacement, dilation and the presence of amniotic fluid. Digital vaginal examination should be avoided if the membranes are ruptured to reduce the risk of introducing infection.

Further history and examination should include determination of the gestational age and presenting part, and elicit symptoms or signs of chorioamnionitis, maternal medical conditions (diabetes, thyrotoxicosis, cardiac disease, hypertension), pregnancy specific disorders (pre-eclampsia) and possible precipitating conditions in the current pregnancy (abruption, placenta praevia, multiple pregnancy, ruptured membranes). Fetal condition and presentation should also be assessed (Table 8.1).

Investigations
General investigations

Specific investigations will be directed by clinical symptoms and signs although urinalysis (to exclude infection) and a full blood count are indicated in the majority of women. A Kleihauer test may provide evidence of feto-maternal

Preterm Labour Managing Risk in Clinical Practice, eds. Jane Norman and Ian Greer. Published by Cambridge University Press. © Cambridge University Press 2005.

Table 8.1. Clinical Assessment of PTL

Fetal and placental conditions
Oligo or polyhydramnios
Abruption, placenta praevia
Intrauterine growth restriction
Intrauterine death
Fetal distress
Multiple pregnancy
Fetal anomaly
Infection
Rupture of the membranes

Maternal conditions
Pre-eclampsia or hypertension
Thyrotoxicosis
Cardiac disease
Diabetes
Systemic illness
Cervical or uterine anomaly

haemorrhage, and serum urea, electrolytes and liver function tests are required if tocolysis is contemplated. Although cardiotocography is poor at assessing contraction strength, it may be helpful for determination of contraction frequency and will provide additional information on the condition of the fetus. If delivery is imminent, the presentation of the fetus should be determined by palpation or ultrasound. In women, in whom delivery is not considered to be imminent, an ultrasound scan may be useful to determine indices of fetal wellbeing, such as fetal size, liquor volume, uterine arterial blood flow and cervical length.

Investigations to confirm or refute the diagnosis of labour

Owing to the difficulties in making the diagnosis of PTL, several diagnostic tools have been developed to confirm the diagnosis. Currently fetal fibronectin and estimation of cervical length are the most promising.

Fetal Fibronectin

Fetal fibronectin (fFn) is a basement membrane protein produced by fetal membranes. Its presence within the vagina beyond 20 weeks' gestation is abnormal and suggests disruption of the extracellular matrix adhering the fetal membranes to the decidua. The presence of fFn in cervico-vaginal secretions has been successfully used as a predictive test for preterm delivery. Recent meta-analysis of over 26 000 women has shown that amongst asymptomatic women the likelihood ratio for a positive result predicting birth before 34 weeks was 4.01 (95% confidence interval (CI) 2.93 to 5.49). The likelihood ratio is defined as the likelihood that a given test result would be expected in a patient with the target disorder (e.g. preterm delivery) compared to the likelihood that the same result would be expected in a patient without the target disorder. The likelihood ratio for a negative result was 0.78 (95% CI 0.72 to 0.84). Amongst symptomatic women (i.e. those presenting with uterine contractions), the likelihood ratio for a positive result predicting birth within 7–10 days of testing was 5.42 (95% CI 4.36 to 6.74), with corresponding ratio for negative results of 0.25 (95% CI 0.20 to 0.31). This suggests that fFn is most accurate in identifying preterm birth in symptomatic women within 7–10 days of testing. (Honest *et al.* 2002). Despite these data, there have been no prospective interventional studies demonstrating a decrease in preterm delivery or improved perinatal outcome using fFn testing. However, there may be selected women in whom fFn may be useful in directing clinical management. Indeed, the American College of Obstetricians and Gynecologists (ACOG) has suggested that a negative fFn may be useful in identifying those with a reduced risk of preterm birth reducing unnecessary interventions (ACOG 2003).

Ultrasound measurements of cervical length

Transvaginal assessment of cervical length is used in some centres as a screening test for prediction of premature labour and is discussed in chapter 5 of this book. Ultrasound measurement of cervical length has also been suggested to be useful as a diagnostic test in threatened PTL. The Society of Obstetricians and Gynaecologists of Canada has suggested that one transvaginal ultrasound assessment of cervical length in this situation improves the identification of those women who subsequently deliver preterm (Van den Hof and Crane 2001). The predictive ability of cervical ultrasound in women presenting with symptoms of preterm labour is also supported by a recent systematic review (Leitich *et al.* 1999). The high negative predictive value could be used to avoid unnecessary interventions in low-risk women. It is difficult based on limited data to make absolute recommendations about the predictive cut-off value for cervical length. Current evidence suggests that in women clinically in PTL, ultrasound measurements of cervical length of $\leq$30 mm will identify 80%–100% of women destined to deliver preterm, and ultrasound identified dilatation of the internal os will identify 70%–90% of women destined to deliver preterm ((Leitich *et al.* 1999). Canadian guidance suggests a cervical length of 30 mm for women with intact membranes prior to 34 weeks' gestation is an appropriate cut off for prediction of those at high risk of preterm delivery.

Differential diagnosis

The differential diagnosis of PTL includes other disorders that result in intermittent abdominal pain. Urinary colic due to infection or stones can present in a similar fashion to PTL, in which case urinalysis may be helpful. These conditions may coexist since infection may precipitate PTL. Gastrointestinal colic may be difficult to differentiate from PTL. Symphysis pubis pain is not usually intermittent but may be difficult to differentiate from preterm contractions associated with abruption (which may be concealed). An adequate history, examination and investigation usually provide the clues to the correct diagnosis.

Outpatient versus inpatient management

There is no definitive evidence on which to recommend one approach in preference to the other. It is suggested that initial management is based on inpatient monitoring but that after 72 hours, selected patients may be suitable for outpatient assessment. Anhydramnios, raised C-reactive protein and positive bacteriology increase the overall risks to the pregnancy and constitute relative contraindications to outpatient management.

Risk benefit analysis of immediate versus delayed delivery

The rationale for the treatment of PTL is based on the premise that an increase in gestational age will confer a benefit to the fetus. Whilst this is true at a population level, it is not possible to be certain for an individual fetus whether prolonging pregnancy and preventing delivery will be of benefit. Preterm labour is sometimes associated with pregnancy complications (such as intrauterine infection or abruption) that are sufficiently severe to compromise fetal wellbeing if delivery does not occur. Clearly in these women delivery should not be delayed.

In the absence of these complicating factors, and where gestational age is very low, the adverse consequences of prematurity far outweigh those associated with the pregnancy continuing and a conservative approach will be most appropriate.

Once the presence or absence of potential complications have been established, the next step is to determine whether tocolysis is indicated. It has been shown that the use of tocolytics to delay delivery does not in itself result in improved neonatal outcome. However, administration of antenatal steroids in order to promote fetal lung maturation or transfer to a unit with specialist neonatal intensive care facilities does have a beneficial effect (Crowley 2002). The current rationale for the use of tocolytics is therefore to delay delivery for 48 hours during which these measures can be implemented.

Tocolysis

The number of drugs available for the acute treatment of PTL is testament to the fact that no tocolytic is completely effective and safe. The major decision, however, is not which drug to administer, but whether or not to instigate tocolysis. This requires a detailed clinical assessment and consideration of the patient specific benefits and risks.

The beneficial effects of tocolysis have been investigated in many randomised controlled trials. However, interpretation of these is confounded by a number of factors.

Firstly, trial methodology should be carefully scrutinised and the inclusion criteria clearly stated. For example, trials that recruit mostly patients at a later gestational age are less likely to show a beneficial effect than those with patients at an earlier stage of pregnancy. For this reason, it may also be inappropriate to group together patients in PTL at different gestational ages. The beneficial or adverse effects of treatment may be gestational age dependent and interpretation of results from a heterogeneous population potentially confounding.

Secondly, 50% of patients with threatened PTL will not deliver preterm, even without treatment. Selection of patients who are more likely to go on to preterm delivery could be improved using measures such as documented cervical change (effacement or dilatation) in association with uterine activity, positive fFn or cervical ultrasound. The use of such investigations makes the study more complex.

Thirdly, the causes of PTL are many and varied, which makes careful patient assessment important prior to recruitment. The management of PTL is dependent upon the cause. As detailed above, tocolysis is inappropriate if prolongation of the pregnancy would have an adverse fetal effect. Inappropriate patient inclusion may be partly responsible for a failure to demonstrate improved fetal outcome using drugs that delay delivery.

Lastly, trial outcome measures are particularly important. Clearly the ultimate aim of treatment is to improve neonatal morbidity and mortality. Unfortunately, since most trials are underpowered to show a change in neonatal outcome data, other surrogate variables may be used, such as delay in delivery, incidence of preterm delivery or increase in fetal weight. These may not accurately reflect mortality or morbidity.

It is on this somewhat tenuous background of evidence that our current assessment of tocolysis is based. With these caveats in mind, the data on the currently available tocolytics are summarised below.

β sympathomimetics

There is little evidence to specifically promote the administration of any particular β_2 sympathomimetic although ritodrine has been extensively studied. All β_2

sympathomimetics are relatively (but not completely) specific for the β_2 rather than the β_1-receptor. There is little doubt that β sympathomimetics, when compared to placebo, reduce the number of deliveries within 48 hours of commencing treatment. However, the aim of treatment is to improve fetal outcome and although more than 1600 women have been studied, there is no documented improvement in neonatal morbidity or mortality (RCOG 2002). The reasons for this could be that: (i) the gestational age at which the majority of women were studied was relatively late and, consequently, adverse fetal outcome comparatively rare. This makes it difficult to demonstrate a beneficial effect of a modest increase in gestational age in the treatment group, (ii) the delay in delivery may not have been used to implement beneficial measures such as transfer to the Neonatal Intensive Care Unit (NICU) or administration of steroids, or (iii) the delay in delivery may have been offset by adverse fetal drug effects or other adverse events. Since there is strong evidence that steroid administration improves preterm fetal outcome and steroids were not given in the majority of the trials, if a β sympathomimetic were to be used it would seem reasonable to delay delivery in the short term, in order to instigate procedures to improve fetal outcome (e.g. administration of steroids or transfer to a unit with NICU facilities). It should be noted that concurrent administration of ritodrine with steroids has not been evaluated in a controlled trial. The long-term administration of ritodrine is not associated with an improved fetal outcome and is therefore not indicated. In conclusion, if ritodrine were to be used, it should only be administered intravenously for the short-term management of uncomplicated PTL in women between 20 and 35 weeks' gestation.

Side effects of ritodrine are common and nausea, vomiting, tremor, palpitations, nervousness and restlessness are frequently reported (Kierse et al. 1989). Such side effects have led to the recent suggestion by the Royal College of Obstetricians and Gynaecologists (RCOG 2002) that β sympathomimetics should no longer be used as the first-line treatment of PTL. A particularly worrying side effect, albeit uncommon, is the development of pulmonary oedema, a complication that has led to a number of maternal deaths (MacLennan et al. 1985, van Iddekinge et al. 1991). The cause is usually fluid overload, which may be precipitated by injudicious hydration prior to, or during tocolytic therapy. A second mechanism is a reduction in renal excretion of sodium, potassium and water due to an antidiuretic effect of ritodrine. The development of pulmonary oedema is more common if there is underlying maternal cardiac disease, multiple pregnancy or multiple drug administration. The problem can be reduced by the administration of ritodrine in 5% dextrose (rather than 0.9% saline which increases fluid retention), the use of low volume infusion pumps and accurate monitoring of fluid input and output.

An increase in maternal heart rate is invariably noted at effective doses of ritodrine and frequently limits the infusion rate. Ritodrine is associated with a fall in diastolic and increase in systolic blood pressure. There is also a fall in peripheral vascular resistance and increase in cardiac output. Myocardial ischaemia and development of (usually benign) arrhythmias has been reported. These may not be important in the majority of young fit women but pre-existing cardiac disease contraindicates the use of β sympathomimetics and it is wise to obtain an ECG prior to instigating therapy in any patient. The β sympathomimetics are associated with marked disturbances in carbohydrate metabolism, increasing blood glucose levels and causing a corresponding rise in insulin levels. Insulin release is also stimulated by a direct $β_2$ effect on the pancreas. Further metabolic effects (acidosis and hypokalaemia) make the administration of β sympathomimetics in diabetic pregnancy hazardous and although administration is not contraindicated, extreme vigilance and close monitoring of blood glucose are required.

Ritodrine crosses the placenta and has similar fetal side effects to those observed in the mother. An increase in fetal heart rate is common although often less pronounced than in the mother. Neonatal blood glucose and insulin may be increased and glucose should be measured following delivery. Follow-up studies have failed to document adverse long-term effects of ritodrine but the data is not particularly robust.

The ritodrine infusion is normally maintained for 24 hours although it can be reduced gradually if uterine activity does not recommence. During infusion, maternal pulse and blood pressure should be recorded every 15 minutes, blood glucose every 4 hours and urea and electrolytes every day. Fluid balance should be noted and the maternal chest auscultated every 4 hours.

Oxytocin receptor antagonists

There is a great deal of evidence to suggest that the oxytocin receptor is involved in the process of labour. In humans the myometrium becomes increasingly sensitive to oxytocin in late pregnancy (Takahashi et al. 1980). The increase in sensitivity is directly related to increased oxytocin receptor density (Fuchs et al. 1984). Similar increases in oxytocin sensitivity have been shown following the onset of preterm labour.

Oxytocin receptor blockade prevents oxytocin-induced activity. Since the latter is likely to mediate labour, administration of an oxytocin antagonist should inhibit myometrial contractility. Atosiban is an oxytocin analogue, marketed and licensed as a tocolytic, that inhibits the effects of oxytocin and vasopressin.

Oxytocin antagonists have been extensively investigated in randomised double blind clinical trials. These have compared atosiban with placebo or comparator (usually β sympathomimetics). Unfortunately it was considered mandatory to include rescue tocolysis in the trial designs, which means that a patient allocated to either group could be given an alternate tocolytic. This makes it difficult to interpret any neonatal benefit and not surprisingly, improved outcomes were not demonstrated. It should be stressed that although the trials cannot provide robust information on this outcome, it does not exclude a neonatal benefit of drug administration. Although comparison atosiban with placebo did not demonstrate an increase in the primary outcome of time from treatment to delivery or therapeutic failure, there was an increase in the number of women remaining undelivered and not requiring an alternative tocolytic at 24 hours, 48 hours and seven days (p < 0.01 for each). This data implies that atosiban can delay delivery compared with placebo although an effect on outcome remains to be demonstrated (Romero *et al.* 2000).

Trials comparing atosiban and ritodrine (Mountquin *et al.* 2000) suggest that the efficacy of the drugs are not dissimilar. There was no difference in numbers of deliveries at 48 hours and seven days. The oxytocin antagonist was however, tolerated much better and the side effects were more common with ritodrine. These results are consistent with trials using β sympathomimetics other than ritodrine. Such evidence has led to the recommendation by the Royal College of Obstetricians and Gynaecologists that if tocolysis is required in uncomplicated threatened preterm labour, atosiban is one of the preferable treatments.

Calcium channel blockers

There are no data from double-blind randomised controlled trials relating to the administration of calcium channel blockers (usually nifedipine) in the acute treatment of PTL. A number of small trials have demonstrated a similar delay in delivery with nifedipine and ritodrine but the trial sizes and/or methodology make definitive statements impossible (Papatsonis *et al.* 1997). Recently, a meta-analysis of the available randomised controlled trials comparing nifedipine with ritodrine for the treatment of PTL was reported (King *et al.* 2002). These data suggest that nifedipine is more effective than ritodrine in delaying delivery and is associated with reduced NICU admission. Unfortunately all of the studies have used surrogate markers for drug effectiveness (e.g. delay in delivery) rather than demonstrating a reduction in neonatal mortality or morbidity. Additionally, the effect of nifedipine has not been compared to placebo. Taken together, the results are promising and suggest that nifedipine may be a reasonable alternative to ritodrine (Lockwood 1997) but until larger robust trials have been performed, and improved fetal outcome has been demonstrated, the drug should be used with caution.

Studies suggest that there are fewer maternal side effects with nifedipine than ritodrine. Maternal effects are mainly dizziness, flushing, headache and oedema due to maternal vasodilatation. Fetal side effects (i.e. acidosis) have been demonstrated in animal studies and may reflect maternal hypotension or a reduction in uterine blood flow. The concerns about fetal safety have, however, not been substantiated in clinical trials.

The RCOG supports the use of nifedipine (RCOG 2002), but it is not licensed as a tocolytic agent and so the responsibility for its use lies with the prescribing doctor.

The dose of nifedipine used in clinical trials has not been standardised. A high-dose regimen of 10 mg nifedipine (repeated to a maximum of 40 mg in the first hour), followed by maintenance of 60–160 mg/day of slow release was used in the largest trial (Papatsonis *et al.* 1997). Most studies have used lower doses and a starting dose of 20 mg followed by 10–20 mg every 4–6 hours may be associated with a reduction in maternal and fetal side effects.

Inhibitors of prostaglandin synthesis

Numerous drugs inhibit prostaglandin formation although data from one drug cannot be extrapolated to another. The most widely investigated drug in this class is the reversible and competitive inhibitor, indomethacin. The quality of data on the effectiveness and side effects of indomethacin is not high but, compared with placebo, indomethacin reduces the incidence of delivery within each of 48 hours and 7–10 days and also before 37 weeks' gestation (Gyetvai *et al.* 1999). The evidence suggests that indomethacin is a more effective tocolytic than the β sympathomimetics. Although a beneficial effect on neonatal outcome has not been demonstrated, meta-analysis of trials comparing indomethacin with placebo or active treatment (Kierse *et al.* 1989) show a trend to a reduction in fetal and neonatal death (relative risk (RR) 0.61; 95% CI 0.33–1.11), which failed to reach statistical significance. Indomethacin is well tolerated by the mother although the side effects of non-steroidal anti-inflammatory agents (peptic ulceration, thrombocytopaenia, nausea, vomiting, diarrhoea, dizziness and allergy) may occur. The major concerns about indomethacin are the fetal effects. The drug crosses the placenta and influences the fetal cardiovascular, renal, haemostatic and gastrointestinal systems. Prostaglandin synthesis is responsible for the maintenance of ductus arteriosus patency and inhibition leads to premature closure, an effect that may be more pronounced at higher gestations (Vermillon *et al.* 1997). Premature ductal closure causes increased fetal pulmonary vascular pressure and smooth muscle hypertrophy, leading to persistent pulmonary hypertension (fetal circulation) in the neonate. The increase in right ventricular and diastolic pressures may also lead to subendocardial ischaemia, particularly in the papillary muscles of the tricuspid valve which is associated with tricuspid regurgitation in the neonate. The effect of indomethacin on fetal renal function is to cause a reversible reduction in urine output (Kirshon *et al.* 1991). This may lead to oligohydramnios although there is no evidence that this, in itself, leads to long-term problems at these gestational ages. The effect of prostaglandin synthesis inhibitors on haemostatic function has been extensively described. The fetal effects are an increase in bleeding time and inhibition of platelet aggregation. The (albeit retrospective) reports of increased intraventricular haemorrhage in neonates delivered to women receiving indomethacin are therefore particularly worrying (Norton *et al.* 1993; Souter *et al.* 1998). The gastrointestinal effects of indomethacin in the fetus are a reduction in intestinal blood flow. This has been linked to necrotising enterocolitis and localised ileal perforation (Norton *et al.* 1993, Fejgin *et al.* 1994).

Although the prostaglandin synthetase inhibitors appear to be effective tocolytics, concerns regarding fetal safety prevent their use in clinical practice. It is believed that some of these unwanted side effects may be mediated through the constitutive type 1 isoform of cyclo-oxygenase (COX-1) as this enzyme is responsible for the unwanted renal and gastric side effects in non-pregnant subjects (Sakamoto 1998). It has been shown that labour is associated with upregulation of COX-2 rather than COX-1 within the uterus. Initial observational studies with nimesulide (10–100 times selective for COX-2) showed it to be highly effective in preventing PTL in high-risk cases (Sawdy *et al.* 1997) and to have no effect on the ductus arteriosus although renal effects occurred (Peruzzi *et al.* 1999). Thus, it was hoped that specific inhibition of COX-2 activity would provide effective tocolysis without the fetal side effects. Unfortunately, a randomised prospective study subsequently showed that nimesulide showed similar short-term adverse fetal effects to indomethacin, with both reducing amniotic fluid index, hourly fetal urine production and ductal blood flow (Sawdy *et al.* 2003). Additionally, preliminary studies of the COX-2 selective inhibitor rofecoxib have not shown it to be effective in preventing preterm delivery (Groom *et al.* 2003).

Magnesium sulphate

Although magnesium sulphate has been used as a tocolytic for more than 30 years, there has been only one randomised trial comparing its effect with placebo in the treatment of PTL. This study of 156 randomised patients failed to demonstrate a beneficial effect on the duration of gestation, fetal weight or neonatal outcome. Comparative studies with other tocolytics have also failed to demonstrate clinical benefits and therefore magnesium is not recommended for the treatment of PTL.

The adverse effects of magnesium sulphate on the mother include pulmonary oedema, impaired reflexes, respiratory depression, altered myocardial conduction and cardiac arrest. The incidence of these side effects may be reduced by careful assessment of plasma magnesium and maternal reflexes since the latter are lost at plasma concentrations below toxic levels. The fetal side effects are those of increased plasma magnesium, drowsiness, hypotonia and hypocalcaemia. Although these are relatively minor, the MAGnet study (to investigate whether magnesium tocolysis reduces cerebral palsy) was terminated due to excess paediatric mortality in the magnesium-exposed group (Mittendorf *et al.* 1997). There is also concern regarding abnormal bone deposition in the early neonatal period as a result of magnesium tocolytic therapy (Matsuda *et al.* 1997). These data indicate that magnesium sulphate should not be used for tocolysis until its safety and effectiveness have been formally evaluated by ongoing randomised trials.

Nitric oxide donors

Nitric oxide (NO) donors act by increasing levels of cGMP in uterine smooth muscle cells and ultimately cause myometrial relaxation. There have been reports of the use of NO donors suggesting that they are effective tocolytics compared to placebo in delaying delivery for 48 hours (Smith *et al.* 1999). However analysis of all the randomised controlled trials showed that NO donors did not delay delivery nor improved neonatal outcome when compared with each of placebo, no treatment or other tocolytic agents (Duckitt and Thornton 2003). There is thus currently insufficient evidence to support the routine administration of NO donors in the treatment of threatened preterm labour.

Other tocolytics

Numerous other drugs, including ethanol, relaxin and progesterone have been used for the treatment of PTL. None have been demonstrated to be effective or improve neonatal outcome.

Emergency cerclage

The role of emergency cervical cerclage in the acute situation is uncertain. There are no randomised trials comparing conservative with surgical management although retrospective reviews have suggested some benefit (Olatunbosun *et al.* 1995). The surgical procedure has a risk of rupture of the membranes and cervical trauma (at the time of insertion or during labour). It would seem unreasonable to consider cerclage for acute treatment on the basis of current evidence unless the cervix is dilated, uterine activity minimal and the gestational age such that neonatal outcome is likely to be poor. The decision should be based on the individual circumstances and the procedure-related risks.

Predelivery interventions to improve neonatal outcome, including steroids

General measures including transfer

The initial management of a woman in preterm labour is to make the diagnosis, determine the cause, ensure that there is no fetal or maternal compromise and instigate treatment to improve neonatal outcome. The latter is usually in utero transfer to a unit equipped to deal with a preterm neonate and administration of steroids with or without tocolysis. Such measures should in no circumstances delay delivery if either the mother or fetus is compromised.

Rarely is the acute management of PTL so urgent that adequate discussion with the parents cannot occur. Many prospective parents are unaware of the outlook for their baby and a compassionate, honest and frank discussion is important. The attendant staff should be familiar with the mortality and morbidity rates adjusted for fetal condition or adverse causative factors. It is helpful to involve the paediatric team as early as possible and, if appropriate, a visit can be organised to the NICU.

Hydration

Immediate hydration has not been demonstrated to be efficacious in the management of preterm labour, and may precipitate maternal pulmonary oedema in conjunction with tocolysis (Stan *et al.* 2002). If (in selected patients) hydration is indicated, a 5% dextrose solution is preferable to 0.9% saline in order to reduce the risk of pulmonary oedema.

Maternal steroid therapy
Single course

Administration of maternal steroids (two doses of betamethasone 12 mg given intramuscularly 24 hours apart or 4 doses of dexamethasone 6 mg given intramuscularly 12 hours apart) is associated with a reduction in neonatal mortality and morbidity (Crowley 2002). There is some evidence from randomised trials, retrospective data and animal experiments suggesting that betamethasone may be safer and more protective of the immature brain than dexamethasone (Whitelaw and Thoresen 2000).

Steroids promote tissue differentiation in a number of organs and reduce the incidence of respiratory distress syndrome (by approximately 50%) and intraventricular haemorrhage (by approximately 70%) (Crowley 2002). A reduction in necrotising enterocolitis has been reported in some, but not all, trials. The effects of maternal steroids are most marked between 24 hours and 7 days after administration. The failure to demonstrate improved outcome in women delivered more than 7 days after steroid administration has led to repeated doses in women who remain undelivered. A recent review suggested that repeated doses of steroids were associated with a lower risk of severe lung disease, compared with a single steroid course (RR 0.64, 95% CI 0.44–0.93). There are, however, concerns about repeated doses of steroids, including increased rates of neonatal and maternal infection as well as decreased birth weight and brain growth restriction in babies of those mothers who were given multiple courses of steroids (Walfisch *et al.* 2001). Several trials are ongoing worldwide to answer the question whether multiple doses of steroids are more beneficial than harmful (Crowther and Harding 2003). Until the results of these trials are available, expert advice is that repeated doses of steroids should be avoided (ACOG 2002; Crowther and Harding 2003).

There are few maternal or fetal contraindications to single maternal steroid administration. Meta-analysis has not confirmed the theoretical risk of an increase in maternal or neonatal infection. There is no reason to withhold administration in women with preterm rupture of the membranes. The association of steroids with maternal pulmonary oedema has not been confirmed and case reports usually describe women who have concurrent administration of a tocolytic. Maternal diabetes is a relative contra-indication to steroid use. Maternal diabetic control is more difficult and a steroid-induced increase in insulin could lead to fetal lung resistance to glucocorticoids. There are currently insufficient data to promote or condemn steroid use in diabetic mothers. In early randomised trials, steroid administration in hypertensive patients was associated with an excess of intra-uterine fetal deaths. Further studies have failed to confirm an association and maternal hypertension should not preclude steroid administration.

Worthy of note is the important but rare complication of adrenal insufficiency, which should be considered in the event of unexplained collapse in the mother or fetus after corticosteroid therapy.

The long-term safety of a single course of steroids has been investigated in trials that have followed survivors for up to 12 years (Smolders-de Haas *et al.* 1990, Banks *et al.* 1999). There was no evidence of adverse effects in steroid-treated individuals.

There has been some debate as to the upper and lower gestational ages at which steroids provide a benefit. At the upper extremes of prematurity (34–37 weeks), the majority of neonates survive without handicap and it is therefore difficult to demonstrate significant benefits. At the lower extremes (24–28 weeks), the prevalence of preterm delivery is low and the numbers of women recruited to trials to date do not allow meaningful analysis. Since a beneficial effect is likely, steroid administration is recommended between 24 and 36 weeks. Multiple pregnancy should not be a contraindication to the use of steroids, although further work is required to assess their role in this scenario.

The recent introduction of surfactant treatment for preterm babies does not diminish the requirement for maternal steroids. The best outcomes have been reported in babies who have received surfactant following maternal administration of steroids.

Thyrotrophin-releasing hormone

Administration of thyrotrophin-releasing hormone (TRH) to women in preterm labour is not associated with improved outcome and infant follow-up to one year of age demonstrates adverse developmental effects (Crowther *et al.* 2002). Maternal TRH therapy should not therefore be used either in conjunction with, or instead of, maternal steroids

Phenobarbital

The antenatal maternal administration of phenobarbital has been suggested to reduce the risk of periventricular haemorrhage in the neonate or infant. There is no good evidence of benefit and phenobarbital administration to women prior to preterm birth cannot be recommended for routine clinical practice (Crowther 2002).

Antimicrobials

Until very recently there was controversy surrounding the use of antibiotics in the treatment of PTL and preterm premature rupture of membranes (pPROM) with no obvious signs of infection. The recently published ORACLE studies assessed 4826 women with pPROM and 6295 women with spontaneous PTL (in the absence of pPROM). Data analysis showed that in singleton pregnancies complicated by pPROM, erythromycin resulted in reduction in delivery at seven days with several neonatal benefits; co-amoxiclav also reduced delivery at seven days but was associated with necrotising enterocolitis (Kenyon *et al.* 2001a). Conversely, with intact membranes neither erythromycin, co-amoxiclav nor both were better than placebo for delaying delivery, preterm delivery rate or neonatal outcome (Kenyon *et al.* 2001b). Antibiotics should not therefore be used routinely for women in uncomplicated preterm labour, unless there is evidence of infection (King and Flenady 2003).

Management of labour and delivery

Intrapartum fetal monitoring

It is important to prevent acute fetal compromise since the prognosis for the preterm infant with hypoxia or acidosis is markedly worse. Adequate assessment of long-term fetal compromise and estimated weight are thus also important. It is reasonable to continuously monitor the fetus if the correct interpretation of the results would alter management. In practice, this requires assessment of viability, prognosis and the maternal risks of intervention. An infant born before 22 weeks' gestation is unlikely to be viable, and monitoring may be distressing whilst failing to improve management. Between 22 and 26 weeks the decision is more difficult and should be individualised, in consultation with the parents and neonatal paediatricians. Above 26 weeks, unless there is marked fetal growth restriction or other overriding circumstances, monitoring is normally carried out although evidence that this improves outcome is lacking. The interpretation of continuous monitoring should be made in conjunction with the gestational age. The effects of immature fetal cardiovascular physiology on the cardiotocograph are marked. Approximately 50% of normal fetuses between 24 and 28 weeks' gestation will have a non-reactive cardiotocograph due to the immaturity of fetal sympathetic innervation (Druzin *et al.* 1985) and experience is required to correctly interpret the results.

Mode of delivery in vertex presentation

The conduct of delivery in women in preterm labour is controversial. There is no compelling evidence favouring abdominal delivery in uncomplicated PTL with a vertex presentation (Grant and Glazener 2002), administration of epidural analgesia or forceps delivery to protect the fetal head (Bottoms 1995). However, the fetal head should be delivered in a controlled manner and an episiotomy may be helpful (although the evidence is not good (Bottoms 1995)).

Mode of delivery in the preterm breech

Breech presentation is more common in preterm than term labour. There is little evidence that abdominal delivery in the uncomplicated preterm breech confers any benefit. The procedure is associated with more maternal disadvantages than the procedure at term since classical or extended uterine incisions are common. The poorly formed lower uterine segment may make delivery of the fetal head difficult and could increase neonatal morbidity. Unfortunately, trials addressing the optimal mode of delivery in preterm infants have failed to recruit adequate numbers (Lumley 2003). Systematic reviews of the trials that have been performed suggest (although not to statistical significance) that babies delivered by elective caesarean section are less likely to have a) respiratory distress syndrome, b) neonatal seizures or c) neonatal death. Maternal morbidity in the caesarean section group was significantly higher (Grant *et al.* 1996; Grant and Glazener 2002). However, these numbers were not significant. Therefore, although there is evidence that caesarean section for breech presentation at term is beneficial (Hannah *et al.* 2000), there is no good evidence to support either vaginal or abdominal delivery for the uncomplicated preterm breech presentation fetus.

Summary

- The causes of PTL and delivery are multifactorial.
- Clinical assessment is a poor guide to the progression of labour.
- Maternal and fetal condition should be evaluated at the time of clinical assessment.

- There is no universally effective test to diagnose preterm delivery.
- Management is dependent upon the cause of PTL.
- Tocolysis should only be administered to enable short-term management (24–48 hours) likely to improve neonatal outcome.
- Atosiban and nifedipine are preferable to ritodrine as tocolytic agents.
- Steroid administration improves fetal outcome.
- The mortality and morbidity risks are principally determined by gestational age at delivery.

REFERENCES

American College of Obstetricians and Gynecologists (ACOG). (2002) ACOG Committee Opinion: Antenatal corticosteroid therapy for fetal maturation. *Obstet. Gynecol.* **99**, 871–3.

(2003) ACOG Committee in Practice Bulletins – Obstetrics. Practice Bulletin no 43 – Management of Preterm labour. *Obstet. Gynecol.* **101**, 1039–48.

Banks, B. A., Cnaan, A., Morgan, M. A. *et al.* (1999) Multiple courses of antenatal corticosteroids and outcome of premature neonates. *Am. J. Obstet. Gynecol.* **181**, 709–17.

Bottoms, S. (1995) Delivery of the premature infant. *Clin. Obstet. Gynaecol.* **38**, 780–9.

Crowley, P. (2002) Prophylactic corticosteroids for preterm birth (Cochrane Review). In *The Cochrane Library,* Issue 4. Oxford: Update Software.

Crowther, C. A. (2002) Phenobarbital prior to preterm birth (Cochrane review). In *The Cochrane Library,* Issue 4. Oxford: Update software.

Crowther, C. A. and Harding, J. (2003) Repeat doses of prenatal corticosteroids for women at risk of preterm birth for preventing neonatal respiratory disease (Cochrane Review) In *The Cochrane Library,* Issue 3. Oxford. Update software.

Crowther, C. A., Alfirevic, Z. and Haslam, R. R. (2002) Antenatal thyrotropin-releasing hormone (TRH) prior to preterm delivery (Cochrane review). In *The Cochrane Library,* Issue 4. Oxford: Update software.

Druzin M. L., Fox A., Kogut E. and Carlson C. (1985) The relationship of the non-stress test to gestational age. *Am. J. Obstet. Gynecol.* **153**, 386–9

Duckitt, K. and Thornton, S. (2003) Nitric oxide donors for the treatment of preterm labour (Cochrane Review). In *The Cochrane Library,* Issue 1. Oxford: Update Software.

Fejgin M. D., Delpino M. L. and Bidiwala K. S. (1994) Isolated small bowel perforation following intrauterine treatment with indomethacin. *Am. J. Perinatol.* **11**, 295–6.

Fuchs, A. R., Fuchs, F., Husslein, P. and Soloff, M. S. (1984) Oxytocin receptors in the human uterus during pregnancy and parturition. *Am. J. Obstet. Gynecol.* **150**, 734–41.

Grant, A. and Glazener, C. M. A. (2002) Elective caesarean section versus expectant management for delivery of the small baby (Cochrane Review). In *The Cochrane Library,* Issue 4. Oxford: Update Software.

Grant, A., Penn, Z. J. and Steer, P. J. (1996) Elective or selective caesarean section for the small baby? A systematic review of the controlled trials. *BJOG* **103**, 1197–200.

Groom, K. M., Shennan, A. H., Jones, B. A., Seed, P. and Bennett, P. (2003) TOCOX – a randomised double-blind placebo-controlled trial of rofecoxib (a cox-2 specific PG inhibitor) for the prevention of preterm delivery in high-risk women. *J. Obstet. Gynaecol* **23**, S19.

Gyetvai, K., Hannah, M. E., Hodnett, E. D. and Ohlsson, A. (1999) Tocolytics for preterm labour: a systematic review. *Obstet. Gynecol.* **94**, 869–77.

Hannah M. E., Hannah W. J., Hewson S. A. *et al.* (2000) Planned caesarean section versus planned vaginal birth for breech presentation at term: a randomised multicentre trial. Term Breech Trial Collaborative Group. *Lancet* **356**, 1375–83.

Honest, H., Bachmann, L. M., Gupta, J. K., Kleijnen, J. and Khan, K. S. (2002) Accuracy of cervico-vaginal fetal fibronectin test in predicting risk of spontaneous preterm birth: systematic review. *BMJ* **325**, 301–11.

Kenyon, S. L., Taylor, D. J. and Tarnow-Mordi, W.; ORACLE Collaborative Group (2001a) Broad-spectrum antibiotics for preterm, prelabour rupture of membranes: the ORACLE I randomised trial. *Lancet* **357**, 979–88.

Kenyon, S. L., Taylor, D. J. and Tarnow-Mordi, W.; ORACLE Collaborative Group (2001b) Broad-spectrum antibiotics for spontaneous PTL: the ORACLE II randomised trial. *Lancet* **357** 989–94.

Kierse, M. J. N. C., Grant, A. and King, J. F. (1989) Preterm labour. In I. Chalmers, M. Enkin and M. J. N. C. Kierse, eds., *Effective Care in Pregnancy and Childbirth.* Oxford: Oxford University Press, pp. 694–745.

King, J. and Flenady, V. (2003) Prophylactic antibiotics for inhibiting preterm labour with intact membranes (Cochrane Review). In *The Cochrane Library,* Issue 3. Oxford: Update Software.

King, J. F., Flenady, V. J., Papatsonis, D. N. M., Dekker, G. A. and Carbonne, B. (2002) Calcium channel blockers for inhibiting preterm labour (Cochrane Review). In *The Cochrane Library,* Issue 4. Oxford: Update Software.

Kirshon, B., Moise, K. J., Mari, G. and Willis, R. (1991) Long-term indomethacin therapy decreases fetal urine output and results in oligohydramnios. *Am. J. Perinatol.* **8**, 86–8.

Leitich, H., Brunbauer, M., Kaider, A., Egarter, C. and Husslein P. (1999) Cervical length and dilatation of the internal cervical os detected by vaginal ultrasonography as markers for preterm delivery: A systematic review. *Am. J. Obstet. Gynecol.* **181**, 1465–72.

Lockwood, C. J. (1997) Calcium channel blockers in the management of preterm labour. *Lancet* **350**, 1339–40.

Lockwood, C. J., Senyei, A. E., Dische, M. R. (1991) Fetal fibronectin in cervical and vaginal secretions as a predictor of preterm delivery. *N. Engl. J. Med.* **325**, 669–74.

Lumley J. (2003) Method of delivery for the preterm infant. *BJOG* **110**, 88–92.

MacLennan F. M., Thomson M. A., Rankin R., Terry P. B. and Adey G. D. (1985) Fatal pulmonary oedema associated with the use of ritodrine in pregnancy. A case report. *BJOG* **92**, 703–5.

Matsuda, Y., Maeda, Y., Ito, M. *et al.* (1997) Effect of magnesium sulfate treatment on neonatal bone abnormalities. *Gynec. Obstet. Invest.* **44**, 82–8.

Mittendorf, R., Covert, R., Boman, J. *et al.* (1997) Is tocolytic magnesium sulphate associated with increased total paediatric mortality? *Lancet* **350**, 1517–18.

Moutquin, J. M., Sherman, D., Cohen, H. *et al.* (2000) Double-blind, randomized, controlled trial of atosiban and ritodrine in the treatment of preterm labour: a multicenter effectiveness and safety study. *Am. J. Obstet. Gynecol.* **182**, 1191–9.

Norton, M. E., Merrill J., Cooper, B. A., Kuller, J. A. and Clyman, R. I. (1993) Neonatal complications after the administration of indomethacin for preterm labour. *N. Engl. J. Med.* **329**, 1602–7.

Olatunbosun, O. A., al-Nuaim L. and Turnell R. W. (1995) Emergency cerclage compared with bed rest for advanced cervical dilatation in pregnancy. *Int. Surg.* **80**, 170–4.

Papatsonis, D. N., Van Geijn H. P., Ader, H. J. *et al.* (1997) Nifedipine and ritodrine in the management of preterm labour: a randomized multicenter trial. *Obstet. Gynecol.* **90** 230–4.

Peruzzi, L., Gianoglio, B., Porcellini, M. G. and Coppo, R. (1999) Neonatal end-stage renal failure associated with maternal ingestion of cyclo-oxygenase-type-1 selective inhibitor nimesulide as tocolytic. *Lancet* **354**, 1615.

Royal College of Obstetricians and Gynaecologists (RCOG). (2002) *Tocolytic Drugs for Women in Preterm Labour RCOG Guideline 1B* http://www.rcog.org.uk/resources/Public/Tocolytic_Drugs_No1(B).pdf

Romero, R., Sibai, B. M., Sanchez-Ramos, L. *et al.* (2000) An oxytocin receptor antagonist (atosiban) in the treatment of preterm labour: A randomised, double-blind, placebo-controlled trial with tocolytic rescue. *Am. J. Obstet. Gynecol.* **182**, 1173–83.

Sakamoto, C. (1998) Roles of COX-1 and COX-2 in gastrointestinal pathophysiology. *J. Gastroenterol.* **33**, 618–24.

Sawdy, R., Slater, D., Fisk, N., Edmonds, D. K. and Bennett, P. (1997) Use of a cyclo-oxygenase type-2-selective non-steroidal anti-inflammatory agent to prevent preterm delivery. *Lancet* **350**, 265–6.

Sawdy, R. J., Lye, S., Fisk, N. M. and Bennett, P. R. (2003) A double-blind randomized study of fetal side effects during and after the short-term maternal administration of indomethacin, sulindac, and nimesulide for the treatment of preterm labour. *Am. J. Obstet. Gynecol.* **188**, 1046–51.

Smith, G. N., Walker, M. C. and McGrath, M. J. (1999) Randomised, double blind, placebo controlled pilot study assessing nitroglycerin as a tocolytic. *BJOG* **106**,736–9.

Smolders-de Haas, H., Neuvel, J., Schmand, B. *et al.* (1990) Physical development and medical history of children who were treated antenatally with corticosteroids to prevent respiratory distress syndrome: a 10 to 12 year follow-up. *Paediatrics* **86**, 65–70.

Souter, D., Harding, J., McCowan L. *et al.* (1998) Antenatal indomethacin- adverse fetal effects confirmed. *Aust. N. Z. J. Obstet. Gynecol.* **38**, 11–16.

Stan, C., Boulvain, M., Hirsbrunner-Amagbaly, P. and Pfister, R. (2002) Hydration for treatment of preterm labour (Cochrane Review). In *The Cochrane Library*, Issue 4. Oxford: Update Software.

Takahashi, K., Diamond, F., Bieniarz, J., Jen, H. and Burd, L. (1980) Uterine contractility and oxytocin. Sensitivity in preterm, term, and posterm pregnancy. *Am. J. Obstet. Gynecol.* **136**, 774–9.

Van den Hof, M. and Crane, J. (2001) Ultrasound cervical assessment in predicting preterm birth. *J. Soc. Obstet. Gynecol. Can.* **23**, 418–21.

Van Iddekinge, B., Gobetz, L., Seaward, P. G. and Hofmeyr, G. J. (1991) Pulmonary oedema after hexoprenaline administration in preterm labour. A report of 4 cases. *S. Afr. Med. J.* **79**, 620–2.

Vermillon, S. T., Scardo, J. A., Lashus, A. G. and Wiles, H. B. (1997) The effect of indomethacin tocorysis on fetal ductus arteriosus constriction with advancing gestational age. *Am. J. Obstet. Gynecol.* **177**, 256–9.

Walfisch, A., Hallak, M. and Mazor, M. (2001) Multiple courses of antenatal steroids: risks and benefits. *Obstet. Gynecol.* **98**, 491–7.

Whitelaw, A. and Thoresen, M. (2000) Antenatal steroids and the developing brain. *Arch. Dis. Child. Fetal Neonatal Ed.* **83** F154–7.

OTHER READING

Anonymous (1995) *PTL. ACOG technical bulletin. 206* (June 1995).

American College of Obstetricians and Gynecologists, Committee on Obstetric Practice (1997). *Fetal fibronectin preterm labour risk test.* ACOG Committee Opinion No. 187. Washington, DC: ACOG.

Howe, D. C. and Calder, A. A. (1998) *PTL. PACE review.* Royal College of Obstetricians and Gynaecologists 98/08.

9

Management of preterm labour with specific complications

Mark Kilby and David Somerset

Birmingham Women's Hospital

Multiple Pregnancy

Aetiology and Incidence

Dizygotic twinning arises when two separate ova are fertilised and implanted. This results in non-identical twins with separate amniotic sacs, chorions and placentae (although the placental masses may fuse together). Monozygotic twinning arises when a single embryo splits to yield genetically identical twins. Depending on the timing of division relative to conception, it may result in diamniotic, dichorionic pregnancy ($\sim$33%), a diamniotic, monochorionic pregnancy ($\sim$66%), a mono-amniotic, monochorionic pregnancy ($\sim$1%) or conjoined twins (rare). Chorionicity may be accurately determined by ultrasound at 11–14 weeks' gestation, but becomes more difficult thereafter. The incidence of monozygotic twinning is relatively stable worldwide at around 3.5 per 1000 births, whilst the incidence of dizygotic twining varies with race and maternal age ($\sim$8.5 per 1000 births in Europe and North America) (Little and Thompson 1988). Dizygotic twinning may also result from assisted conception techniques, leading to a higher incidence in some centres. For the UK as a whole, the incidence of multiple births has increased from 10.4 per 1000 maternities in 1985 to 14.4 per 1000 in 1997, with higher-order pregnancies tripling from 0.14 to 0.45 per 1000, reflecting the increasing use of assisted conception techniques (Taylor and Fisk 2000).

Preterm delivery is considered the most important complication of multiple pregnancy and it is responsible for the majority of the increased perinatal morbidity and mortality. The Scottish Twins Study (Patel *et al.* 1984) reported delivery before 37 completed weeks in 44% of twins (vs. 6% of singletons), and delivery before 32 completed weeks in 10%. A large American multicentre study involving 33 873 pregnancies reported delivery before 37 completed weeks in 54% (vs. 9.6% of singletons), with twins accounting for 2.6% of neonates but 12.2% of preterm infants (Gardner *et al.* 1995). Another huge epidemiological study of over 750 000

Preterm Labour Managing Risk in Clinical Practice, eds. Jane Norman and Ian Greer. Published by Cambridge University Press. © Cambridge University Press 2005.

Table 9.1 Gestational age at delivery for pregnancies progressing beyond 20 weeks from a series of 142 conceptions following ovulation induction with gonadotrophins

Number of fetuses	N	Mean gestation at delivery (completed weeks)
Singleton	82	39
Twins	21	35
Triplets	5	33
Quadruplets	3	29

Caspi *et al.* (1976)

pregnancies in New York State reported twins delivering an average of 19 days earlier than singletons (Caspi *et al.* 1976; Kiely 1990). Higher-order multiple births tend to deliver even more prematurely (Table 9.1) (Caspi *et al.* 1976).

The increased incidence of preterm labour associated with multiple gestations is generally attributed to uterine over-distension leading to an increase in the frequency and strength of contractions. However, there is little objective evidence to support this assertion. Two epidemiological studies show similar birthweight specific perinatal mortality for twins and singletons weighing less than 1500 g at birth, but a lower risk of perinatal death for twins weighing between 1500 g and 2500 g compared to singletons (relative risk (RR) 0.4–0.45) (Fabre *et al.* 1988; Kiely 1990). Somewhat surprisingly, both these studies also showed an increased risk of perinatal death for twins weighing greater than 2500 g compared to singletons. Whilst these data were corrected for birthweight as opposed to gestational age, the two variables are related. Therefore, they indicate that whilst there is no advantage to twins in being born extremely premature, they do appear to be at some advantage to singletons when born slightly early (although intrauterine growth restriction may account for some of this variation).

Prediction

As discussed above, multiple pregnancy is in itself a significant risk factor for both preterm delivery and extremely pre-term delivery, with risk being directly proportional to the number of fetuses present (Table 9.1). In addition, data from the Scottish morbidity record (1992–97) identified nulliparity and maternal short stature as independent risk factors for preterm labour in twins (Smith *et al.* 2002). Further stratification of risk may be possible using methods discussed in detail in Chapter 5. Briefly:

Ultrasound

Ultrasound assessment of the cervix between 18 and 28 weeks may be useful in predicting risk. Both cervical funnelling and cervical length less than 25–30 mm have been reported as carrying relative risks of between 2- and 7-fold for preterm delivery in twin pregnancies (Goldenberg *et al.* 1996; Wennerholm *et al.* 1997; Yang *et al.* 2000). However, these studies were not consistent in their ability to predict extremely preterm birth, or in the predictive power of funnelling. A single study has addressed an intervention (cervical cerclage) following cervical ultrasound in twin pregnancy, and this showed no benefit of cerclage in the group found to be high risk (Newman *et al.* 2002).

Home uterine activity monitoring

Trials of home uterine activity monitoring have been exclusive to the USA, and their conclusions of usefulness inconsistent. There is some evidence to suggest that such monitoring may benefit those women with reduced access to midwifery/ medical supervision by facilitating early referral, but little evidence of benefit in women with good access to antenatal care (Dyson *et al.* 1991, 1998; CHUMS Group 1995; Wapner *et al.* 1995).

Fetal fibronectin

The detection of fetal fibronectin in cervical secretions has also been shown to increase the risk of preterm labour in twin pregnancies. In particular, two studies have reported a positive test at 28 weeks' gestation to increase the relative risk of delivery before 32 weeks by 9-fold (95% confidence interval (CI) 1–68-fold) (Goldenberg *et al.* 1996) and before 35 weeks by 6-fold (95% CI 3–15-fold) (Wennerholm *et al.* 1997); however, the confidence intervals from these studies were wide. Furthermore there have been no studies addressing whether widespread use of such testing has any benefit in either twin or higher-order pregnancy.

Preventative strategies

Given the high incidence of preterm labour in multiple pregnancies, many strategies of been advocated to reduce this risk. The use of randomised controlled trials over the last two decades has shown that at best, most interventions are harmless and at worst, some may increase the risk of premature delivery.

Prenatal care

Recent studies in the USA have confirmed the importance of good antenatal care in reducing the risks of preterm labour in twin gestations, with an adjusted odds ratio (OR) of 0.45 (95% CI 0.30–0.68) (Luke *et al.* 2003; Vintzileos *et al.* 2003).

Bed rest

Observational studies from the 1950s identified improved perinatal outcomes in twin pregnancies amongst middle-class women, leading to the suggestion that all mothers carrying twins be admitted "at the 30th week in order by diet and rest to tide them over the danger period" (Newman *et al.* 2002). A Cochrane meta-analysis of 6 trials involving over 600 women and 1400 babies reported (Crowther 2001):

1. Routine bed rest in hospital for multiple pregnancy did <u>not</u> reduce the risk of preterm birth or perinatal mortality.
2. For women with otherwise uncomplicated twin pregnancy, routine admission to hospital for bed rest was associated with a significant *increase* in the risk of very preterm birth (<34 weeks) (OR 1.84; 95% CI 1.01–3.34)
3. Routine hospitalisation for bed rest of women with triplet pregnancies suggests beneficial effects including prolonged gestation, but the numbers were too small (19 women) to reach statistical significance.
4. Routine hospitalisation for bed rest of women with twin pregnancies complicated by cervical effacement and dilatation prior to labour did <u>not</u> reduce the risk of preterm birth or perinatal mortality.

A major limitation of this meta-analysis is that four of the six trials were carried out in Harare, Zimbabwe and all the trials were published between 1984 and 1991 (when the use of ultrasound may not have been routine). Thus the results may not be generalisable to a twenty first century healthcare system with different racial groups and routine use of high-resolution ultrasound. Nevertheless, the evidence as it stands does not support routine admission to hospital for bed rest of women with twin pregnancies and in fact, suggests that it may be harmful. However, routine admission for bed rest of women with higher-order pregnancies during the third trimester may be beneficial (Crowther *et al.* 1991).

Cervical cerclage

There is no current evidence to support routine cervical cerclage in twin or higher-order pregnancy (Grant 1989; Mordel *et al.* 1993; Strauss *et al.* 2002). The indications for placement of a suture are therefore the same as those in a singleton pregnancy (Chapter 5). Furthermore a recent American study, using cervical length <25 mm (measured using ultrasound) at between 18 and 26 weeks as a screening test, failed to show any advantage to routine cervical cerclage even in this high-risk group of twin pregnancies (Seki *et al.* 2000).

Tocolysis

There is no current evidence to support the use of prophylactic tocolytic agents in twin or higher-order pregnancy. Trials have been conducted using a variety of oral betamimetic drugs, including isoxuprine, ritodrine, salbutamol and terbutaline. The results have been consistent in showing no effect in prolonging gestation (Keirse *et al.* 1989).

Corticosteroids

The use of maternally administered corticosteroids to reduce perinatal morbidity and mortality due to complications of prematurity is fully discussed in Chapter 8. Of note, however, no significant beneficial effect has been demonstrated in multi-fetal pregnancies (Crowley 2000). Whilst it is assumed that this is because of the small numbers involved in the trials, the lack of effect could theoretically be due to sub-therapeutic drug levels due to increased plasma volume expansion or the effects of a larger feto-placental unit. Notwithstanding, it is generally assumed that the beneficial effects in multifetal pregnancies will be similar to that in singletons and it is unlikely that any further placebo-controlled trials would be acceptable.

Since the meta-analysis of the effect of corticosteroids (Crowley 2000) identified a statistically beneficial effect only if delivery took place within seven days of administration, a practice has evolved whereby some obstetricians institute weekly or fortnightly repeat courses of steroid injections to cover the "at risk" period for women carrying twin or higher-order pregnancies. Concerns have been raised about the theoretical complications of such treatment (Brocklehurst *et al.* 1999), and a retrospective cohort study from Bristol (Murphy *et al.* 2002) has failed to show any advantage to such a policy in terms of reduced incidence of respiratory distress (OR 0.7, 95% CI 0.2–2.0) but did demonstrate a significant reduction in mean birthweight at term (129 g, 95% CI 33–218 g). Thus prophylactic repeat courses of antenatal corticosteroids cannot be recommended.

Investigation and treatment of threatened pre-term labour

Most complications of pregnancy are commoner in twin and higher-order gestation, and some of these problems may precipitate pre-term labour (Table 9.2). Thus it is important to rapidly assess both fetal and maternal wellbeing as fully as possible before deciding on management. An initial set of observations and investigations is suggested in Table 9.3.

Table 9.2 Complications of multiple pregnancy that may be associated with preterm labour

Chorioamnionitis following an invasive procedure (e.g. amniocentesis)
Intrauterine death
Intrauterine growth restriction
Placental abruption
Pre-eclampsia
Polyhydramnios secondary to twin to twin transfusion syndrome
Polyhydramnios secondary to other causes
Vaginal or urinary tract infection

Table 9.3 Initial observations and investigations

Maternal temperature, pulse, blood pressure and urine analysis

Abdominal palpation

Sterile speculum examination to assess cervix and take swab for culture

Digital or ultrasound assessment of cervix if not seen clearly on speculum
examination

Fetal cardiotocograms (CTGs) if gestational age >26 weeks

Ultrasound assessment of fetal presentation, growth and wellbeing, and liquor
volume

Full blood count +/− Group and Save +/− pre-eclampsia profile (urea and
electrolytes, liver function tests, Urate)

Pre-eclampsia, a large abruption, tense polyhydramnios and chorioamnionitis should be swiftly excluded by maternal observations and examination. Fetal well-being should be confirmed by auscultation of the fetal heart rate (Cardiotocogram (CTG) if sufficiently mature) and active labour/membrane rupture excluded by a sterile speculum examination. A high vaginal swab should be sent for culture, and the cervical assessment clarified by digital or ultrasound examination if required. A fetal fibronectin test should be performed if available. A midstream urine sample should be tested for the presence of protein, blood, nitrites and leukocyte esterase before sending for formal microscopy and culture. Blood should be taken for a full blood count and if required, Group and Save and pre-eclampsia profile (renal function, liver function and serum urate). Wide-bore intravenous access should be established if intravenous tocolysis is being considered, if labour is thought to be established, or if there has been vaginal bleeding or suspicion of an abruption. If possible, fetal assessment by high resolution ultrasound should be performed. The purpose of this examination is to confirm fetal presentation and exclude intrauterine growth restriction, polyhydramnios and in monochorionic pregnancy, twin–twin transfusion syndrome. If not previously documented, placenta previa should be excluded.

In all instances prior to 36 weeks' gestation, excepting acute chorioamnionitis, corticosteriods should be administered to the mother to promote fetal lung maturity, if this has not already been done (Chapter 7). It should be noted that within the trials included in the Cochrane Collaboration meta-analysis there were too few multiple pregnancies to assess any benefit separately from singletons; however, there is no theoretical reason to believe the effect will be any less (Crowley 2000). Whether a further course should be administered if a previous course has been given more than seven days previously is not currently known. The authors' practice is to administer a second course if the gestational age is less than 34 weeks, the previous course was given more than 14 days previously and the risk of premature labour considered high (e.g. regular uterine contractions and some evidence of cervical change).

The complications of pre-eclampsia and intra-uterine growth restriction are discussed later in this chapter.

Acute chorioamnionitis

Acute chorioamnionitis should be treated as for a singleton pregnancy: broad spectrum antibiotics and urgent delivery are indicated. Caesarean section may be indicated depending on gestation, if there is fetal compromise or malpresentation.

Placental abruption

Placental abruption should be managed as for a singleton pregnancy. Tocolysis is contraindicated (Chapter 7) and delivery by caesarean section may be required if there is fetal compromise or a malpresentation (see below). Given the larger placental mass, increased maternal-placental perfusion and tendency for postpartum uterine atony associated with multiple gestations, the risk of massive haemorrhage is increased.

Genital tract infection

Genital tract infection is associated with premature labour as in singleton pregnancies (Chapter 5). If infection is suspected on examination, then targeted antibiotic treatment is indicated. The choice of antibiotic should be guided by local prescribing guidelines.

Intrauterine death

Intrauterine death of both twins should be treated as for a singleton pregnancy. Labour should be allowed to proceed naturally with augmentation if necessary. The risk of disseminated intravascular coagulation (DIC) due to the release of thromboplastic substances into the maternal circulation is low, but becomes significant three to four weeks after fetal demise (Sutton *et al.* 1971; Howie 1995). A clotting screen should be carried out in all cases involving an intrauterine death, and should be repeated regularly (e.g. weekly) if the pregnancy remains on going. The management of preterm labour when only one fetus has died and the other remains alive is more problematic. In monochorionic pregnancy, the chance of the live fetus surviving the death of its co-twin and remaining neurologically intact is only around 30% (probably due to the presence of placental anastomosis causing an episode of profound hypotension as the first twin dies) (Bajoria *et al.* 1999). Brain damage, should it occur, is likely to be immediate and therefore urgent delivery is unlikely to be advantageous. In these circumstances, if the surviving twin remains well, it may well be best to attempt to delay delivery at least until corticosteroids have been administered, and if possible until sufficient time has passed to allow for ultrasound assessment of possible neurological damage (two to four weeks). Prior knowledge of neurological damage in the surviving twin allows parents the choice of termination of pregnancy or declining intervention for fetal distress during labour, should they so wish. Intrauterine death of a dichorionic twin should not affect the survivor adversely, except by precipitating premature delivery. Thus, so long as the surviving twin remains well and there is no contra-indication, tocolysis at least until cortico-steroids have been administered should be advantageous.

Polyhydramnios

Polyhydramnios may be secondary to twin–twin transfusion syndrome in a monochorionic pregnancy, or any of the other causes found in singleton preg-nancy (non-immune hydrops, diabetes, rhesus disease (immune hydrops), unex-plained). Expert guidance should be sought if time permits. Therapeutic amnio drainage may reduce uterine distension and thereby diminish uterine contrac-tions, but is itself associated with premature labour. The risk (from amnio drainage) is in the order of 1% in an asymptomatic mother, but is likely to be much higher if she is already contracting. An alternative approach would be to use an antiprostaglandin such as indomethacin (e.g. 25 mg p.o. tds) or sulindac (e.g. 200 mg p.o. bd) (Peek et al. 1997). As well as acting as tocolytics (Chapter 7), these agents reduce fetal urine output thus reducing the polyhydramnios. Sulindac has theoretical advantages in that it may be both less nephrotoxic and less likely to cause premature closure of the ductus arteriosus (Rasanen and Jouppila 1995).

Tocolysis

Tocolysis is indicated for threatened preterm labour in multiple pregnancy to allow for administration of corticosteroids and facilitate intrauterine transfer. As with the evidence for corticosteroids, there are insufficient numbers of multiple pregnancies included in the trials to analyse efficacy separately. Concerns have also been raised about a possibility of increased susceptibility of mothers with multiple pregnancy to betamimetic-induced pulmonary oedema, but these have not been reported with either calcium channel blockers such as nifedipine, or the oxytocin antagonist atosiban, which are thus to be preferred (Chapter 8).

Intrauterine transfer

Intrauterine transfer to a unit with sufficient neonatal cots is an unfortunately common event currently, even in tertiary referral centres (Bennett et al. 2002). This is even more of a problem with higher-order pregnancies as few neonatal care units nationally have three or more ventilator spaces vacant at any one time. Thus early liaison with neonatal colleagues is vital to ensure that facilities to receive and care for multiple premature babies are available (for instance, even if the cots are available, extra senior paediatricians may need to be called in to make sure of sufficient expertise for *each* baby at birth). If cots are not available locally, a long transfer may be required. This should be discussed at Consultant Obstetric and Paediatric level, since unnecessary transfer is disruptive and distressing for the mother but late transfer may be disastrous, with delivery occurring before arrival.

Mode of Delivery

The huge New York epidemiological study performed by Kiely (1990) reported that perinatal mortality for twins presenting by the vertex and delivering vaginally was around twice that of those delivered by caesarean section. For twins presenting by the breech and delivering vaginally, mortality was around threefold higher than those delivered by caesarean section. However, when these results were stratified by birthweight the figures look very different, because the twins delivered vaginally were much smaller than those delivered by caesarean section. Thus, for twins presenting by the vertex with birth weights between 1001–2500 g, vaginal delivery was actually associated with a slightly lower perinatal mortality rate (although the confidence intervals span unity: RR 0.81, 95% CI 0.55–1.18). Interestingly, caesarean section did appear to offer some protection for birthweights above 3000 g, but the confidence intervals were wide due to the small numbers of larger twins (relative risk of perinatal death for vaginal birth vs. caesarean section: RR 4.22, 95% CI 1.10–27.7). As with most epidemiological studies, birthweight rather than gestational age was recorded; however, this huge study certainly suggests that elective caesarean section carries no benefit for premature twins presenting by the vertex. Unfortunately, the birthweight specific analysis was not performed for those presenting by the breech. A historical review of twin deliveries at McGill University (Canada) from 1963 to 1984 demonstrated no improvement in neonatal condition at birth from a rise in the Caesarean section rate from 3.2% to 50.8% (reaching 92% for non-cephalic presentation) (Bell *et al.* 1986). There was a reduction in neonatal morbidity and mortality from respiratory distress syndrome in the later part of the study, but this was more likely to be due to improvements in neonatal care than mode of delivery. Again, this study did not analyse preterm deliveries separately. Smith *et al.* (2002) investigated risks to the second twin from intended vaginal breech birth in 1438 premature (<36 weeks) twin deliveries in Scotland between 1992 and 1995. This comprehensive population study showed no difference in mortality between first and second twins within this population, and again confirmed that the majority of deaths were due to complications of prematurity, not intrapartum anoxia.

Diamniotic; very low birthweight/very preterm; first twin cephalic

There are some fairly consistent observational data regarding mode of delivery in low birthweight twins (500–1499 g). This group represents only 10%–12% of all twin deliveries, but about 75% of twin neonatal morbidity and mortality (Patel *et al.* 1984; Oconnor and Hiadzi 1996). As with the epidemiological studies, most paediatric follow-up studies have tended to report birthweight rather than gestational age, but this group roughly equates to very preterm births (<32 weeks' gestation). One early report was that of Barrett *et al.* (1982), who reported higher morbidity in second twins born vaginally, as opposed to Caesarean section, weighing between 1000 g and 1499 g, and higher mortality in those weighing between 500 g and 999 g. The authors recommended a policy of routine Caesarean section for all twins with an estimated weight of less than 1500 g, but more contemporary studies have failed to demonstrate any advantage to such a policy. Doyle *et al.* (1988) reported on 124 sets of twins born over a 9 year period, with a 27% Caesarean section rate. They showed no neonatal advantage from Caesarean section once gestational age and birthweight had been taken into account. Morales *et al.* (1989) reported on 156 twin pairs weighing less than 1500 g, including details of presentation. Again, following multivariate analysis correcting for birthweight and gestational age, no advantage from Caesarean section was demonstrated, even for breech presentation. In a longer term Swedish follow-up study examining deliveries over a 10 year period (1973–83), during which the Caesarean section rate rose from 7.7% to 68.9%, Rydhstrom (1990) showed that 8%–9% of twins weighing less than 1500 g had cerebral palsy or mental retardation when followed up for at least 8 years. They found no reduction in this prevalence with time, despite the 9-fold increase in Caesarean section rate, and no advantage to Caesarean section in twins presenting by the breech. However, more recently, Davison *et al.* (1992) reported on 54 second twins delivered vaginally by breech extraction and weighing between 750 g and 2000 g. Whilst they needed more days of mechanical ventilation and oxygen therapy than their first-born (cephalic) siblings, when compared to 43 gestation-matched second twins where both were delivered by Caesarean section there were no significant differences in neonatal morbidity, including severe grades of interventricular haemorrhages, respiratory distress or necrotising enterocolitis. The limitation of all these studies is that, other than birthweight, they do not allow for the clinical condition of the babies before birth. Thus, it may be that a significant number of Caesarean sections were performed because the fetuses were already compromised, and thus would have been expected to do worse in the neonatal period irrespective of the mode of delivery. In conclusion, there is no clear evidence of an advantage to routine Caesarean section for very low birthweight/very premature twins. On the other hand, the evidence that there is very clearly points to an advantage in increasing gestational age. Thus, prolonging pregnancy is likely to be far more important in terms of improving perinatal morbidity and mortality than mode of delivery.

Diamniotic; preterm, first twin breech (any gestation)

With regard to breech presentation in twin pregnancies, the Royal College of Obstetricians and Gynaecologists (RCOG) guideline (2001) states that "there is insufficient evidence to support Caesarean section for the delivery of the first or second twin". This guideline observes that the Term Breech Trial studied neither multiple pregnancies nor preterm deliveries (Hannah *et al.* 2000). It was also noted that the risk of "locked twins" (where the presenting twin is breech, the second twin is cephalic and their heads lock above the pelvic inlet preventing delivery of the first twin) is felt to be rare (1/817). However, lack of evidence for a benefit does not infer evidence for a lack of benefit: most obstetricians in the UK would recommend elective Caesarean section at term where the presenting twin was breech (Green and Wilkinshaw 2002). Given the lack of any compelling evidence of best practice at term, it must be appreciated that there is no good evidence on which to base practice preterm. It should be clear from the studies discussed above, that for very preterm birth (<32 weeks), gestational age and birthweight are of overriding importance, minimalising any possible advantage to caesarean birth. Decisions regarding mode of delivery at this gestation should therefore be guided by the condition of the fetuses, and involve full discussion with the parents and attending paediatric and obstetric staff (RCOG 2001). Between 32 and 37 weeks' gestational age becomes less important and it is the authors' usual practice to recommend delivery by caesarean section at this gestation.

Monoamniotic

There are unique risks associated with the vaginal delivery of monoamniotic pregnancies. Most notable of these is cord entanglement, which is associated with intrauterine death, intrapartum hypoxia, and even premature division of the second twin's cord due to mistaken identity as the first is delivered. Entanglement appears to be ubiquitous with survival rates as low as 50% reported historically (Nyberg *et al.* 1984). "Locked" twins and other compound presentations are also thought to be more frequent than in diamniotic pregnancy. To avoid further risks of cord entanglement and the risk of "locking" it is recommended that monoamniotic twins be delivered by caesarean section (Taylor and Fisk 2000).

Triplets and higher-order pregnancies

Even allowing for gestational age, the risk of cerebral palsy increases with each additional fetus. The risk for at least one child from a triplet pregnancy developing cerebral palsy is 8.0%, and from a quadruplet pregnancy is 42.9% (O'Connor *et al.* 1979). Observational series suggest higher Apgar scores and lower perinatal mortality associated with caesarean section for higher-order pregnancy (Crowther and Hamilton 1989; Collins and Bley 1990), although some authors still advocate vaginal

Table 9.4. Risks of preterm Caesarean section for multiple pregnancy

- Poorly formed lower uterine segment requiring midline uterine incision
- Increased incidence of low-lying placenta complicating incision
- Increased incidence of malpresentation complicating delivery
- Uterine entrapment of after-coming head with breech extraction
- Fetal surgical laceration with oligohydramnios
- Increased incidence of postpartum haemorrhage
- Iatrogenic prematurity (given that most women presenting in threatened preterm labour will not deliver immediately see Chapter 4)

delivery in carefully selected cases (Dommergues *et al.* 1995). Potential complications during vaginal delivery include difficulty in monitoring all fetuses, malpresentations, cord entanglement if monoamniotic, and "locking". It is common practice in the UK to deliver higher-order pregnancies by Caesarean section so long as a reasonable chance of fetal survival exists (see below), and this has the advantage of ensuring that an adequate paediatric team can be assembled (Taylor and Fisk 2000).

Delivery at the limits of viability

Survival for infants alive at the onset of labour is below 50% for fetuses weighing less than 750 g at 26 weeks' gestation, or 500 g at 27 weeks' gestation (Draper *et al.* 1999). Even amongst those that survive, long periods of neonatal intensive care will be required and the majority will suffer some form of long-term morbidity. Against this background it is difficult to justify exposing the mother to the not inconsiderable risks of caesarean section at this gestation (Table 9.4). It is also worth considering case reports of interval delivery of fetuses in higher-order pregnancy, with the aim of gaining further time in utero for the undelivered siblings (Taylor and Fisk 2000). Both emergency cervical cerclage and conservative management have been reported, but such a policy is not without risk. The authors' experience includes a case of ascending infection leading to chorioamnionitis, uncontrollable postpartum haemorrhage and hysterectomy.

Medical staffing issues

Given the unpredictable risks associated with both vaginal and abdominal delivery of multiple pregnancies (Tables 9.4 and 9.5), an experienced obstetrician should be present to supervise delivery in all cases. It is usual to have a midwife and an experienced neonatologist (some units use neonatal nurses skilled in intubation/resuscitation) for each baby present at delivery.

Table 9.5. Risks of preterm vaginal delivery for multiple pregnancy

- Difficulty in monitoring all fetuses
- Increased risk of intrapartum hypoxia
- Increased risk of malpresentation, especially with the non-presenting fetus(es)
- Risk of 'locking' for breech-cephalic combinations
- Risk of Caesarean section for the second twin
- Increased risk of postpartum haemorrhage (vs. singletons)
- Risk of cord entanglement (monoamniotic only)

Pre-eclampsia

Definition and aetiology

The International Society for the Study of Hypertension in Pregnancy (ISSHP) defines pre-eclampsia as "*de novo hypertension after 20 weeks gestation, returning to normal postpartum, and proteinuria*" (Brown *et al.* 2001). Hypertension is defined as systolic blood pressure ≥140 mmHg and/or diastolic blood pressure ≥90 mmHg. Proteinuria is defined as ≥300 mg per 24 hours or ≥30 mg protein/mmol creatinine on spot test. For clinical purposes a looser definition is required, since women with essential hypertension or renal disease are at significantly higher risk of developing superimposed pre-eclampsia (Higgins and de Swiet 2001). Furthermore, approximately 20% of eclamptic patients and 15% of patients with HELLP syndrome (haemolysis, elevated liver enzymes and low platelets) are normotensive (Anumba and Robson 1999). Thus when there is clinical suspicion of pre-eclampsia, serial blood tests (including haemoglobin, platelet count, serum urate, renal function and liver function) may be required to confirm or refute the diagnosis.

It is almost 90 years since Zweifel called toxaemia "the disease of many theories" (Zweifel 1916). Pre-eclampsia only occurs in the presence of a placenta, and resolves within a few days of delivery. Multi-organ dysfunction (primarily vascular, renal and hepatic) underlie the maternal manifestations of the disease, and endothelial damage is thought to be primarily responsible for these problems. Current opinion suggests that abnormal placentation, characterised by failure of spiral artery conversion leading to placental bed hypoxia, predates maternal systemic symptoms (Walker 1998; Heikkila *et al.* 2001). It is hypothesised that a soluble factor released from this hypoxic placental bed causes the endothelial damage. However, failure of spiral artery conversion does not always lead to maternal symptoms, and it is also independently associated with intrauterine growth restriction (Sheppard and Bonnar 1981). Furthermore, pre-eclampsia is also known to be associated with a large placental mass in the absence of spiral artery pathology (e.g. multiple pregnancy, molar pregnancy, rhesus disease) (Walker 1998).

Incidence of PTL

It is a commonly held belief in obstetrics that pre-eclampsia is associated with premature labour, but there is no convincing evidence to support this. Since early onset pre-eclampsia is associated with intrauterine growth restriction (Long et al. 1980), it may be that an earlier generation of obstetricians and paediatricians assumed that these infants were premature as opposed to growth-restricted.

Management of PTL in a patient with pre-eclampsia

The primary cause of maternal morbidity and serious mortality from pre-eclampsia are cerebro-vascular accidents, which are associated with severe hypertension (Neilson 2001). The primary cause of neonatal mortality and morbidity in pre-eclampsia is prematurity (Long et al. 1980; Paruk and Moodley 2000). Since the only cure for pre-eclampsia/eclampsia is delivery of the placenta (i.e. delivery), it can be readily appreciated that at gestations of less than 34 weeks balancing the interests of mother and unborn child can be difficult.

Due to the associated risk of placental insufficiency leading to intrauterine growth restriction in patients with pre-eclampsia, there is an increased risk of fetal distress during labour. Ultrasound assessment of growth, liquor volume and Doppler velocimetries may assist in quantifying this risk, and continuous electronic fetal heart rate monitoring is advised during labour.

Gestation greater than 34 weeks

At gestations of greater than 34 weeks there is no doubt that delivery is in the best interests of the mother and carries little risk to fetus (given adequate neonatal care facilities). Thus labour should be allowed to continue, with close monitoring and attention to blood pressure and fluid balance.

Gestation up to 34 weeks

At gestations of less than 34 weeks, if a pre-eclamptic patient presents with preterm labour, tocolysis may be considered to enable administration of corticosteroids to enhance fetal lung maturity, or to allow transfer to a centre with appropriate neonatal intensive care facilities. However, severe pre-eclampsia (see Table 9.6) would be a contra-indication to the use of tocolysis, primarily because any significant delay in delivery will increase the risks of major complications in the mother (and thereby to her baby). Furthermore, severe pre-eclampsia is associated with pulmonary oedema, which may be exacerbated by the use of atosiban or beta-adrenergic drugs such as ritodrine. It is also worth remembering that onset of pre-eclampsia before 34 weeks is

Table 9.6. Criteria for severe pre-eclampsia

1. Systolic BP > 160 mmHg or Diastolic BP > 110 mmHg on 2 occasions, atleast 6 hours apart
2. Proteinuria > 5g/24 hours
3. Oligouria (< 400 ml/day)
4. Neurological signs or symptoms (headache, scotomata, visual blurring, altered consciousness)
5. Pulmonary oedema/cyanosis
6. Epigastric pain
7. Deranged liver function tests
8. Liver rupture/subcapsular liver haematoma
9. Thrombocytopenia < $100 \times 10^9/l$
10. HELLP syndrome

Paruk and Moodley (2000).

associated with rates of placental abruption of between 5% and 10% (Long *et al.* 1980). Abruption may not be clinically apparent but may precipitate preterm labour, and would be a further contra-indication to the use of tocolysis.

Thus in clinical practice, the use of tocolysis to attempt to delay delivery in pre-eclamptic patients with PTL is rare, and any such decision should be made at Consultant level.

Steroids

Corticosteroids to enhance fetal pulmonary maturity should be given to preterm patients with pre-eclampsia. There are no documented adverse effects on the disease process. In fact it is well recognised that a short course of high dose corticosteroids will improve the maternal platelet count and liver function, and this has been recommended as a therapeutic avenue for patients with HELLP syndrome with severe thrombocytopenia (Tompkins and Thiagarajah 1999; Isler *et al.* 2001).

Magnesium sulphate

Magnesium sulphate ($MgSO_4$) has been shown to reduce the risk of eclampsia in pre-eclamptic patients as well as reducing the incidence of recurrent fits in eclamptic patients, with a significant reduction in both maternal fetal morbidity and mortality (The Collaborative Eclampsia Trail Group 1995; The Magpie Trial Collaboration Group 2002). However, it also has a tocolytic action of similar efficacy to beta-adrenergic drugs (Macones *et al.* 1997). Thus it should be born in mind when treating pre-eclamptic patients with magnesium sulphate that it may delay spontaneous vaginal delivery. Furthermore, the use of magnesium sulphate and corticosteroids has been associated with pulmonary oedema, necessitating the need for low volume infusions and close clinical monitoring of patients (Elliott *et al.* 1979; Yeast *et al.* 1993).

Iatrogenic preterm delivery

The commonest reason for preterm delivery in pre-eclampsia is elective delivery because of concerns regarding fetal or maternal wellbeing. After 34 weeks' gestation, delivery will usually be in the best interests of mother and baby. Mode of delivery (induction of labour or elective Caesarean section) will depend on both fetal and maternal condition, past obstetric history and maternal preference. Prior to 34 weeks several small trials comparing expectant management vs. early delivery in women with severe pre-eclampsia have demonstrated a fetal advantage from expectant management at no detriment to maternal health (Sibai *et al.* 1985; Odendaal *et al.* 1987, 1990; Moodley *et al.* 1993).

A recent authoritative review suggested that the following categories of patients with pre-eclampsia be delivered within 48 hours irrespective of gestation (Paruk and Moodley 2000):

1. Thrombocytopenia $< 50 \times 10^9/l$
2. Aspartate aminotransferase/alarine aminotransferases more than twice normal range
3. Epigastric pain
4. Persistent headaches/visual disturbances
5. Pulmonary oedema
6. Rapidly deteriorating renal function tests
7. Impending eclampsia
8. Uncontrollable hypertension
9. Oliguria not responding to fluid administration
10. Severe fetal growth restriction
11. Fetal heart rate abnormalities

Delivery under these circumstances will usually be by Caesarean section given the difficulty of inducing labour at early gestation and the high incidence of fetal compromise.

Intrauterine growth restriction (IUGR)

Definition and aetiology

A growth-restricted fetus may be defined as one that has failed to reach its true growth potential. Its growth may have been impaired by hypoxia, starvation, infection, structural malformation or aneuploidy (Bobrow *et al.* 1998). For clinical purposes it is useful to divide small for gestational age (SGA) fetuses identified prospectively by ultrasound biometry into three groups:

1. Normal small fetuses (normal anatomy, normal chromosomes, normal liquor volume and normal umbilical artery end diastolic blood flow)
2. Abnormal small fetuses (structural abnormality or aneuploidy)
3. Growth-restricted fetuses (structurally and chromosomally normal, with reduced liquor volume and impaired umbilical artery end diastolic blood flow)

The first group constitute the 10% of normal fetuses whose birthweight lies below the 10th percentile. They are not growth-restricted, but remain at increased risk of perinatal morbidity and mortality (Draper et al. 1999). The second and third groups consist of pathologically small fetuses, but not all cases of intrauterine growth restriction will fulfil all these criteria. Growth restriction not associated with fetal abnormality may be due to placental insufficiency, maternal disease (including starvation) or toxins (including drugs, smoking and infection). However, only those cases associated with placental insufficiency or fetal hypoxia would be expected to show abnormalities of liquor volume or umbilical artery blood flow. Where there is doubt, serial ultrasound measurements will identify a reduced growth velocity pathognomonic of true growth restriction (Chang et al. 1993).

Incidence of PTL

Undoubtedly, proportionally more growth-restricted fetuses are delivered preterm than term, but this is primarily due to iatrogenic intervention. There are no good data to confirm a higher incidence of spontaneous PTL associated with growth-restricted fetuses.

Management of PTL associated with IUGR

Diagnosis

It may be that when a patient presents in threatened preterm labour, the fetus is already known to be growth-restricted. However, where possible all women presenting in threatened preterm labour should have an ultrasound assessment including fetal presentation, biometry (estimated fetal weight), liquor volume and umbilical artery Doppler. The more information available regarding fetal size and condition, the more informed the choices that can be made regarding management. If the fetus falls into the second diagnostic group (structural or chromosomal abnormality), then the parents may not wish for fetal monitoring or intervention.

Tocolysis

Neonatal morbidity and mortality are critically dependent on gestation (e.g. survival for a 500 g fetus born at 26 weeks is around 40%, rising to around 60% at 28 weeks) (Draper et al. 1999); thus prolonging gestation where possible is vitally important. However, the usual contra-indications to tocolysis apply (Chapter 7), and given that many growth-restricted fetuses will have associated mal-placentation there are increased risks of both placental abruption and fetal distress (Krebs *et al.* 1996).

Steroids

Corticosteroids to enhance fetal pulmonary maturity should be given (Chapter 7).

Monitoring

Growth-restricted fetuses are at increased risk of intrapartum fetal distress, hypoxia, neonatal encephalopathy and stillbirth (Lin *et al.* 1991; Confidential Enquiry into Stillbirths and Deaths in Infancy 1995; Krebs *et al.* 1996; Badawi *et al.* 1998). Using cordocentesis it has been demonstrated that 31% of small for gestational age fetuses with normal umbilical and uterine artery blood flow are hypoxic prior to labour, rising to 63% if either the umbilical or uterine artery waveforms are abnormal, with 86% hypoxic if both uterine and umbilical artery waveforms are abnormal (Nicolaides *et al.* 1989). It is well recognised that labour itself causes relative hypoxia and acidosis in a normal term fetus (Boylan and Parisi 1994), and the effects of this may be catastrophic in a preterm growth-restricted fetus that is already hypoxic (Westgren *et al.* 1984). Prematurity compounds the adverse effects of fetal hypoxia, with neonatal mortality (23% vs. 3%) and major neurological deficit at 1 year (27% vs. 13%) significantly higher in acidotic preterm babies than in non-acidotic babies matched for birthweight and gestation (Low *et al.* 1992).

Thus continuous electronic fetal heart rate monitoring is mandatory during PTL with a growth-restricted fetus (RCOG Clinical Effectiveness Support Unit 2001). Cardiotocography using an ultrasound transducer is the usual method for monitoring the fetal heart rate, though use of a fetal scalp electrode is not contra-indicated. Abnormal (suspicious) fetal heart rate monitoring is an indication for urgent delivery. Prior to 34 weeks' gestation there is no place for fetal scalp blood sampling, since in the one study which reported on its use, it was associated with a delay in delivery and increased rates of cerebral palsy (Luthy *et al.* 1987; Shy *et al.* 1990). Furthermore, in pregnancies where the fetus is already known to be at significant risk of hypoxia (i.e. abnormal umbilical artery blood flow) it would be reasonable to offer elective caesarean section prior to the occurrence of fetal heart rate abnormalities.

Transfer to a unit with neonatal intensive care facilities

Growth restriction compounds the problems associated with prematurity, such as hypoglycaemia, hypoxic ischaemic encephalopathy and necrotising enterocolitis. Availability of paediatric assessment and resuscitation at delivery and access to neonatal intensive care is therefore extremely important. If possible, in utero transfer is preferable to extra-uterine transfer, given the problems of transporting tiny ventilated infants.

Mode of delivery

As discussed above, preterm growth-restricted infants are at extremely high risk of neonatal morbidity and mortality, and these risks may be increased as a result of intrapartum hypoxia. For these reasons, there should be a low threshold for delivery by caesarean section, especially prior to 34 weeks' gestation. This recommendation is based on expert opinion, since no trial has specifically compared mode of delivery and outcome in growth-restricted preterm infants, The caesarean section itself may be technically challenging, with a poorly formed lower segment, oligohydramnios and frequent malpresentation. At the extremes of viability (less than 28 weeks), the poor prognosis for a growth-restricted infant irrespective of mode of delivery should be discussed with the parents (Draper *et al.* 1999). At such early gestation, the likely need for a midline uterine incision that may seriously compromise the future reproductive performance of the mother should preclude operative delivery in most cases.

Iatrogenic PTD

Most growth-restricted fetuses that are identified antenatally will be delivered electively once there is evidence of fetal compromise. Given the difficulty of successfully inducing labour preterm and the risks of labour to the fetus outlined above, elective delivery will usually be by caesarean section. Timing the delivery to achieve the best perinatal outcome remains controversial, however, the findings of the Growth Restriction Intervention Trial (GRIT) Study Group (2003) suggest that (at least within the trial) obstetricians were judging timing of delivery correctly. It is clear from the survival data from the Trent region that for any given birthweight, survival increases with maturity to 32 weeks (Draper *et al.* 2003). Thus so long as there is not evidence of acute fetal compromise, it is likely that prolonging gestation to at least 32 weeks is beneficial.

Conclusions

i. Multifetal pregnancy is a major cause of preterm labour, and the incidence is increasing due to the increasing use of assisted reproductive technologies. Good antenatal care has been shown to reduce preterm delivery rates and improve neonatal outcomes. Screening tests based on ultrasound measurements of cervical length or on the detection of fetal fibronectin in cervical secretions are effective in predicting increased risk, but no interventional studies based on these screening tests have been shown to improve outcome. Investigation and treatment of threatened preterm labour is similar to that in singleton pregnancies. A policy of routine Caesarean delivery does not improve outcomes, and there is evidence that prophylactic repeat courses of antenatal corticosteroids may be detrimental to neonatal outcome.

ii. There is no evidence to support the commonly held notion that pre-eclampsia is associated with an increased incidence of spontaneous preterm labour. Tocolysis may be indicated to allow time for corticosteroids to promote fetal lung maturity, but in practice either the fetal or maternal manifestations of the disease process are usually a contra-indication.

iii. There is no good evidence to suggest that IUGR is associated with an increased risk of spontaneous preterm labour. However, it has been demonstrated that both SGA and IUGR fetuses are at significant risk of intrauterine hypoxia, which will be exacerbated by the effects of labour. Prematurity significantly worsens the prognosis for such fetuses, in terms of both perinatal mortality and neurological outcome. Prolonging pregnancy beyond 30 completed weeks may provide significant outcome benefits for a severely growth-restricted fetus; however, delivery by Caesarean section may be indicated where significant concern exists regarding fetal wellbeing.

REFERENCES

Anumba, D. O. and Robson, S. C. (1999) Management of pre-eclampsia and haemolysis, elevated liver enzymes, and low platelets syndrome. *Curr. Opin. Obstet. Gynecol.* **11**, 149–56.

Badawi, N., Kurinczuk, J. J., Keogh, J. M. *et al.* (1998) Antepartum risk factors for newborn encephalopathy: the Western Australian case-control study. *BMJ* **317**, 1554–8

Bajoria, R., Wee, L. Y., Anwar, S. and Ward, S. (1999) Outcome of twin pregnancies complicated by single intrauterine death in relation to vascular anatomy of the monochorionic placenta. *Hum. Reprod.* **14**, 2124–30.

Barrett, J. M., Staggs, S. M., Van Hooydonk, J. E. *et al.* (1982) The effect of type of delivery upon neonatal outcome in premature twins. *Am. J. Obstet. Gynecol.* **143**, 360–7.

Bell, D., Johansson, D., McLean, F. H. and Usher, R. H. (1986) Birth asphyxia, trauma, and mortality in twins: has Cesarean section improved outcome? *Am. J. Obstet. Gynecol.* **154**, 235–9.

Bennett, C. C., Lal, M. K., Field, D. J. and Wilkinson, A. R. (2002) Maternal morbidity and pregnancy outcome in a cohort of mothers transferred out of perinatal centres during a national census. *BJOG* **109**, 663–6.

Bobrow, C., Holmes, R. and Soothill, P. W. (1998) Aetiology of small for gestational age fetuses. In J. Studd, ed. *Progress in Obstetrics and Gynaecology 13*. Edinburgh: Churchill Livingstone, pp. 113–26.

Boylan, P. C. and Parisi, V. M. (1994) Fetal acid-base balance. In R. K. Creasy and R. Resnik, eds., *Maternal Fetal Medicine*. Philadelphia: W. B. Saunders, pp. 349–58.

Brocklehurst, P., Gates, S., McKenzie-McHarg, K., Alfirevic, Z. and Chamberlain, G. (1999) Are we prescribing multiple courses of antenatal corticosteroids? A survey of practice in the UK. *BJOG* **106**, 977–9.

Brown, M. A., Lindeheimer, M. D., de Suite, M., Van Assche, A. and Moutquin, J-M. (2001) The classification and diagnosis of hypertensive disorders of pregnancy: statement from the International Society for the Study of Hypertension in Pregnancy (ISSHP). *Hypertens. Pregnancy* **20**, ix–xiv.

Caspi, E., Ronen, J., Schreyer, P. and Goldberg, M. D. (1976) The outcome of pregnancy after gonadotrophin therapy. *BJOG* **83**, 967–73.

Chang, T. C., Robson, S. C., Spencer, J. A. and Gallivan, S. (1993) Identification of fetal growth retardation: comparison of Doppler waveform indices and serial ultrasound measurements of abdominal circumference and fetal weight. *Obstet. Gynecol.* **82**, 230–6.

Collins, M. S. and Bley, J. A. (1990) Seventy-one quadruplet pregnancies: management and outcome. *Am. J. Obstet. Gynecol.* **162**, 1384–91.

Confidential Enquiry into Stillbirths and Deaths in Infancy. (1995) Annual report for 1993. London: Dept. of Health.

Crowley, P. (2000) Prophylactic corticosteroids for preterm birth. *Cochrane Database Syst. Rev.* 2, CD000065.

Crowther, C. A. and Hamilton, R. A. (1989) Triplet pregnancy: a 10-year review of 105 cases at Harare Maternity Hospital, Zimbabwe. *Acta Genet. Med. Gemellol. (Roma)* **38**, 271–8.

Crowther, C. A. (2001) Hospitalisation and bed rest for multiple pregnancy. *Cochrane Database Syst. Rev.* 1, CD000110.

Crowther, C. A., Verkuyl, D. A., Ashworth, M. F., Bannerman, C. and Ashurst, H. M. (1991) The effects of hospitalization for bed rest on duration of gestation, fetal growth and neonatal morbidity in triplet pregnancy. *Acta Genet. Med. Gemellol. (Roma)* **40**, 63–8.

Davison, L., Easterling, T. R., Jackson, J. C. and Benedetti, T. J. (1992) Breech extraction of low-birthweight second twins: can cesarean section be justified? *Am. J. Obstet. Gynecol.* **166**, 497–502.

Dommergues, M., Mahieu-Caputo, D., Mandelbrot, L. *et al.* (1995) Delivery of uncomplicated triplet pregnancies: is the vaginal route safer? A case-control study. *Am. J. Obstet. Gynecol.* **172**, 513–17.

Doyle, L. W., Hughes, C. D., Guaran, R. L., Quinn, M. A. and Kitchen, W. H. (1988) Mode of delivery of preterm twins. *Aust. N. Z. J. Obstet. Gynaecol.* **28**, 25–8.

Draper, E. S., Manktelow, B., Field, D. J. and James, D. (2003) Tables for predicting survival for preterm births are updated. *BMJ* **327**, 872.

Dyson, D. C., Crites, Y. M., Ray, D. A. and Armstrong, M. A. (1991) Prevention of preterm birth in high-risk patients: the role of education and provider contact versus home uterine monitoring. *Am. J. Obstet. Gynecol.* **164**, 756–62.

Dyson, D. C., Danbe, K. H., Bamber, J. A. (1998) Monitoring women at risk for preterm labour. *N. Engl. J. Med.* **338**, 15–19.

Elliott, J. P., O'Keeffe, D. F., Greenberg, P. and Freeman, R. K. (1979) Pulmonary edema associated with magnesium sulfate and betamethasone administration. *Am. J. Obstet. Gynecol.* **134**, 717–19.

Fabre, E., Gonzalez de Aguero, R., de Agustin, J. L., Perez-Hiraldo, M. P. and Bescos, J. L. (1988) Perinatal mortality in twin pregnancy: an analysis of birthweight-specific mortality rates and adjusted mortality rates for birthweight distributions. *J. Perinat. Med.* **16**, 85–91.

Gardner, M. O., Goldenberg, R. L., Cliver, S. P. *et al.* (1995) The origin and outcome of preterm twin pregnancies. *Obstet. Gynecol.* **85**, 553–7.

Goldenberg, R. L., Iams, J. D., Miodovnik, M. *et al.* (1996) The preterm prediction study: risk factors in twin gestations. National Institute of Child Health and Human Development Maternal-Fetal Medicine Units Network. *Am. J. Obstet. Gynecol.* **175**, 1047–53.

Grant, A. (1989) Cervical cerclage to prolong pregnancy. In I. Chalmers, M. Enkin and M. J. N. C. Keirse, eds., *Effective Care in Pregnancy and Childbirth.* Oxford: Oxford University Press, pp. 633–45.

Green, P. M. and Wilkinshaw, S. (2002) Management of breech deliveries. *The Obstetrician and Gynaecologist* **4**, 87–91.

Hannah, M. E., Hannah, W. J., Hewson, S. A. (2000) Planned Caesarean section versus planned vaginal birth for breech presentation at term: a randomised multicentre trial. Term Breech Trial Collaborative Group. *Lancet* **356**, 1375–83.

Heikkila, A., Makkonen, N., Heinonen, S. and Kirkinen, P. (2001) Elevated maternal serum hCG in the second trimester increases prematurity rate and need for neonatal intensive care in primiparous preeclamptic pregnancies. *Hypertens. Pregnancy* **20**, 99–106.

Higgins, J. R. and de Swiet, M. (2001) Blood-pressure measurement and classification in pregnancy. *Lancet* **357**, 131–5.

Howie, P. W. (1995) The coagulation and fibrinolytic systems, and their disorders in obstetrics and gynaecology. In C. R. Whitfield, ed., *Dewhurst's Textbook of Obstetrics and Gynaecology for Postgraduates.* Oxford: Blackwell Science Ltd., pp. 510–26.

Isler, C. M., Barrilleaux, P. S., Magann, E. F., Bass, J. D. and Martin, J. N., Jr. (2001) A prospective, randomized trial comparing the efficacy of dexamethasone and betamethasone for the treatment of antepartum HELLP (hemolysis, elevated liver enzymes, and low platelet count) syndrome. *Am. J. Obstet. Gynecol.* **184**, 1332–7.

Keirse, M. J. N. C., Grant, A. and King, J. F. (1989) Preterm labour. In I. Chalmers, M. Enkin and M. J. N. C. Keirse, eds., *Effective Care in Pregnancy and Childbirth.* Oxford: Oxford University Press, pp. 694–749.

Kiely, J. L. (1990) The epidemiology of perinatal mortality in multiple births. *Bull. N. Y. Acad. Med.* **66**, 618–37.

Krebs, C., Macara, L. M., Leiser, R. *et al.* (1996) Intrauterine growth restriction with absent end-diastolic flow velocity in the umbilical artery is associated with maldevelopment of the placental terminal villous tree. *Am. J. Obstet. Gynecol.* **175**, 1534–42.

Lin, C. C. Su, S. J. and River, L. P. (1991) Comparison of associated high-risk factors and perinatal outcome between symmetric and asymmetric fetal intrauterine growth retardation. *Am. J. Obstet. Gynecol.* **164**, 1535–41.

Little, J. and Thompson, B. (1988) Descriptive epidemiology. In I. MacGillivray, D. M. Campbell and B. Thompson, eds., *Twinning and Twins*. Chichester: John Wiley, pp. 37–66.

Long, P. A., Abell, D. A. and Beischer, N. A. (1980) Fetal growth retardation and pre-eclampsia. *BJOG* **87**, 13–18.

Low, J. A., Galbraith, R. S., Muir, D. W. *et al.* (1992) Mortality and morbidity after intrapartum asphyxia in the preterm fetus. *Obstet. Gynecol.* **80**, 57–61.

Luke, B., Brown, M. B., Misiunas, R. *et al.* (2003) Specialized prenatal care and maternal and infant outcomes in twin pregnancy. *Am. J. Obstet. Gynecol.* **189**, 934–8.

Luthy, D. A., Shy, K. K., van Belle, G. *et al.* (1987) A randomized trial of electronic fetal monitoring in preterm labour. *Obstet. Gynecol.* **69**, 687–95.

Macones, G. A., Sehdev, H. M., Berlin, M., Morgan, M. A. and Berlin, J. A. (1997) Evidence for magnesium sulfate as a tocolytic agent. *Obstet. Gynecol. Surv.* **52**, 652–8.

Moodley, J., Koranteng, S. A. and Rout, C. (1993) Expectant management of early onset of severe pre-eclampsia in Durban. *S. Afr. Med. J.* **83**, 584–7.

Morales, W. J. O'Brien, W. F., Knuppel, R. A., Gaylord, S. and Hayes, P. (1989) The effect of mode of delivery on the risk of intraventricular hemorrhage in nondiscordant twin gestations under 1500 g. *Obstet Gynecol.* **73**, 107–10.

Mordel, N., Zajicek, G., Benshushan, A. *et al.* (1993) Elective suture of uterine cervix in triplets. *Am. J. Perinatol.* **10**, 14–16.

Murphy, D. J., Caukwell, S., Joels, L. A. and Wardle, P. (2002) Cohort study of the neonatal outcome of twin pregnancies that were treated with prophylactic or rescue antenatal corticosteroids. *Am. J. Obstet. Gynecol.* **187**, 483–8.

Neilson, J. P. (2001) Hypertensive diseases of pregnancy. In G. Lewis, ed., *Why Mothers die 1997–1999. The Fifth Report of the Confidential Enquiries into Maternal Deaths in the United Kingdom.* London: RCOG Press, pp. 76–93.

Newman, R. B., Krombach, R. S., Myers, M. C. and McGee, D. L. (2002) Effect of cerclage on obstetrical outcome in twin gestations with a shortened cervical length. *Am. J. Obstet. Gynecol.* **186**, 634–40.

Nicolaides, K. H., Economides, D. L. and Soothill, P. W. (1989) Blood gases, pH, and lactate in appropriate- and small-for-gestational- age fetuses. *Am. J. Obstet. Gynecol.* **161**, 996–1001.

Nyberg, D. A., Filly, R. A., Golbus, M. S. and Stephens, J. D. (1984) Entangled umbilical cords: a sign of monoamniotic twins. *J. Ultrasound Med.* **3**, 29–32.

O'Connor, M. C., Murphy, H. and Dalrymple, I. J. (1979) Double blind trial of ritodrine and placebo in twin pregnancy. *BJOG* **86**, 706–9.

Oconnor, R. A. and Hiadzi, E. (1996) The intrapartum management of twin pregnancies. In J. Studd, ed., *Progress in Obstetrics and Gynaecology*, vol. 12. Edinburgh: Churchill Livingstone, pp. 121–34.

Odendaal, H. J., Pattinson, R. C. and du Toit, R. (1987) Fetal and neonatal outcome in patients with severe pre-eclampsia before 34 weeks. *S. Afr. Med. J.* **71**, 555–8.

Odendaal, H. J., Pattinson, R. C., Bam, R., Grove, D. and Kotze, T. J. (1990) Aggressive or expectant management for patients with severe preeclampsia between 28–34 weeks' gestation: a randomized controlled trial. *Obstet. Gynecol.* **76**, 1070–5.

Paruk, F. and Moodley, J. (2000) Treatment of severe pre-eclampsia/eclampsia syndrome. In J. Studd, ed., *Progress in Obstetrics and Gynaecology 14*. Edinburgh: Churchill Livingstone, pp. 102–19.

Patel, N., Barrie, W., Campbell, D. *et al.* (1984) Scottish twin study; preliminary report. Glasgow, University of Glasgow.

Peek, M. J., McCarthy, A., Kyle, P., Sepulveda, W. and Fisk, N. M. (1997) Medical amnioreduction with sulindac to reduce cord complications in monoamniotic twins. *Am. J. Obstet. Gynecol.* **176**, 334–6.

Rasanen, J. and Jouppila, P. (1995) Fetal cardiac function and ductus arteriosus during indomethacin and sulindac therapy for threatened preterm labour: a randomized study. *Am. J. Obstet. Gynecol.* **173**, 20–5.

Royal College of Obstetricians and Gynaecologists (RCOG) (2001) *RCOG Guideline No 20: The management of breech presentation*. London: RCOG.

Royal College of Obstetricians and Gynaecologists (RCOG) Clinical Effectiveness Support Unit. (2001) *The use of electronic fetal monitoring: the use and interpretation of cardiotocography in intrapartum fetal surveillance*. London: RCOG Press.

Rydhstrom, H. (1990) Prognosis for twins with birthweight less than 1500 gm: the impact of cesarean section in relation to fetal presentation. *Am. J. Obstet. Gynecol.* **163**, 528–33.

Seki, H., Kuromaki, K., Takeda, S. and Kinoshita, K. (2000) Prophylactic cervical cerclage for the prevention of early premature delivery in nulliparous women with twin pregnancies. *J. Obstet. Gynaecol. Res.* **26**, 151–2.

Sheppard, B. L. and Bonnar, J. (1981) An ultrastructural study of utero-placental spiral arteries in hypertensive and normotensive pregnancy and fetal growth retardation. *BJOG* **88**, 695–705.

Shy, K. K., Luthy, D. A., Bennett, F. C. *et al.* (1990) Effects of electronic fetal-heart-rate monitoring, as compared with periodic auscultation, on the neurologic development of premature infants. *N. Engl. J. Med.* **322**, 588–93.

Sibai, B. M., Taslimi, M., Abdella, T. N. *et al.* (1985) Maternal and perinatal outcome of conservative management of severe pre-eclampsia in midtrimester. *Am. J. Obstet. Gynecol.* **152**, 32–7.

Smith, G. C., Pell, J. P. and Dobbie, R. (2002) Birth order, gestational age, and risk of delivery related perinatal death in twins: retrospective cohort study. *BMJ* **325**, 1004–9.

Strauss, A., Heer, I. M., Janssen, U. *et al.* (2002) Routine cervical cerclage in higher-order multiple gestation - does it prolong the pregnancy? *Twin Res.* **5**, 67–70.

Sutton, D. M. C., Hauser, R., Kulapong, P. and Bachmann, F. (1971) Intravascular coagulation in abruptio placentae. *Am. J. Obstet. Gynecol.* **109**, 604–14.

Taylor, M. J. O. and Fisk, N. M. (2000) Multiple pregnancy. *The Obstetrician and Gynaecologist* **2**, 4–10.

The Chums Group. (1995) A multicenter randomized controlled trial of home uterine monitoring: active versus sham device. The Collaborative Home Uterine Monitoring Study (CHUMS) Group. *Am. J. Obstet. Gynecol.* **173**, 1120–7.

The Collaborative Eclampsia Trial Group. (1995) Which anticonvulsant for women with eclampsia? Evidence from the Collaborative Eclampsia Trial. *Lancet* **345**, 1455–63.

The GRIT Study Group. (2003) A randomised trial of timed delivery for the compromised preterm fetus: short term outcomes and Bayesian interpretation. *BJOG* **110**, 27–32.

The Magpie Trial Collaboration Group. (2002) Do women with pre-eclampsia, and their babies, benefit from magnesium sulphate? The Magpie Trial: a randomised placebo-controlled trial. *Lancet* **359**, 1877–90.

Tompkins, M. J. and Thiagarajah, S. (1999) HELLP (hemolysis, elevated liver enzymes, and low platelet count) syndrome: the benefit of corticosteroids. *Am. J. Obstet. Gynecol.* **181**, 304–9.

Vintzileos, A. M., Ananth, C. V., Smulian, J. C. and Scorza, W. E. (2003) The impact of prenatal care on preterm births among twin gestations in the United States, 1989–2000. *Am. J. Obstet. Gynecol.* **189**, 818–23.

Walker, J. J. (1998) Current thoughts on the pathophysiology of pre-eclampsia/eclampsia. In J. Studd, ed., *Progress in Obstetrics and Gynaecology 13*. Edinburgh: Churchill Livingstone, pp. 177–90.

Wapner, R., Cotton, D., Artal, R., Librizzi, R. and Ross, M. (1995) A randomized multicenter trial assessing a home uterine activity monitoring device used in the absence of daily nursing contact. *Am. J. Obstet. Gynecol.* **172**, 1026–34.

Wennerholm, U. B., Holm, B., Mattsby-Baltzer, I. (1997) Fetal fibronectin, endotoxin, bacterial vaginosis and cervical length as predictors of preterm birth and neonatal morbidity in twin pregnancies. *BJOG* **104**, 1398–404.

Westgren, M., Hormquist, P., Ingemarsson, I. and Svenningsen, N. (1984) Intrapartum fetal acidosis in preterm infants: fetal monitoring and long-term morbidity. *Obstet. Gynecol.* **63**, 355–9.

Yang, J. H., Kuhlman, K., Daly, S. and Berghella, V. (2000) Prediction of preterm birth by second trimester cervical sonography in twin pregnancies. *Ultrasound Obstet. Gynecol.* **15**, 288–91.

Yeast, J. D., Halberstadt, C., Meyer, B. A., Cohen, G. R. and Thorp, J. A. (1993) The risk of pulmonary edema and colloid osmotic pressure changes during magnesium sulfate infusion. *Am. J. Obstet. Gynecol.* **169**, 1566–71.

Zweifel, P. (1916) Eclampsie. In A. Doderlein, ed., *Handbuch der Gerburtshilfe, II*. Wiesbarden: Bergman, pp. 672–6.

10

Anaesthetic issues in preterm labour, and intensive care management of the sick parturient

Anne May and Chris Elton

Introduction

The anaesthetist is an essential part of the team caring for a woman who is to undergo a preterm delivery of her baby or babies. The anaesthetist is also involved in managing sick women and women who are at risk of a preterm delivery, and it is therefore important that the anaesthetist is involved in the care of these women early and that communication is excellent. This is a stressful time for the woman and her family and they are usually extremely anxious and are subjected to information from many sources. Inconsistency in this information can be disastrous. There are many situations where the obstetric team focus on preventing preterm labour and may be unwilling to discuss the scenario "what if this delivery is inevitable?" with the woman and her family. Management of the labour and delivery from the analgesic and anaesthetic point of view may become rushed, suboptimal and without adequate discussion of risks and benefits.

It is worthwhile mentioning the anaesthetic risks of pregnant women and, in particular, the increased risks associated with emergency general anaesthesia, especially when the woman is sick. Though the number of direct deaths due to anaesthesia has fallen as documented in successive Reports on the Confidential Enquiries into Maternal Deaths (CEMD) (Department of Health 1998, 2001) there are a significant number of indirect deaths where anaesthesia has contributed. There are an increasing number of women with significant intercurrent medical problems who become pregnant and many of those are at risk of a preterm delivery. The anaesthetic risks for these women are high and team planning early in pregnancy is essential. The anaesthetic chapter entitled "Obstetric Anaesthesia – Delays and Complications" in the 7th Annual Report of the Confidential Enquiry into Stillbirths and Deaths in Infancy (CESDI) (Maternal and Child Health Research Consortium 2000) discusses many anaesthetic problems that are particularly relevant in the care of women delivering preterm and also the morbidity that may be associated with general anaesthesia.

Preterm Labour Managing Risk in Clinical Practice, eds. Jane Norman and Ian Greer. Published by Cambridge University Press. © Cambridge University Press 2005.

Work to date on the 27/28 CESDI project (Macintosh 2003) supports the assertion that the analgesic and anaesthetic management of women delivering at this gestation is far from ideal. A recent special report (Holdcroft *et al.* 2003) on small babies and substandard anaesthesia highlighted that in one in ten deliveries there was a failure of anaesthetic management with a significant number of these deliveries classed as needing immediate delivery.

The aim of this chapter is to highlight the areas where the anaesthetist should be involved as part of the team and where anaesthetic expertise can improve the outcome for both mother and baby. It will also explain the limitations of anaesthetic intervention and/or support.

Though the focus of the chapter will be on women in whom delivery is inevitable, there are other areas where the anaesthetist is involved and, therefore, we will review these accordingly.

1. Where there is an increased risk of precipitating labour.
   - Trauma
   - Coincidental surgery
   - Cervical cerclage (rescue).
2. Planned preterm delivery.
   - Fetal reasons
   - Maternal health reasons.
3. Where the delivery is inevitable.

Situations where there is an increased risk of precipitating labour

The specific problems and considerations of non-obstetric emergencies in pregnant women are often ignored. The incidence of emergency surgery in pregnant women is around 2% (Brodsky *et al.* 1980). In addition pregnant women will present with medical emergencies. The most common problems are:

- Trauma
- Obstetric interventions such as cervical cerclage
- Acute abdomen, e.g. ovarian cyst, cholycystitis, appendicitis.
- Biopsy of a suspicious mass, e.g. lymph glands, breast lump.
- Resuscitation, e.g. attempted suicide, convulsions, infection and other medical emergencies.
- Investigations, e.g. computed tomography and magnetic resonance imaging scans.

Routine surgery is delayed for pregnant women wherever possible and therefore those women who have surgery are often seriously ill. In particular, in the Accident and Emergency department, the physiological changes of pregnancy, the effects of drugs that are administered, and the risk of premature delivery and miscarriage may be overlooked, as many of these women are looked after by a team that has no specialist knowledge of pregnancy.

Obstetricians should ensure that they are involved in the care of these women and that anaesthetic involvement should be by an obstetric anaesthetist or someone with significant training in obstetric anaesthesia.

The main areas of concern are the maintenance of the normal physiology of pregnancy, in particular that normal cardiovascular and respiratory physiology are maintained wherever possible. There are three areas where the obstetrician can give invaluable support and advice to these patients.

- Fetal monitoring
- The risk of premature delivery and the use of tocolytic drugs
- Drug treatments, in particular analgesics.

Fetal monitoring

Surgery and anaesthesia may alter uterine activity and placental perfusion and this will affect the condition of the fetus. The use of fetal monitoring is to be recommended for a viable fetus, though monitoring during a surgical procedure is controversial and may be difficult to perform. Pre- and post-operative monitoring is to be recommended. For intraoperative monitoring a transvaginal ultrasound probe may be used (Rosen 1999). Erroneous interpretation of the cardiotocograph (CTG) has led to unnecessary delivery by Caesarean section (Immer-Bansi *et al.* 2001) as loss of beat-to-beat variability and baseline fetal heart rate (FHR) due to anaesthetic drugs cause difficulties in interpretation.

It is important to avoid hypoxia and hypotension and to ensure that aorto-caval compression is avoided at all times.

Risk of premature delivery and miscarriage

Miscarriage or premature delivery may be a direct result of the medical emergency or the treatment administered. As described above the risks and benefits of any drug treatment need to be assessed. The anxiety and stress of the disease will also play an important part and the risks can be minimised by optimising the maternal and fetal wellbeing. Catecholamines are increased by pain and anxiety and high catecholamine levels adversely affect uterine blood flow (Shnider *et al.* 1979). Fetal loss is highest with lower abdominal surgery.

Indomethacin, magnesium sulphate and β-sympathomimetic drugs may be used to prevent preterm labour though there is no conclusive evidence as to their effectiveness (see Chapter 8). It may be more important to reduce the levels of endogenous catecholamines circulating in the mother and anxiolytics such as benzodiazepines should be considered.

Drug treatment

The effects of drugs on the fetus are divided according to the stage of the fetal development and the time of preterm delivery falls into the fetal phase. At this stage most organs are fully formed though the cerebral cortex, cerebellum and urogenital tract are still continuing to develop. Drugs administered during this time may affect the growth of the fetus or the functional development within specific organs (Anonymous 1996).

A clear understanding of physiology and pharmacology will ensure that drugs are administered carefully to pregnant women.

The following are affected by pregnancy:

- Absorption: both the oral and inhalational route are affected. The oral route may be affected by the nausea and vomiting associated with pregnancy and the reduced gastric pH. Absorption of inhalational agents is more rapid due to the increased minute ventilation and cardiac output.
- Distribution: there is a greater volume for distribution as well as the altered plasma protein profile. The fetus also represents another compartment for the distribution of drugs.
- Transfer to the fetus: this depends on the lipid solubility, pKa and protein binding of the drug.
- Metabolism: some drugs are metabolised by plasma cholinesterase (e.g. suxamethonium) and the levels of this decrease in pregnancy thus reducing metabolism. The liver functions normally in pregnancy unless the woman develops a disease affecting the liver, the most common disease being HELLP (haemolysis, elevated liver enzymes and low platelet count) which is associated with pre-eclampsia.
- Elimination: increased renal and respiratory elimination of drugs.

There is a reluctance to administer drugs to the pregnant woman despite the importance of treating the underlying medical or surgical condition. In balancing the risks and benefits of treatment we should ensure that the mother's condition is correctly treated. The excellent review by Rathmell *et al.* (1997) on the management of pain during pregnancy and lactation discusses the risks and benefits of commonly used drugs in the treatment of pain. The three groups of drugs commonly used in the treatment of pain are opioids, non-steroidal anti-inflammatory drugs (NSAIDs) and local anaesthetics. The use of opioids in the short-term management of post-operative pain is very different from the use of opioids in the drug-abusing mother. It is important to remember the alterations in fetal heart rate patterns that occur and the difficulties in using the CTG as a reassurance of fetal wellbeing. Standard post-operative treatment of pain should not be withheld from pregnant mothers and the use of intramuscular or patient controlled analgesia using morphine should be an integral part of their care. There has been a reluctance to use NSAIDs in pregnancy due to the risks of decrease in amniotic fluid and closure of the ductus arteriosus in the fetus, though they are excellent drugs in the treatment of musculoskeletal and post-operative pain. The United States Food and Drug Administration (FDA) pregnancy risk classification categories for medications used in pain management grades is useful when assessing the risks and benefits of treatment for the pregnant patient.

Local anaesthetics may be used as an integral part of the treatment and this will include the use of regional analgesia and anaesthesia. Local anaesthetics may be combined with opioids and administered by the epidural or spinal route.

The specific anaesthetic requirements for this group of patients are the same as any pregnant woman though there are additional factors that should be considered. All these women are very anxious and need a sympathetic approach from the anaesthetist. The preoperative discussion should include the risks and benefits of the various anaesthetic techniques and the anaesthetist needs to be aware of specific anxieties of the woman and, wherever possible, to reassure her. When the surgery can be performed under local or regional anaesthesia this is the method of choice; however, there are many major surgical procedures where general anaesthesia is essential. In these cases standard techniques to minimise the risks of general anaesthesia in pregnancy must be adhered to. Epidural analgesia should be considered as an integral part of the anaesthetic management allowing the epidural to be used for postoperative analgesia.

Laparoscopic surgery is increasingly used and there are special problems that should be considered. The use of carbon dioxide to provide a pneumoperitoneum has led to concern that maternal and fetal acidosis may develop with detrimental effects on both mother and fetus. There has been concern that capnography underestimates the maternal ventilation as it does not adequately monitor carbon dioxide levels and the work by Cruz et al. (1996) on pregnant ewes recommended that maternal carbon dioxide levels should be monitored using an arterial line. However, work using data from the Swedish Health Registry (Reedy et al. 1997) would not support routine arterial blood gas monitoring and this is endorsed by Steinbrook and Datta (1997). The use of the lowest pressure pneumoperitoneum to minimise aorto-caval compression should be used.

Planned preterm delivery

This may be as a result of:
- Fetal reasons
- Maternal health reasons.

A significant number of preterm deliveries are planned induction of labour or Caesarean section. Early delivery may be as a result of fetal deterioration, maternal deterioration or a combination of the two. Increasing numbers of women become pregnant with medical conditions that in the past were not associated with survival to adult life, and these conditions such as pulmonary hypertension may deteriorate during pregnancy, which may in turn cause fetal compromise. Alternatively, disorders of the fetus, placenta or uterus may cause fetal compromise, necessitating delivery. In practice most common disorders that require early delivery affect both mother and fetus (e.g. pre-eclampsia). Team planning is paramount to improve outcome and this care is best provided by teams of obstetricians (feto-maternal medicine consultants), neonatologists and obstetric anaesthetists, with physician, radiological, surgical and intensive care input where appropriate. Not all delivery units will have such teams at their disposal suggesting the need at least for discussion if not referral to a regional centre. Societies such as the Obstetric Anaesthetists Association (UK) and the Society of Obstetric Anesthesia and Perinatology (USA) have a role in establishing high-risk databases of previous cases.

Planned preterm delivery for fetal reasons

Assessment of the fetus in utero is discussed in Chapters 7 to 9. In general fetal wellbeing is commonly assessed by cardiotocography, growth assessment, fetal movement, Doppler ultrasound and limited invasive investigation of the fetus. On a simple level the decision to deliver is based on the apparent nutrition and oxygenation of the fetus or evidence of impending fetal jeopardy (e.g. presence of reversed end diastolic umbilical flows). It is important that the anaesthetist understands the effects of labour, pain of labour and anaesthetic interventions on the fetus. A compromised feto-placental unit will respond adversely to decreased blood flow to the placenta, which may be caused by pain-induced catecholamine release, changes in carbon dioxide concentration and the haemodynamic changes induced by regional neuronal blockade.

Planned preterm delivery for maternal reasons

Maternal illness may be congenital or acquired, or the illness may be unique to pregnancy, may only be clinically apparent in pregnancy or be exacerbated by pregnancy. Some maternal illnesses may even be improved by pregnancy. The mainstay of feto-maternal medicine is that once a decision is made to continue with pregnancy, then expectant management occurs in an attempt to continue the pregnancy to as late a gestation as possible. (In many countries terminating the pregnancy because it constitutes a threat to the mother's life is an option.) Liaison with the anaesthetic team is important during this management because necessary anaesthesia or analgesia for delivery may dramatically lead to a deterioration in the clinical condition, even when the woman has relatively mild symptoms (e.g. aortic stenosis).

There is an increasing trend to view childbirth as a physiological process that should be managed by midwifery staff without medical intervention. Women are treated as "low risk" by default unless they or their midwife identify features which merit medical attention. Inevitably, for a variety of reasons, severe illness is often not identified until late in pregnancy, if at all. This may be because the staff involved do not understand the woman's illness, or that the woman herself feels she is "cured" of a prior problem such as lymphoma, leukaemia, kyphoscoliosis or congenital heart disease, when the illness and its previous treatment can have major implications. This is compounded by a common hospital problem of failure to find past hospital records.

Cardiac disease

Early in pregnancy, oestradiol concentrations rise, inducing vasodilatation, a fall in systemic vascular resistance, fall in pulmonary vascular resistance and rise in cardiac output. Circulating blood volume rises and colloid osmotic pressure falls. The developing uterus may partially obstruct vena-caval flow in the supine position inducing a fall in cardiac output, blood pressure and uterine perfusion.

In general the physiological response to pregnancy serves to improve oxygen delivery to the fetus. In disease states an understanding of these changes helps to predict the effect of the pregnancy on disease symptomatology and, conversely, an understanding of the disease helps to predict the effect of the disease on fetal wellbeing.

Women with cardiac disease should be managed by a multidisciplinary consultant team, as discussed above. Patients with "grown up" congenital heart disease and pulmonary hypertension will need specialist input from supraregional centres. In some women, serial echocardiography and cardiac catheterisation may be necessary in pregnancy.

In some cases admission to intensive care for establishment of invasive monitoring (such as pulmonary arterial lines) and optimisation may be useful prior to operative delivery.

Combined procedures where Caesarean section is followed by immediate coronary revascularisation or valve replacement may be necessary, which means that obstetricians, anaesthetists and neonatologists have to be prepared to deliver in specialist cardiac centres. The practical aspects of caring for a labouring woman on a cardiac intensive care unit surrounded by patients recovering from cardiac surgery should not be overlooked.

Where possible a "stress-free" labour with careful epidural analgesia and monitoring is preferable to operative delivery but this is not possible at all gestations.

Didactic rules about type of anaesthesia such as the contraindication of spinal anaesthesia in aortic stenosis are less important than the expertise of the anaesthetist and refinement of the technique used (Van de Velde *et al.* 2003).

In general terms spinal and epidural analgesia causes vasodilatation with minimal decrease in myocardial contractility. When used for anaesthesia, the tendency for reflex tachycardia is decreased by reduction in cardiac sympathetic outflow. Spinal drugs cause more immediate and significantly more effective anaesthesia with concomitant cardiovascular change. These cardiovascular changes are improved using low dose epidural and spinal analgesia and combined spinal epidural techniques for anaesthesia and analgesia. Anaesthetists traditionally use ephedrine, a drug with direct and indirect sympathetic action, as a positive inotrope, chronotrope and vasoconstrictor to reduce cardiovascular changes induced by spinal and epidural blockade. The actions of ephedrine may be harmful in some conditions and pure vasoconstrictors such as phenylephrine may be a better choice where tachycardia and/or an increase myocardial work is detrimental (e.g. aortic stenosis).

General anaesthesia causes profound and complex cardiovascular changes. At induction, myocardial depression and vasodilatation occur followed by a catecholamine surge at intubation. At institution of positive pressure ventilation, decreased venous return and increased pulmonary pressures occurs. General anaesthetics cause uterine relaxation with increased bleeding and greater requirement of the use of oxytocics such as syntocinon, ergometrine and prostaglandins, which in themselves have profound cardiovascular side effects. At extubation a further surge in catecholamines occurs.

Hypertension

Hypertension is the most common cause of planned preterm delivery. Hypertension may be chronic, be induced by pregnancy (gestational hypertension) or be associated with proteinuria or other stigmata of pre-eclampsia see Table 10.1. Pre-eclampsia may complicate chronic hypertension.

Modern management is based on expectant management that can normally extend gestation by around two weeks. The decision to deliver is complex but is based on its likely effects on fetal and maternal wellbeing (Churchill and Duley 2002)

Induction of labour and vaginal delivery is preferable but is not always possible, in which case planned Caesarean section is an alternative. Before delivery, stabilisation of blood pressure, control of coagulopathy and treatment of eclampsia is essential. The peripartum care of women with pre-eclampsia should occur in areas with facilities for high dependency care. This should include invasive and non-invasive monitoring of blood pressure, blood gases continuous oxygen saturation

Table 10.1. Clinical features of pre-eclampsia

De novo hypertension arising after 20 weeks, gestation and normalising within three months postpartum with one or more of the following:

Proteinuria >300 mg/day or dipstick persistently > 1 g/l

Renal insufficiency, plasma creatinine > 0.10 mmol/l

Liver disease, aspartate transaminase > 40 IU/l and/or severe epigastric-right upper quadrant pain

Neurological problems, convulsions (eclampsia), hyperreflexia with clonus, severe headaches with hyperreflexia

Haematological disturbances, thrombocytopenia, haemolysis

Fetal growth retardation

Source: (after Magee *et al.* 1999, Brown and Buddle 1997)

and urine output, easy access to laboratory investigations and blood products in addition to on site intensive care facilities.

Acute hypertensive control can be with labetolol (oral or intravenous), hydralazine (intravenous) or nifedipine (oral, modified release). All of these drugs are vasodilators and can cause a precipitous fall in blood pressure with significant effects on an already compromised fetal circulation. It is common to give a 500 ml colloid preload during induction of normotension. Following this, however, fluid should be restricted to a basal infusion of Hartmanns solution or normal saline.

If oliguria occurs then early central venous pressure (CVP) monitoring using the antecubital fossa route is useful. Subclavian and internal jugular vein cannulation has been associated with significant morbidity and mortality, particularly in the presence of coagulopathy. A low CVP (<4 mmHg) indicates hypovolaemia; however, a CVP greater than 7 mmHg is not helpful in assessing volume status. The reports of the UK CEMD (Department of Health 1998, 2001) has criticised aggressive uncoordinated volume expansion in pre-eclampsia, pointing out that renal failure is rare, usually reversible and rarely fatal whilst volume overload is a common cause of pulmonary oedema and may increase risk of the acute respiratory distress syndrome (ARDS), a relatively common cause of death in pre-eclampsia. Pulmonary oedema may occur following delivery in pre-eclampsia when excess extravascular fluid is reabsorbed, and in the presence of renal impairment, low colloid osmotic pressure and increased pulmonary pressures, when fluid floods across the damaged endothelium of alveoli. Mild pulmonary oedema may cause dyspnoea with increased respiratory rate followed by arterial desaturation that can then develop into classic frank pulmonary oedema with blood

Table 10.2. Absolute and relative maternal and fetal indications for delivery of the fetus in severe pre-eclampsia

Absolute	Relative
Maternal	*Maternal*
Convulsion	Severe hypertension
Cerebral irritability	Right upper quadrant abdominal pain
Heart failure	Heavy proteinuria
Oliguria with urine output < 20 ml/hr	
Uncontrollable hypertension	
Rising serum creatinine (>50%)	
Thrombocytopenia	
Disseminated intravascular coagulation	
Clinical placental abruption	
Fetal	*Fetal*
Fetal distress	Intrauterine growth retardation

stained frothy sputum. Early oedema may respond to diuretic therapy but severe disease may require endotracheal intubation, positive pressure ventilation and invasive monitoring of arterial blood pressure, CVP, pulmonary capillary wedge pressure and cardiac output on an intensive care unit. Delayed transfer to an appropriate intensive care unit was a criticism of care in successive reports of the UK CEMD.

Magnesium is the treatment of choice in eclampsia but has only been recently acknowledged as a safe and effective treatment in pre-eclampsia (Magpie Collaborative Group 2002), where it halves the incidence of eclamptic seizure. In this study magnesium was not associated with harmful neonatal effects and there was a decreased mortality in the magnesium group. Nevertheless, magnesium is associated with significant cardiac, respiratory, renal and neurological toxicity, and clinical monitoring and dose adjustment, if necessary, is essential.

Pre-eclampsia may be complicated by a coagulopathy with disseminated intravascular coagulation and thrombocytopaenia. This may be combined with haemolysis and elevated liver enzymes (the HELLP syndrome). Although the latter is probably part of the spectrum of endothelial disease seen in pre-eclampsia its presence is particularly sinister and indicates a protracted recovery and increased morbidity and mortality (Haddad *et al.* 2000).

Significant coagulopathy may preclude regional analgesia or anaesthesia because of the risk of epidural haematoma and consequent cord compression. Given that the coagulopathy of pre-eclampsia can occur rapidly following normal coagulation tests, there are relatively few case reports of epidural haematoma in the literature. Where thrombocytopaenia is an isolated feature a platelet count of greater than 75–100 per litre is considered acceptable (Beilin *et al.* 1997).

If anaesthesia is required for Caesarean section then regional anaesthesia is favoured. Traditionally, subarachnoid regional anaesthesia has been avoided because of the theoretically rapid onset of sympathetic blockade and hypotension. In comparison with epidural anaesthesia there seems little difference in maternal hypotension (Hood and Curry 1999). However, hypotension seems less of a problem if the patient has been treated with antihypertensives. The use of a combined spinal epidural with a relatively low dose of anaesthetic solution in the subarachnoid space with epidural top ups may be a further solution to this problem. Whilst similar effects on maternal blood pressure may be seen using epidural or subarachnoid anaesthesia, the effects on the fetus may not and comparative studies have not been large enough to detect differences in fetal outcome between regional techniques. Nevertheless, there is a clear difference in effectiveness between subarachnoid and epidural anaesthesia that results in a high failure rate of epidural anaesthesia.

General anaesthesia is occasionally required in severe pre-eclampsia where the dangers of an oedematous airway and the pressor response to intubation/extubation must not be forgotten. Potential treatments for the pressor response, in addition to a generous dose of induction agent, include:

$MgSO_4$ 2 g (decrease or omit dose of non-depolarising muscle relaxant)
Alfentanil 1–2 mg
Fentanyl 200 µg
Remifentanil 0.5 µg/kg
Labetolol 20 mg
Esmolol 1.5 mg/kg – extubation only

Following delivery there is usually a rapid resolution of organ dysfunction which occurs usually over around 24 hours in pre-eclampsia but can take in excess of 72 hours in the HELLP syndrome.

Cardiac arrest

Cardiopulmonary resuscitation in pregnancy with external cardiac compression is less effective in pregnancy than in non-pregnant women. Distorted anatomy such as elevation of the liver can lead to a high risk of maternal trauma and in addition aorto-caval compression restricts venous return. The effects of aorto-caval compression can be reduced by left-sided tilt of the women (e.g. with a Cardiff Wedge). Unless there is rapid return of maternal circulation Caesarean section is indicated and the Caesarean delivery should be considered an essential stage in the resuscitation of the woman rather than an attempt to save the fetus. Caesarean section may facilitate internal cardiac compression. If necessary, direct current cardioversion should be performed as far away from the uterus as practicable (Whitty 2002).

Brain death

There have been a number of case reports of brain death with delayed delivery of the fetus, which were usefully reviewed in 2003 (Powner and Bernstein 2003). Pregnancy has been continued for as long as 107 days following maternal brain death (from 15 to 32 weeks, of gestation) in intensive care requiring intermittent positive pressure ventilation, inotropic support with careful control of blood pressure and temperature, treatment of sepsis with hormone and endocrine replacement (Powner and Bernstein 2003).

Thromboembolic disease

Women with actual or potential for thromboembolic (thrombophilia) disease require coordinated care for delivery. Anticoagulation can increase the risk of abruption and postpartum haemorrhage and increase bleeding during operative procedures in addition to increasing the risk of epidural haematoma. Where anticoagulation cannot be stopped for delivery, epidural analgesia or anaesthesia is contraindicated. It can take as long as 8–12 hours after a prophylactic dose of low molecular weight heparin for coagulation to become acceptably normal to insert a spinal or epidural needle. Anticoagulant therapy should be delayed for two hours following insertion or removal of an epidural needle or catheter.

Where patients are receiving therapeutic doses of anticoagulant then this needs to be stopped for a variable time (at least 24 hours) prior to anaesthesia if regional anaesthesia is required, with monitoring of anti-Xa activity if available.

Respiratory disease

Asthma

Asthma may improve, deteriorate or remain the same in pregnancy (Bhatia and Bhatia 2000). Severe asthmatics may experience deterioration in late pregnancy. It is rare for asthma to influence timing of delivery. In acute asthma it must be remembered that the pCO_2 is normally low (3.5–4 kPa) and therefore a rise to a "normal" pCO_2 of 5–5.5 kPa may represent significant decompensationis.

Restrictive lung disease

Women with restrictive lung disease often deteriorate in pregnancy due to greater oxygen demand, increased minute volume and splinting of the diaphragm (Bhatia and Bhatia 2000). In general a forced vital capacity of less than one litre or 50% of capacity is predictive of a poor outcome. Kyphoscoliosis, in particular, may deteriorate in the third trimester because of the normal reliance on diaphragmatic breathing. Associated pelvic problems may preclude normal delivery, necessitating Caesarean delivery. General anaesthesia may be difficult because of problems with intubation and ventilation and post-operative respiratory failure. Regional anaesthesia may be difficult because of distorted anatomy, unpredictable epidural and subarachnoid anatomy making dose assessments difficult. Dramatic changes in respiratory muscle function may occur as segmental anaesthesia is induced and regional anaesthesia may need to be converted to general anaesthesia if respiratory function is compromised. Patients may require a period of post-operative ventilation. Of course treatment with internal fixation such as Harrington rods may make attempts at needle insertion impossible.

Renal disease

Renal plasma flow rises early in pregnancy with concomitant increase in glomerular filtration rate and creatinine clearance. Hence, urea and creatinine fall. Renal dysfunction may deteriorate further in pregnancy with hypertension and proteinuria. Renal disease is associated with spontaneous abortion, pre-eclampsia, polyhydramnios intrauterine growth retardation, fetal death and preterm delivery. A high creatinine before pregnancy is associated with worse maternal outcome, worsening renal disease and poor fetal outcome.

Chronic haemodialysis is associated with subfertility and fetal loss. In pregnancy, maternal anaemia worsens, dialysis requirement is greater and anticoagulation during haemodialysis may be a problem. Fetal problems often necessitate early delivery and the usual problems of anaesthesia in dialysis patients are seen (hypertension, vascular access, fluid and electrolyte status, anticoagulation, avoidance of fluid loading) but do not preclude regional anaesthesia (Luciani *et al.* 2003).

Transplanation

Advances in transplantation of hearts, lungs, kidneys and livers means that there are published series of cases were successful pregnancies have followed transplantation. The effects of immunosuppression, physiological alteration and effect of the underlying disease may influence premature delivery and consequent anaesthetic input.

Immunosuppressive treatment with cyclosporin and disease itself (e.g. renal disease) may cause hypertension and be associated with pre-eclampsia (McGrory *et al.* 2003). Risk of thromboembolism may be increased. Renal transplants are usually sited in the iliac fossae, which needs to be remembered in planning surgical incision.

Cardiac transplantation is associated with high risk to mother and fetus. The incidence of Caesarean section is high. Adequate preload is essential during anaesthesia. Denervation of the heart means that drugs such as atropine are ineffective. Adrenergic drugs may not have a predictable action and silent ischaemia can be present (Scott *et al.* 1993).

Where the delivery is inevitable

A clear understanding of the problems and limitations that face the anaesthetist caring for women in whom preterm delivery is inevitable should improve the overall care given to these women and this will be discussed under three headings:
- Risk factors
- The anaesthetic implications of the treatment of preterm labour
- Timely and appropriate provision of analgesia and/or anaesthesia.

Risk factors for preterm delivery

There are risk factors associated with preterm delivery and many of these have relevance to the anaesthetist. In particular, underlying maternal disease, surgery and trauma have been discussed in the previous sections, but also there may be problems associated with young maternal age, smoking and drug abuse. A careful and sympathetic medical assessment is essential to optimise the care for these patients. It is also important that the anaesthetist is told about obstetric and fetal problems including uterine or placental abnormality, or multiple pregnancy and any fetal abnormalities. Ideally the anaesthetist will be acquainted with the woman and her history during ward rounds. One of the specific problems is chorioamnionitis that is common in this group of preterm labouring women. There has been considerable debate about the placement of epidural catheters in women with chorioamnionitis, and also the association of maternal pyrexia with epidural analgesia. Chorioamnionitis may be associated with systemic maternal infection and the patient may exhibit one or more of the following: fever, tachycardia, uterine tenderness, foul smelling amniotic fluid and maternal leucocytosis. The raised temperature is likely to be over 38.5° C. Such a rise in temperature is significant and is likely due to an underlying infection rather than epidural analgesia. It is important to consider the rise in maternal temperature associated with epidural analgesia. The first serious look at this association was in a prospective controlled study that showed a clear association between epidural analgesia and hyperthermia (Fusi *et al.* 1989). Perhaps more important is the lack of rise in temperature demonstrated by the control group who were administered opioids (meperidine), as opioids have been demonstrated to inhibit the febrile response (Negishi *et al.* 2001). The study by Vinson *et al.* (1993) showed an association between epidural analgesia and rise in maternal temperature, with the duration of the epidural correlating with a rise of temperature of 0.07° C per hour exposure to epidural analgesia. However the study by Lieberman *et al.* (1997) looked at the impact of the rise in temperature associated with epidural analgesia on the fetus and the use of neonatal sepsis evaluations. The media coverage of this study caused considerable problems to obstetric anaesthetists and this prompted the study by Philip *et al.* (1999) and was accompanied by an editorial by Camann (1999). At the present time it is accepted that epidural analgesia is associated with a rise in maternal temperature after an epidural has been running for greater than five hours though the mechanism is uncertain (Mercier and Benhamou, 1997). This must be differentiated from the rise in maternal temperature seen in mothers who have a systemic infection. We can be reassured that the use of epidural analgesia in labour does not compromise the neonate by resulting in the need for a neonatal sepsis workup or the unnecessary administration of antibiotics. The anaesthetist who is asked to administer an epidural to a woman who is ill with chorioamnionitis has a dilemma. The anaesthetist is concerned that the woman will suffer from cardiovascular compromise or cause a spread of the infection to the epidural space or meninges. In these circumstances it is sensible to optimise the patients condition and administer intravenous antibiotics before the epidural is performed. For the patient with a localised infection epidural analgesia is generally felt to be safe with antibiotic cover. Prompt action by the obstetrician can therefore avoid unnecessary delays in providing epidural analgesia.

The anaesthetic implications of the treatment of preterm labour

The main treatments used in preterm labour are:
- Steroids
- Tocolytics

Steroids

The use of dexamethasone is well recognised to reduce the incidence of respiratory distress syndrome (RDS) in the preterm neonate and the benefit has been shown to be greatest in the 30–32 week gestation period. Ideally, two doses given 12 to 24 hours apart are recommended with delivery greater than 24 hours after the second dose. The exacerbation of pregnancy-induced hypertension and diabetes and the potential masking of infection are all relevant to the anaesthetist. It is also important that the anaesthetist is aware of the optimum time of delivery.

Tocolytics

The use of tocolytics is to reduce the myometrial contractility and subsequent fetal distress. The efficacy of tocolytic therapy is controversial and is discussed in Chapter 7. The most important uses of tocolytic agents may be to allow time for treatment with dexamethasone, or allow time for an in utero transfer or a neonatal cot to become available. The main groups of drugs used are:

- β-adrenergic agents
- Magnesium sulphate
- Prostaglandin synthetase inhibitors
- Calcium channel blockers
- Oxytocin antagonists such as atosiban.

The β-adrenergic agents have both β_1 and β_2 actions and it is the β_2 effects that relax uterine muscle whereas the β_1 action stimulates heart muscle and increases heart rate and cardiac output. Ritodrine is the most commonly used β-sympathomimetic agent and it is administered orally or intravenously. The side effects include cardiac arrythmias, hypotension, pulmonary oedema and cerebral vasospasm and death. These drugs relax uterine muscle by activating adrenyl cyclase that stimulates the conversion of adenosine triphosphate (ATP) to cyclic adenosine monophosphate (cAMP). Cyclic AMP also acts on the ion transport across the cell membrane so that sodium ions are pumped out of the cells and potassium ions are pumped into the cells. There is increased antidiuretic hormone secondary to the β-adrenergic drugs and sodium is reabsorbed at the renal tubules, leading to a significant risk of fluid overload. The β_2-positive chronotropic and ionotropic actions increase heart rate, stroke volume and left ventricular ejection fraction, leading to an increase in cardiac output. Pulmonary oedema is a well-recognised complication of β-adrenergic therapy especially where there has been inappropriate use of intravenous fluids or where the woman has cardiac disease. The changes associated with sodium and potassium ion movement enhance the likelihood of arrythmias. The metabolic changes associated with ritodrine increase blood glucose levels rapidly and concurrent treatment with dexamethasone can have serious consequences. Careful fluid management, monitoring of urea, electrolytes and blood sugar, blood pressure and pulse rate and, where appropriate, electrocardiogram (ECG) monitoring are all essential to ensure the safety of the mother and fetus in preterm labour. Before administering anaesthesia or analgesia to women receiving β-adrenergic agents, the anaesthetist should undertake a careful history and examination and will want the results of all these investigations available. Ideally, the anaesthetic intervention should be delayed until the cardiovascular effects of ritodrine are wearing off and the tachycardia is subsiding. In practice, this may not be possible as the half-life of ritodrine may be as long as 120 minutes with a second peak at 6–8 hours (Yentis 1990). There may also be a persisting tachycardia relating to stress and anxiety that confuses the issue. Potassium is driven into the cells while ritodrine is administered and extracellular potassium levels would suggest a hypokalaemia. After the ritodrine infusion is ceased the potassium leaves the cells and sodium re-enters and a lethal rebound hyperkalaemia has been reported 60 to 150 minutes after the ritodrine was stopped. Six patients were described who developed ECG changes diagnostic of hyperkalaemia and were found to have serum potassium levels of more than 7.0 mmol/l in the peri-operative period (Kotani *et al.* 2001). All these patients had general anaesthesia for an emergency Caesarean delivery though none received succinylcholine. Succinylcholine is recognised to cause a rise in serum potassium even in healthy patients (Hood and Curry 1999). Previous case reports had warned of the use of succinylcholine in women who had received magnesium and ritodrine therapy combined with bed rest to prevent preterm labour (Sato *et al.* 2000). In this series one patient suffered a cardiac arrest and in another two significant ECG changes associated with hyperkalaemia were seen. These case reports highlight the increased risks of general anaesthesia that women treated with ritodrine plus or minus magnesium are exposed to. All these case reports show the diagnostic importance of the ECG and the increased risks associated with general rather than regional anaesthesia. The drugs used to safely conduct a general anaesthetic in an emergency situation may cause a rise in potassium levels to dangerous levels. Though the underlying electrolyte disturbance is still present, regional anaesthesia carries less risk to the patient. The risk of the development of pulmonary oedema is to be remembered and careful fluid management is essential.

The initiation of regional anaesthesia and, to a lesser extent, analgesia may be associated with hypotension and the routine treatment of this hypotension is intravenous fluid and ephedrine. The anaesthetist may be reluctant to administer ephedrine to a patient who already has a significant tachycardia and in these circumstances may prefer to use phenylephrine.

Magnesium sulphate

The tocolytic effects of magnesium sulphate were first described in 1959 (Hall 1959). Magnesium sulphate probably acts through its calcium antagonist action and magnesium and ritodrine may be equally effective in preventing preterm labour. The main implications of magnesium therapy for the anaesthetist are the potentiation of non-depolarising relaxants and the exaggerated hypotensive effect that may occur with regional anaesthesia (James 1998).

Prostaglandin synthetase inhibitors

Most of the work has been done on indomethacin and the main concerns are fetal and have already been described in Chapters 6 and 8. Indomethacin, naproxen and aspirin may affect platelet function, however, this effect has been shown not to be a contraindication to regional analgesia or anaesthesia (Urmey and Rowlingson 1998).

Calcium channel blockers

Nifedipine is the most widely used and may be administered by the oral route. The patient may experience headaches and nausea and there may be a drop in blood pressure associated with dizziness.

Atosiban

The oxytocin antagonist atosiban has gained increasing popularity for the treatment of preterm delivery though there is no anaesthetic literature relating to its use to date. The Royal College of Obstetincians and Gynaecologists guideline on Tocolytic Drugs for Women in Preterm Labour (RCOG 2002) gives a useful discussion of the use of tocolytic agents in clinical practice.

Timely and appropriate provision of analgesia and/or anaesthesia

Analgesia or anaesthesia will almost certainly be required for labour or Caesarean delivery. The difficulties arise in ensuring that analgesia and anaesthesia is appropriate and timely. The deterioration of the maternal or fetal health may be acute, and labour may become inevitable at any time while trying to stop the labour. In planning the appropriate anaesthetic management of these women, the risk factors and the anaesthetic implications of the treatment of preterm labour as well as the normal risks of anaesthesia associated with pregnancy plus the added risks for the preterm baby should be considered.

In planning the mode of delivery, maternal and fetal factors should be considered.

The main reasons for delivery are as follows:

- There is deterioration in maternal health; this may either be pre-existing (cardiac disease) or pregnancy related (pre-eclampsia).
- Evidence of significant fetal compromise as shown by routine monitoring. (e.g. Doppler).
- Preterm labour becomes inevitable despite treatment.
- In labour, when the condition of the fetus deteriorates as shown by routine monitoring.

If the delivery is necessary due to the deterioration of maternal health the medical condition should be stabilised before delivery. The mode of delivery and analgesia or anaesthesia required will depend on the maternal condition, and the balance of risks and benefits to both the mother and the fetus. Ideally, time should be spent planning the delivery and wherever possible this should be a semi-elective or elective delivery. Generally, regional analgesia or anaesthesia is preferred for these cases.

The routine monitoring of the fetus may show that the fetus is not growing or that the in utero condition is deteriorating and in these circumstances early delivery is required. In this situation it is usually possible to deliver the baby electively, and many of these babies are delivered by Caesarean section at a time to suit the whole team and so that maternal health is not compromised by the mother being poorly prepared for anaesthesia. Regional anaesthesia is recommended as for all pregnant women, but in this situation it is especially important that the mother is awake to experience the birth and see her baby. She and her partner will then have the opportunity to take part in the decision making for their baby. If the delivery is before 24 weeks, gestation the lower uterine segment may not be well formed so a classical incision may need to be made in the uterus; this, and a need to exteriorise the uterus necessitates an excellent regional block. It is helpful if the anaesthetist is made aware of these possibilities before the anaesthetic is administered.

The main area to be considered is when preterm labour becomes inevitable despite treatment. There are several questions that arise and it is helpful to consider each in turn.

- At what time does the woman need analgesia?
- When does the labour become inevitable?
- What are the specific problems of preterm labour?
- What are the neonatal physiological considerations?
- What is the best mode of delivery?
- What is the ideal analgesic or anaesthetic?

At what time does the woman need analgesia?

It is common for there to be no anaesthetic involvement with a women in preterm labour until the delivery becomes inevitable and this often leads to the use of inappropriate analgesia, with women denied of the benefits of regional analgesia for labour. It is understandable that attention is focused on preventing the labour but, equally, the need for pain relief is present whether the labour is inevitable or not. It is common that women are given pethidine or other opioid analgesia at this time and this is inappropriate for the reasons that will be set out below. It could be argued that epidural analgesia should be provided to all women in suspected preterm labour even if labour does not establish.

When does the labour become inevitable?

This is always the most difficult question to answer and the reason that so many women are given inappropriate or no analgesia. If it was always certain when labour was established, planning analgesia would be easier though there is no excuse for denying a woman who is in pain analgesia.

What are the specific problems of preterm labour?

The main problems have already been discussed in the sections on the risk factors associated with preterm labour and the anaesthetic implications of the treatment of preterm labour, in addition to the neonatal physiological considerations (see below). During the latent phase of labour the woman needs emotional support and analgesia. It is important to remember that the active phase of the first stage of labour may be rapid and this may lead to a precipitate delivery. The preterm baby is small and may be delivered through a cervix that is not fully dilated, for example, at around 7 cm dilatation. It is often at this late stage that the anaesthetist is called to provide epidural analgesia. At this stage the woman is usually distressed, both physically and emotionally, and it may be difficult for the professionals to provide a controlled environment for the delivery of the preterm infant.

What are the neonatal physiological considerations?

It is generally accepted that the preterm infant is vulnerable to the stress of labour and delivery. There are several reasons for this including the lower haemoglobin concentration leading to a reduced oxygen carrying capacity in the neonate. There is a relative deficiency in clotting factors and this combined with the soft bone structure covering the brain means these neonates are more susceptible to intra-cranial haemorrhage than a full term baby.

What is the best mode of delivery?

These factors may influence the mode of delivery aiming to minimise intracranial trauma, ensuring that a vaginal delivery is not precipitate or if a Caesarean section is thought to be the delivery of choice that the neonate is handled gently, and this may lead to the consideration of a classical Caesarean section rather than a lower segment incision especially where the lower segment is poorly formed.

What is the ideal analgesic or anaesthetic?

In thinking about the ideal analgesic it is important to consider the safety of the mother and the baby. The maternal risk factors of pregnancy and those specific to any underlying disease or treatment of the preterm labour have already been discussed above. It is also important to remember that there may have been a sudden change of plan from preventing the preterm delivery to accepting it as inevitable, and, therefore, there may be considerable distress on behalf of the mother and her partner. Emotional support is essential as well as ensuring that appropriate analgesia and anaesthesia are provided. There has been a reluctance to give analgesia to the mother due to the poor handling of, in particular, opiate analgesia by the neonate. During the intra-partum phase the administration of opiates to the mother results in poor beat to beat variability in the fetal heart rate, and this may make the assessment of fetal wellbeing difficult. There is less protein available for binding to drugs that cross the placenta and there is also a poor blood–brain barrier, therefore, there is a danger of higher opiate levels in the fetal central nervous system. The immature enzyme systems mean that there is less ability to metabolise and excrete drugs in the neonate. It is therefore wise to avoid opiate drugs though these are commonly given and in repeated doses during the treatment of preterm labour (Macintosh 2003). There is good justification to administer epidural analgesia to women in preterm labour even if the labour is stopped and the epidural needs to be removed. There seems to be a reluctance to involve anaesthetists early in the management of these women and leaving anaesthetic involvement until the delivery becomes inevitable. Chestnut (Muir *et al.* 1999) recommends to his residents: " If you do not occasionally discontinue epidural analgesia in a preterm patient whose labour has stopped, you probably are not starting epidural analgesia sufficiently early in your preterm patients." Early epidural analgesia avoids the problem of the anaesthetist being asked to put in an epidural when a vaginal delivery is imminent. Without early involvement it is difficult to achieve rapid analgesia and to reduce the likelihood of a precipitate delivery of the neonate through a cervix dilated to about 7 cm. In such an event a spinal or combined spinal epidural is possibly the best way to provide excellent rapid analgesia and a relaxed pelvic floor that will reduce the uncontrollable need to push when the baby is felt in the birth canal. A low dose spinal using 1ml of 0.25% bupivacaine (plain) and 25 μg of fentanyl will achieve this without reduction of motor power. The main advantage of using regional analgesia is that the woman is pain free and in control both physically and mentally. She is able to be involved in the delivery and see her baby, and be involved in any decision-making that may be necessary in the immediate post-delivery period. If an epidural is placed the onset of action is a little longer and the sacral roots may not be reached as efficiently as they are with a spinal anaesthetic. Combining the epidural and spinal gives the best chance of achieving good analgesia and the flexibility to use the epidural should a Caesarean section be indicated or further analgesia required. Epidural analgesia reduces maternal catecholamines and therefore placental perfusion will improve to the benefit of the neonate; therefore epidural analgesia should be thought of as an integral part of intrauterine neonatal resuscitation of the preterm infant.

Good communication is essential if the preterm baby is to be delivered by Caesarean section and the use of the four-point classification of the urgency of Caesarean section is to be recommended (Lucas *et al.* 2000). This classification has been recommended by the Royal College of Obstetricians and Gynaecologists and used in the data collection for the Sentinel Caesarean Section Audit (RCOG 2001), and has been shown to help clinicians differentiate between those Caesarean deliveries that should be immediate as there is a threat to the life of the mother or fetus and those where they need to deliver the baby less quickly.

Grade	Definition
1. Emergency	1. Immediate threat to life of mother or fetus
2. Urgent	2. Maternal or fetal compromise that is not immediately life threatening
3. Scheduled	3. Needing early delivery but no maternal or fetal compromise
4. Elective	4. At a time to suit the woman and maternity team

The importance of a clear indication of the urgency of delivery is to be able to avoid general anaesthesia wherever possible as despite the reduction in maternal mortality, as shown by successive reports of the CEMD (Department of Health 1998, 2001) and the CESDI 7th report on general anaesthesia (Maternal and Child Health Consortium 2000), there are still significant risks associated with general anaesthesia.

There will be a small percentage of preterm deliveries that fall into the grade 1 category and depending on the efficiency of the team involved in the Caesarean delivery and the experience and seniority of the anaesthetist general anaesthesia may be avoided. In the grade 2 and 3 categories regional anaesthesia should be the anaesthetic of choice unless there are medical contraindications.

The choice of regional anaesthetic depends if there is an epidural already *in situ* or whether the block needs to be sited de novo. Wherever possible the epidural should be topped up for the Caesarean delivery and anaesthesia may be achieved in 10 minutes though it is usually within 30 minutes. If anaesthesia is needed where there is no epidural running then the choice of regional block lies with the anaesthetist. In most units a spinal or combined spinal epidural anaesthetic will be used though there are clinical situations where an epidural may be the anaesthetic of choice. The use of a spinal anaesthetic or a combined spinal epidural anaesthetic has an onset time of around ten minutes. The major delays in the decision to delivery interval are in transferring the woman to theatre, mobilising the theatre team and, in some cases, the initiation of regional anaesthesia (Maternal and Child Health Research Consortium 2000; Tuffnell *et al.* 2001). It is also important to remember that really fast delivery may not always be in the interest of the neonate as discussed in the paper by MacKenzie and Cooke (2001), where those babies delivered quickest had the poorest cord pH values. Maternal stress may be excessive where the delivery is preceded by a high-speed dash down the corridor to theatre followed by the rapid induction of general anaesthesia.

In conclusion, we should aim for timely anaesthetic involvement in the care of women in preterm labour so that epidural analgesia can be placed in good time and the anaesthetic choice should fit with the degree of urgency of the delivery. The delivery of the neonate to a mother who has regional analgesia or anaesthesia is most likely to ensure the gentle delivery of the baby to an awake mother who is able to take part in the birth of her baby.

Summary

The anaesthetic issues in preterm labour, and intensive care management of the sick parturient require excellent communication between all members of the team caring for the woman and her baby. A clear understanding within the team of the specific problems facing each of the healthcare professionals should improve the standard of care given to this group of patients.

REFERENCES

Anonymous (1996) Pre conception pregnancy and prescribing. *Drug zTher. Bull.* **34**, 25–7.

Beilin, Y., Zahn, J. and Comerford, M. (1997) Safe epidural analgesia in thirty parturients with platelet counts between 69,000 and 98,000 mm(-3). *Anesth. Analg.* **85**, 385–8.

Bhatia, P. and Bhatia, K. (2000) Pregnancy and the Lungs. *Postgrad. Med. J.* **76**, 683–6.

Brodsky, J. B., Cohen, E., Brown, B. J., Wu, M. and Whitcher, C. (1980) Surgery during pregnancy and fetal outcome. *Am. J. Obstet. Gynecol.* **138**, 1165–7.

Brown, M. A. and Buddle, M. L. (1997) What's in a name? Problems with the classification of hypertension in pregnancy. *J. Hypertens.* **15**, 1049–54.

Camann, W. (1999) Intrapartum epidural analgesia and neonatal sepsis evaluations. a casual or causal association? *Anesthesiology* **90**, 1250–2.

Churchill, D. and Duley, L. (2002) Interventionist versus expectant care for severe pre-eclampsia before term. *Cochrane Database Syst. Rev.* **3**, CD003106.

Cruz, A. M., Southerland, L. C., Duke, T. *et al.* (1996) Intraabdominal carbon insufflation in the pregnant ewe: uterine blood flow, intraamniotic pressure, and cardiopulmonary effects. *Anesthesiology* **85**, 1395–402.

Department of Health. (1998) *Why Mothers Die. Report on Confidential Enquiries into Maternal Deaths In the United Kingdom 1994–1996.*

  (2001) *Why Mothers Die. Report on Confidential Enquiries into Maternal Deaths In the United Kingdom, 1997–1999.*

Fusi, L., Steer, P. J., Maresh, M. J. and Beard, R. W. (1989) Maternal pyrexia associated with epidural analgesia in labour. *Lancet* **i**, 1250–2.

Haddad, B., Barton, J. R., Livingston, J. C., Chahine, R. and Sibai, B. M. (2000) Risk Factors for adverse maternal outcomes among women with HELLP (hemolysis, elevated lives enzymes, and low platelet count) syndrome. *Am. J. obstet. Gynecol.* **183**, 444–8.

Hall, D. (1959) The effects of magnesium therapy on the duration of labor. *Am. J. Obstet. Gynecol.* **78**, 27–32.

Holdcroft, A., Konje, J. C. and May, A. (2003) Special report. Small babies and substandard anaesthesia: the Confidential Enquiries into Stillbirths and Deaths in Infancy 27/28 report. *Int. J. Obstet. Anesth.* **12**, 271–4.

Hood, D. D. and Curry, R. (1999) Spinal versus epidural anesthesia for cesarean section in severely preeclamptic patients: a retrospective survey. *Anesthesiology* **90**, 1276–82.

Immer-Bansi, A., Immer, F. F., Henle, S., Sporri, S. and Petersen-Felix, S. (2001) Unnecessary emergency Caesarean section due to silent CTG during anaesthesia? *Br. J. Anaesth.* **87**, 791–3.

James, M. F. M.(1998) Magnesium in obstetric anaesthesia. *Int. J. Obstet. Anesth* **7**, 115–23.

Kotani, N., Kushikata, T., Hashimoto, H. *et al.* (2001) Rebound perioperative hyperkalaemia in six patients after cessation of ritodrine for premature labor. *Anesth. Analg.* **93**, 709–11.

Lieberman, E., Lang, J. M., Frigoletto, F. Jr. *et al.* (1997) Epidural analgesia, intrapartum fever, and neonatal sepsis evaluation. *Pediatrics* **99**, 415–19

Lucas, D. N., Yentis, S. M., Kinsella, S. M. *et al.* (2000) Urgency of Caesarean Section: a new classification. *J. R. Soc. Med.* **93**, 346–50.

Luciani, G., Bossola, M., Tazza, L. *et al.* (2003) Pregnancy during chronic haemodialysis. a single dialysis-unit experience with five cases. *Ren. Fail.* **24**, 853–62

McGrory, C. H., McCloskey, L. J., DeHoratius, R. J. *et al.* (2003) Pregnancy outcomes in female renal recipients: a comparison of systemic lupus erythematosus with other diagnoses. *Am. J. Transplant* **3**, 35–42.

Macintosh, M. (Ed.) (2003 *Project 27/28 CESDI. An Enquiry into Quality of Care and its Effects on the Survival of Babies Born at 27–28 weeks.* London: The Stationary Office.

MacKenzie, I. Z. and Cooke, I. (2001) Prospective 12 month study of 30 minute decision delivery intervals for "emergency" Caesarean section. *BMJ* **322**, 1334–5.

Magee, L. A., Ornstein, M. P. and von Dadelszen, P. (1999) Fortnightly review: Management of hypertension in pregnancy. *BMJ* **318**, 1332–6.

Magpie Collaborative Group. (2002) Do women with pre-eclampsia, and their babies, benefit from magnesium sulphate. The Magpie Trial: a randomised placebo controlled trial. *Lancet* **359**, 1877–90.

Maternal and Child Health Research Consortium. (2000) *Confidential Enquiry into Stillbirths and Deaths in Infancy, 7th Annual Report.* Available at www.cemach.org.uk/publications

Mercier, F. J. and Benhamou, D. (1997) Hyperthermia related to epidural analgesia in labour. *Int. J. Obstet. Anesth.* **6**, 19–24.

Muir, H. A., McGrath, J. M. and Chestnut, D. H. (1999) Preterm delivery and labour. In D. H. Chestnut, ed., *Obstetric Anaesthesia Principles and Practice*, 2nd edn. Mowsby, pp. 665–93.

Negishi, C., Lenhardt, R., Ozaki, M. *et al.* (2001) Opioids inhibit febrile responses in humans, whereas epidural analgesia does not: an explanation for hyperthermia during epidural analgesia. *Anesthesiology* **94**, 218–22.

Philip, J., Alexander, J. M., Sharma, S. K. *et al.* (1999) Epidural analgesia during labor and maternal fever. *Anesthesiology* **90**, 1271–5.

Powner, D. J. and Bernstein, I. M. (2003) Extended somatic support for pregnant women after brain death. *Crit. Care Med.* **31**, 1241–9.

Rathmell, J., Viscomi, C. and Ashburn, M. (1997) Management of non obstetric pain during pregnancy and lactation. *Anesth Analg.* **85**, 1074–87

Reedy, M. B., Kallen, B. and Kuehl, T. J. (1997) Laparoscopy during pregnancy: a study of fetal outcome parameters with use of the Swedish Health Registry. *Am. J. Obstet. Gynecol.* **177**, 673–9.

Rosen, M. A. (1999) Management of anaesthesia for the pregnant surgical patient. *Anesthesiology* **91**, 1159–63.

Royal College of Obstetricians and Gynaecologists Clinical Effectiveness Support Unit. (2001) *National Sentinel Caesarean Section Audit Report.* London: RCOG.

Royal College of Obstetricians and Gynaecologists. (2002) Tocolytic Drugs for women in Preterm Labour clinical guideline. London: RCOG

Sato, K., Nishiwaki, K., Kuno, N. *et al.* (2000) Unexpected hyperkalaemia following succinylcholine administration in prolonged immobilised parturients treated with magnesium and ritodrine. *Anesthesiology* **93**, 1539–41.

Scott, J. R., Wagoner, L. E., Olsen, S. L., Taylor, D. O. and Renlund, D. G. (1993) Pregnancy in heart transplant recipients: management and outcome. *Obstet. Gynecol.* **82**, 324–7.

Shnider, S. M., Wright, R. G., Levinson, G. *et al.* (1979) Uterine blood flow and plasma norepinephrine changes during maternal stress in the pregnant ewe. *Anesthesiology* **50**, 524–7.

Steinbrook, R. A. and Datta, S. (1997) Increase in the arterial-to-end-tidal gradient (intraabdominal carbon dioxide insufflation in the pregnant ewe). *Anesthesiology* **87**, 1596.

Tuffnell, D. J., Wilkinson, K. and Beresford, N. (2001) Interval between decision and delivery by Caesarean section- are current standards achievable? Observational case series. *BMJ* **322**, 1330–3.

Urmey, W. F. and Rowlingson, J. C. (1998) Do antiplatelet agents contribute to the development of perioperative spinal hematoma? *Reg. Anesth. Pain Med.* **23 Suppl**, 146–51.

Van de Velde, M., Budts, W., Vandermeersch, E. and Spitz, B. (2003) Continuous spinal analgesia for labour pain in a parturient with aortic stenosis. *Int. J. Obstet. Anesth.* **12/1** 51–4.

Vinson, D. C., Thomas, R. and Kiser, T. (1993) Association between epidural analgesia during labour and fever. *J. Fam. Pract.* **36**, 617–22

Whitty, J. E. (2002) Maternal cardiac arrest in pregnancy. *Clin. Obstet. Gynecol.* **45**, 377–92.

Yentis, S. M. (1990) Suxamethonium and hyperkalaemia. *Anaesth. Intensive Care* **18**, 92–101.

11

Management of the preterm neonate

Richa Gupta[1] and Michael Weindling[2]

[1] Liverpool Women's Hospital
[2] University of Liverpool and Liverpool Women's Hospital

Immediate resuscitation of the preterm neonate

Introduction

The importance of a planned and coordinated approach to the initial resuscitation, stabilisation and subsequent management of babies born between 27 and 28 completed weeks' gestation was emphasised in the Confidential Enquiries of Stillbirths and Deaths in Infancy (CESDI) Project 27/28 Enquiry (Mackintosh 2003). This chapter covers many of the aspects of care that the report highlighted as contributing to optimising the care of the premature infant. More than 90% of the babies studied for the CESDI report required resuscitation. Having a resuscitation system based on the needs of infants is the recommended approach. The resuscitation guidelines used by the neonatal life support course have been formalised for the term neonate based on combined evidence from the limited pool of resuscitation trials, consensus views on best practice and experimental animal models (Kattwinkel *et al.* 1999; Niermeyer *et al.* 2000). The basic approach to resuscitating a preterm neonate is similar to that of the term neonate with emphasis on maintaining body heat and possible earlier progression to advanced manoeuvres to stabilise the airway and administer exogenous surfactant.

Anticipation

Communication forms a cornerstone of the management of imminent preterm deliveries. Liaison between the delivery suite and the Neonatal Intensive Care Unit (NICU) is thus essential to ensure that potential problems are anticipated and that appropriate cot spaces are available. Obstetric staff and midwifery staff usually initiate the counselling of parents and it is then usual for a member of the paediatric team to have a discussion with the prospective parents. This is an opportunity to outline resuscitation measures, subsequent management and possible outcomes, depending on the gestational age of the fetus. It is helpful to have information leaflets to provide parents with relevant data; in Liverpool, we show

Preterm Labour Managing Risk in Clinical Practice, eds. Jane Norman and Ian Greer. Published by Cambridge University Press. © Cambridge University Press 2005.

parents survival charts based on the unit's experience over the last three years. Prospective parents are also offered the opportunity to visit the NICU to meet staff and see its layout.

The improved survival and long-term outcome of extremely low birthweight (ELBW) babies has changed attitudes towards resuscitation of these babies. In 1986, a survey of American paediatric residents showed that as residents became more experienced, there was an increasing reluctance to resuscitate high-risk infants; this lack of enthusiasm was considered to be due to the high subsequent mortality (Berseth *et al.* 1986). A more recent survey of American paediatricians showed that 96% of physicians questioned offered full resuscitation to these babies. There were various reasons: a sense of an obligation to treat, uncertainty about the true gestational age and a desire to defer withholding of treatment decisions until admission to the neonatal unit. This apparent increase in willingness to resuscitate may also be a reflection of a more positive attitude towards survival and outcome due to improved treatment strategies. There is, however, no doubt that optimising the outcome at resuscitation is a key element in determining healthy survival.

Preparation

Personnel

All staff, who attend deliveries, should have regular formal training in resuscitation such as attendance at a neonatal life support course. Very preterm infants should ideally be delivered during normal working hours when there is senior cover available on-site, enabling optimal supervision of interventions and decision-making. These are high-risk deliveries, which should be attended by the most experienced neonatal medical and nursing staff.

Equipment

Equipment should be fully re-stocked after each delivery and checked daily. Ideally, "Parabags" containing essential items for resuscitation should be ready and accessible on both the delivery suite and the neonatal unit. When multiple births are expected, a full set of equipment for each baby is required. An example of core equipment required is illustrated in Figure 11.1 and shown in box 11.1.

Resuscitation

Prevention of hypothermia

Hypothermia is a major factor in causing problems in resuscitation and subsequent stabilisation of premature neonates. It contributes to metabolic acidosis and reduced arterial oxygen tension, which in turn inhibits surfactant production and causes pulmonary hypertension leading to right-to-left shunting. Very small babies, who are severely hypothermic with core temperatures below 32.9 °C on

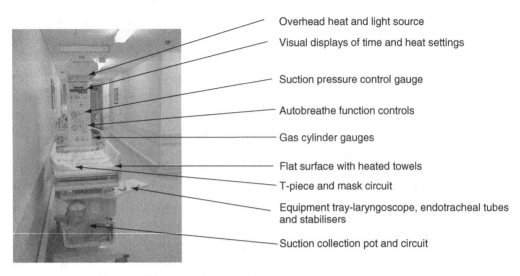

Overhead heat and light source

Visual displays of time and heat settings

Suction pressure control gauge

Autobreathe function controls

Gas cylinder gauges

Flat surface with heated towels

T-piece and mask circuit

Equipment tray-laryngoscope, endotracheal tubes and stabilisers

Suction collection pot and circuit

Figure 11.1 Example of modern Resuscitaire equipment

Box 11.1   Equipment for immediate resuscitation of preterm infants at birth

Temperature regulation:	Overhead heater, flat surface for resuscitating
	Pre-warmed towels/ blankets/Gamgee
Airway:	Laryngoscopes, preferably with size 0 or 00 straight blades
	Endotracheal tubes, sizes 2.0, 2.5, 3.0 for premature babies and babies $< 2.5\,kg$
	Stabilisers for endotracheal tubes
	(Geudel airways)
	Suction catheters and controlled suction
Breathing:	Bag and mask with pressure limited valve or T-piece for delivering breaths
	Oxygen delivery and concentration regulating system
	Stethoscope
Circulation:	Umbilical lines
	Fluid
	Dextrose
Drugs:	Adrenaline
	Sodium bicarbonate
	Surfactant

Transportation:	Mobile resuscitaire with automated ventilation facility or neonatal transport incubator with ventilating facility
Monitoring:	Arterial oxygen saturation, heart rate, temperature

---

Box 11.2   Algorithm for neonatal life support (Resuscitation Council UK, 2001)

NEWBORN LIFE SUPPORT

Dry the baby, remove any wet cloth & cover
↓
Initial Assessment at Birth
Start the clock or note the time
Assess COLOUR, TONE, BREATHING, HEART RATE
↓
If not breathing . . .
↓
Control the airway
Head in the neutral position
↓
Support the breathing
If not breathing – FIVE INFLATION BREATHS (each 2–3 seconds duration)
Confirm a response:- increase in HEART RATE or visible CHEST MOVEMENT
↓
If there is no response
Double check head position and apply JAW THRUST
5 inflation breaths
Confirm a response:- increase in HEART RATE or visible CHEST MOVEMENT
↓
 If there is still no response
a) Use a second person (if available) to help with airway control and repeat inflation breaths
b) Inspect the oropharynx under direct vision (is suction needed?) and repeat inflation breaths
*[c) Insert an oropharyngeal (Geudel) airway and repeat inflation breaths]

Box 11.2 (cont.)

Consider intubation

Confirm a response:- increase in HEART RATE or visible CHEST MOVEMENT

↓

When the chest is moving

Continue the ventilation breaths if no spontaneous breathing

↓

Check the heart rate

If the heart rate is not detectable or slow (less than 60 bpm) and NOT increasing

↓

Start chest compressions

First confirm the chest movement – if not moving return to airway

3 chest compressions to 1 breath for 30 seconds

Reassess heart rate

If improving – stop chest compressions, continue ventilation if not breathing

If heart rate still slow, continue ventilating and chest compressions

Consider venous access and drugs at this stage

AT <u>ALL</u> STAGES, ASK . . . DO YOU NEED HELP?

*[ ] not advisable for extremely low birthweight babies – see main text

©Resuscitation Council UK; Design courtesy of Laerdal

Box 11.3   Summary of approach to newborn resuscitation

Dry and cover the baby

Assess the situation

Airway

Breathing

Chest compressions

Drugs

---

admission to a neonatal unit, have 80% mortality (Stanley and Alberman 1978). In the CESDI Project 27/28 Enquiry (Mackintosh 2003), 73% of the babies who died had temperatures below 36 °C on admission to the neonatal unit, as did 59% of the survivors. This is not an unexpected finding as maintaining a premature infant's temperature at an optimal level, such as 36 °C is difficult.

Because of their large surface area to volume ratio, premature babies are particularly vulnerable to heat loss. There are four modalities by which heat loss occurs, evaporation, convection, conduction and radiation. *Evaporative losses* occur through transfer by the latent heat of evaporation due to the presence of amniotic fluid, which transfers heat from the body to the air as it dries. Prompt removal of this fluid by wiping the baby gently with a warm dry towel or sheet helps prevent this. Resuscitation equipment should be placed away from doors or windows, which may allow draughts to cause heat loss through *convection*. Ensuring that the neonate is placed on a pre-warmed flat surface once it has been wiped dry can prevent *conductive heat losses*. Wrapping or covering the baby, especially the head, reduces heat loss through *radiation*. The use of clear plastic food bags has become widespread in facilitating reduction in heat loss. Placing the baby under an overhead heater helps to maintain a warm environment and has a similar effect.

Assessment of initial condition

Basic observations of skin colour, muscle tone, respiratory effort and heart rate can be done quickly whilst the neonate is being dried and wrapped. Many premature infants will appear peripherally pale or cyanosed, and it is therefore important to check the lips and tongue for central cyanosis.

Muscle tone is assessed by the degree of limb flexion and spontaneous movement, both of which may be lacking in many premature babies of early gestations who may be initially floppy and limp.

Premature infants may have an initial few gasps but then have difficulty in establishing regular spontaneous and effective breathing. The breathing pattern must be closely observed for rate and regularity. Indrawing of the intercostal muscles or grunting noises indicate respiratory distress, which requires prompt action.

The heart rate should be confirmed by auscultation of the apex beat. This is important because palpation for peripheral pulses or at the base of the umbilical cord are not reliable when the pulse is weak or slow.

Airway

Confirmation of a patent airway is a priority during resuscitation; without this, breathing will be ineffective. Premature neonates, especially those of lower gestations have poor pharyngeal tone that predisposes them to mechanical obstruction of the airway by the soft tissues of the oro-pharynx and the tongue. Placing the head and neck in a neutral position usually provides a clear airway. Occasionally mucus or blood may obstruct the airway, and these can be removed by gentle suction under direct vision. Airway opening manoeuvres such as chin lift or a jaw thrust may be required in larger babies, but care must be take to avoid pressure on the soft tissues around the lower jaw and neck.

It is rare to need an airway adjunct such as a Geudel airway for premature babies, but this should be considered if there is a structural airway problem such as a cleft palate. The lack of appropriately sized apparatus may limit its use, and intubation may be more appropriate if there is a significant compromise to maintaining airway patency.

There is interest in the use of a laryngeal mask to stabilise the difficult airway in neonates but this has yet to be fully evaluated.

Breathing

The provision of breathing support at the resuscitation of newborn premature infants is one of the most controversial areas in neonates. Babies who have not shown signs of spontaneous breathing, or whose heart rate has not increased to greater than 100 beats per minute (bpm) after being dried and having their airway cleared, should conventionally have five rescue breaths. It is now advised that each of these breaths should provide a sustained inflation for 2–3 seconds. The aim of these breaths is to provide sufficient distending pressure to inflate the lungs, aiding clearance of lung fluid and hence enabling oxygenation. The optimal device for delivering inflations should be able to provide a regulated positive inspiratory pressure as well as helping to maintain airway patency in expiration, i.e. positive end expiratory pressure.

The delivery mechanism for these breaths has traditionally been a bag and mask device attached to an oxygen delivery circuit. The bag should have a pressure-limited blow-off valve set to 30 cm of water, attached to a pressure monitoring device. Alternative methods, such as a T-piece connected to a pressure-regulated continuous gas flow, have also been used. There is some evidence that the latter type of device may allow better delivery of controlled sustained breaths with positive end expiratory pressure than either self-inflating bags or anaesthetic bags, independently of operator ability (Finer *et al.* 2001). This interesting study compared two types of anaesthetic bag with a 'Neopuff' flow-controlled pressure-limited device for neonatal resuscitation carried out by nurses and physicians of varying experience. Regardless of operator experience or ability, the Neopuff was better at delivering the desired airway pressures while maintaining more consistent airway patency. A larger randomised controlled trial to investigate this would be useful, but its usefulness would be limited by having to be non-blinded to the device used.

The minimum pressure required to inflate the lungs is that which produces detectable movement of the chest wall with an improvement in colour and heart rate. In premature babies, who have surfactant deficient lungs, there is reduced lung compliance and the lungs are stiff. In practice, pressures of 20–25 cm of water are usually required in smaller premature infants to minimise barotrauma. This is rather less than the pressures used for term infants (up to 30 cm of water). Cautious use of higher pressures up to 30 cm of water may be required for premature babies if the lungs are very stiff.

Air versus oxygen

An important aspect of respiratory support to consider is what concentration of oxygen to use. Resuscitation at delivery has conventionally involved the liberal use of oxygen, but premature babies are vulnerable to the effects of hyperoxia because they are unable to deal effectively with the oxygen free radicals that may form. Free radicals probably contribute to damage to retinal vessels, may play a part in the pathogenesis of retinopathy of prematurity and increase the risk of developing chronic lung disease. Sudden hyperoxia during resuscitation may also lead to vasoconstriction, reducing cerebral blood flow and increasing the risk of cerebral ischaemic damage (Nijima *et al.* 1988; Lundstrom *et al.* 1995).

Measures to monitor and limit inspired oxygen during resuscitation seem to be a sensible approach to avoiding these problems. Three studies have investigated the use of air versus oxygen in resuscitation, neither proving any overwhelming benefit to the use of oxygen, nor showing that using air is detrimental (Ramji *et al.* 1993; Saugstad *et al.* 1998; Vento *et al.* 2001). However, all three studies showed a delayed time to first breath and time to first cry in the babies resuscitated with 100% oxygen compared with those resuscitated in room air. In the Saugstad multi-centre study there was 5% less mortality in the babies resuscitated in room air than in the oxygen group. These studies mainly involved asphyxiated term newborn infants, so results of randomised controlled trials using limited amounts of oxygen in resuscitation of premature newborn babies are awaited (Tan *et al.* 2002).

Intubation versus continuous positive airway pressure (CPAP)

Further controversy lies in the area of advanced airway support. Continuous positive airway pressure (CPAP) has been advocated as a means of splinting open the upper airway of premature babies (Morley 1999). As we are now in the era of antenatal steroids and exogenous surfactant, severe respiratory distress syndrome caused by pure surfactant deficiency is becoming less common (Crowley 1999). Concern is now growing regarding the pressure effects of mechanical ventilation on the developing lung, so alternative strategies such as CPAP are being explored. Jobe *et al.* (2002) used premature lambs, which had received antenatal glucocorticoids, to compare the effects of no ventilation, conventional ventilation or CPAP (Jobe *et al.* 2002). Neutrophil numbers and hydrogen peroxide levels from alveolar washings were used as markers of lung injury.

Both were significantly increased in the lambs that were ventilated conventionally, compared with those that received CPAP; neutrophil numbers were over six times higher in the conventional ventilation group than the CPAP group. This supports the notion that administering CPAP from birth may reduce the incidence of chronic lung disease in ELBW babies. A cohort study suggested that babies <1501 g who were greater than 27 weeks' gestation with respiratory distress syndrome (RDS) could be managed effectively from birth using early nasal CPAP (Jonsson *et al.* 1997). Systematic review of prophylactic CPAP (Subramaniam *et al.* 2000) revealed only one randomised controlled trial before the routine use of antenatal steroids and surfactant. This compared early CPAP with headbox oxygen in the treatment of RDS. It showed an increased need for ventilation in the CPAP group. Further randomised controlled trials comparing outcomes between CPAP and intubation for ELBW babies at birth using current treatment regimes are awaited. Although there is enthusiasm for commencing CPAP shortly after birth in ELBW babies, published data to support this practice is lacking.

Circulation

Chest compressions

If the heart rate does not increase in response to adequate ventilation, it is necessary to start chest compressions. Chest compressions are a mechanical means of propelling blood from the heart to the coronary arteries and to the lungs to allow oxygenation. The latter process can only be fulfilled if the lungs are being aerated, so it is imperative that chest movement is confirmed with each assisted breath before chest compressions are started.

The person doing the chest compressions can stand at either end of the baby. In practice standing at the baby's feet allows another resuscitator to manage the airway. To give chest compressions, two hands should encircle the chest with the fingers underneath the back and the thumbs placed in the midline over the lower third of the sternum. Care must be taken to maintain this position and not allow the thumbs to stray to either side to avoid damaging the ribs or internal organs. The chest is gently compressed to a depth of one-third towards the spine. A ratio of three chest compressions to every one breath should be given for 30 seconds. The recommended rate is to achieve 30 cycles of 3:1 compressions to breaths in one minute; not easy to achieve effectively in practice. After 30 seconds the heart rate should then be checked to detect any response. If it is over 100 bpm, chest compressions can be discontinued and airway and breathing support should continue as necessary. A heart rate of less than 60 bpm or no audible heart sounds requires continuation of full cardiopulmonary resuscitation and consideration of drug treatment (Resuscitation Council UK 2001).

Drugs
Surfactant

Administration of surfactant falls into the grey area between resuscitation and beginning of stabilisation and definitive treatment for RDS. Endogenous surfactant lowers surface tension in the lung, easing inflation. As production of this lipoprotein does not start until after 24 weeks' gestation, premature babies are unable to aerate the lungs effectively. Extremely low birthweight babies are therefore at high risk of developing RDS.

With improved survival, the approach towards care of the ELBW baby is to prevent the development of problems causing long-term morbidity. Ameliorating lung injury due to RDS from the outset reduces respiratory complications. Meta-analysis of trials studying selective early or prophylactic surfactant administered as soon after birth, compared to delayed treatment has shown significant reductions in pneumothorax (typical relative risk (RR) 0.70, 95% confidence interval (CI) 0.59 to 0.82) and pulmonary interstitial emphysema (typical RR 0.63, 95% CI 0.43 to 0.93, Yost and Sol 2002). There was also a trend towards reduction in mortality in the groups receiving early treatment (typical RR 0.87, 95% CI 0.77 to 0.99, Yost and Sol 2002). There are some advocates of administering surfactant immediately post-intubation before giving any positive pressure breaths (Thompson and Kempley 1999). The skill and certainty of the resuscitator in correctly placing the endotracheal tube (ETT) limit this practice. A pragmatic approach that is generally used is that surfactant is given after confirmation by auscultation that the ETT has been correctly placed, whilst in the delivery room.

The type of surfactant used has also been subjected to scrutiny. Several randomised controlled trials have compared the efficacy of artificial surfactants to natural surfactants. Systematic review with meta-analysis of 11 trials showed natural surfactants gave a significant reduction in risk of pneumothorax compared to synthetic surfactant (typical RR 0.63, 95% CI 0.53 to 0.75) (Soll and Blanco 2003). A reduction in mortality with natural surfactants (typical RR 0.87, 95% CI 0.76 to 0.98) was seen most dramatically in a study comparing poractant alfa (mortality 14%) with the synthetic pumactant (mortality 31%) (Ainsworth *et al.* 2000).

This was borne out in the findings of the CESDI report (Mackintosh 2003) where there was almost a twofold increase in mortality in infants receiving synthetic rather than natural surfactant (*odds ratio (OR) 1.88, 95% CI 1.14–3.11 (*adjusted for sex, birthweight <5th centile and baby's condition at 5 minutes of age)). Natural surfactants are derived from bovine or porcine sources and have hydrophobic surfactant proteins SP-B and SP-C that may contribute towards the greater efficacy in improving lung compliance and more rapid onset of effect.

Adrenaline (Epinephrine)

Drug administration is one of the aspects of neonatal resuscitation that has relied heavily on extrapolation from animal, adult and paediatric studies. Limited clinical opportunity and ethical considerations constrain the undertaking of controlled interventional studies using drugs in preterm neonates.

As the need for cardiopulmonary resuscitation in very preterm babies is usually related to problems with establishing effective ventilation, drugs are rarely given. When required, the main drugs used in neonatal resuscitation are adrenaline (epinephrine), sodium bicarbonate and naloxone. The latter drug is mainly used to reverse the effects of respiratory depression caused by intrapartum maternal opioid analgesia, and it is therefore rarely used in preterm neonates.

There is little evidence for any effectiveness of adrenaline in improving the outcome of resuscitation in neonates, particularly in preterm infants. In a retrospective study of 5 years of potential adrenaline use during resuscitation at delivery, O'Donnell *et al.* (1998) reported its actual use in 0.2% of deliveries. Survival in term infants was 67%. Only 30% of infants below 29 weeks' gestation survived, of which 50% had no congenital abnormalities. However, 78% of this premature group died or had a detectable neurodevelopmental disability. Another retrospective study supports the view that extreme prematurity and asystole were associated with a poor outcome both at delivery and during the first week of life (Sims *et al.* 1994).

The dosing regimes and mode of administration of adrenaline that are recommended have been derived from animal models and paediatric data, with no direct evidence to confirm safety or efficacy in neonates (Wyckoff *et al.* 2001). The current guidelines for neonatal use are that adrenaline is indicated if there is asystole or a bradycardia (heart rate less than 60 bpm) despite adequate ventilation for 30 seconds. The dose should be 0.1 to 0.3 ml of a 1:10 000 solution (0.01 to 0.03 mg/kg) given intravenously or via an ETT, every 3 to 5 minutes whilst continuing cardiopulmonary support (Niermeyer *et al.* 2000). Controlled trials to evaluate the safety and efficacy of adrenaline in neonatal resuscitation are needed, but, as stated above, difficult to conduct in practice.

Sodium bicarbonate

Acidosis develops quickly in the presence of the hypoxia and decreased coronary and cerebral perfusion that occur during cardiopulmonary arrest and prolonged resuscitation. Usually this is a mixed respiratory and metabolic acidosis, which compromises myocardial function. Theoretically, the administration of sodium bicarbonate should act as a buffer, enabling the clearance of CO_2. This is, however, only effective if there is adequate ventilation. Otherwise there is free diffusion of CO_2 across cell membranes causing paradoxical intracellular acidosis. Conversely, a metabolic alkalosis may develop, which causes a left shift of the oxyhaemoglobin dissociation curve, resulting in increased O_2 affinity for haemoglobin and reducing tissue uptake of O_2. Again, data for sodium bicarbonate use have been gathered from animal models and there is no direct evidence to support its use in brief neonatal resuscitation. It is thus only recommended for use in prolonged cardio-pulmonary resuscitation where the clinical situation is refractory to adequate ventilation. Doses of 1 to 2 mEq/kg of a 0.5 mEq/kg (4.2% solution) of sodium bicarbonate are given as a slow bolus.

Antenatal steroids

The twin strategies of the introduction of antenatal steroids to augment endogenous surfactant production and the administration of exogenous surfactant have both helped reduce the severity of RDS (Crowley 1995, 1999; Soll and McQueen 1992).

Summary

Neonatal resuscitation is an evolving area. There are growing concerns that some of the therapeutic approaches based on adult and paediatric practice are not suitable or safe for the needs of newborn babies. In particular, the organs of premature babies are immature and vulnerable. They may suffer damage during resuscitation, compromising survival and long-term outcomes. In particular, the use of 100% oxygen is being questioned. There is no evidence to support its use, yet hyperoxia is associated with many of the problems neonatologists are keen to prevent. This current critical approach to resuscitation may prompt further clinical studies under controlled conditions to continue improving the care that premature newborn babies receive from the early minutes following birth.

Management until discharge from the neonatal unit

Introduction

Because of advances in antenatal and postnatal care, the clinical management of premature babies is dynamic and evolving. It is not possible to cover the entire scope of management of preterm infants in this chapter. However, we will in this short section, outline current management strategies that are being used or developed to care for premature infants, and the evidence for them.

Admission and stabilisation on the neonatal unit

The first 24–48 hours after admission to a NICU are critical for preterm infants. The main priorities are maintaining effective airway and ventilatory support, whilst stabilising the circulation and protecting the infant from heat loss and infection.

On admission, to the neonatal unit, the baby is weighed. Weighing is essential, forming a basis for accurate fluid management and the prescription of drugs. Thereafter, electrodes and transducers are applied to monitor physiological variables: heart rate, blood pressure, respiratory rate, oxygen saturation and temperature. Peripheral veins (and sometimes arteries) and the umbilical artery (and sometimes the umbilical vein) are cannulated. All ventilated infants have a chest X-ray to ascertain the underlying diagnosis – not all respiratory distress is due to surfactant deficiency – and to ensure that the ETT is appropriately positioned. Abdominal X-rays are taken to check the position of umbilical catheters.

An audit of outcome of preterm admissions to Liverpool Women's Hospital showed that the highest mortality was – as expected – amongst babies born less than 28 weeks' gestation. The time to stabilise babies was shortest when they were admitted by more senior medical and nursing staff (specialist registrars and Advanced Neonatal Nurse Practitioners). This is an important consideration as handling and exposure should be minimised in newborn premature infants, especially those who are sick, to avoid additional stress.

Thermal environment

Premature ELBW babies start to lose heat from the moment they emerge from the womb. After the baby has been dried, heat is mainly lost through the skin. This is because the epidermis is only two to three cell layers thick and dermal integrity is poor during the first week after birth. There is therefore little protection against transepidermal water losses due to passive diffusion, and this can lead to profound weight loss of up to one-fifth of body weight in normal (20%) humidity. Increasing humidification and regulating the temperature of the infant's environment can effectively reduce these losses. Double-walled incubators with high (80%) ambient humidity can reduce weight loss to one-twentieth of body weight (Hammarlund and Sedin 1979).

Low birthweight babies need to be nursed in a thermoneutral environment because this is the temperature at which the energy required to maintain body temperature is minimal (Sinclair 2002). The body temperature of premature infants can be maintained by the use of servo-controlled incubators; alternatively, the incubator air temperature needs to be adjusted frequently by hand. The incubator temperature should be set to achieve an anterior abdominal wall temperature of 36 °C.

Respiration
Surfactant

Surfactant is now routinely given to premature babies requiring intubation and ventilation for respiratory distress syndrome. Natural surfactants have a more rapid onset of action than artificial surfactants, and this is reflected in reduced

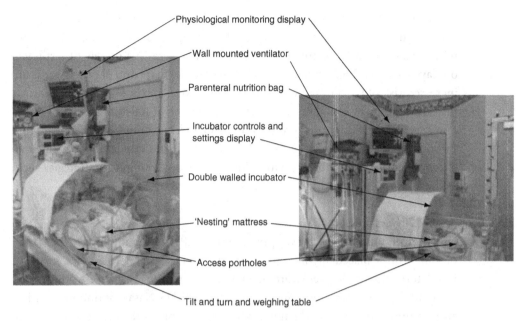

Physiological monitoring display

Wall mounted ventilator

Parenteral nutrition bag

Incubator controls and
settings display

Double walled incubator

'Nesting' mattress

Access portholes

Tilt and turn and weighing table

Figure 11.2 Example of modern incubator, equipment and environment in a Neonatal Intensive Care Unit caring for a preterm infant – taken and reproduced with parental permission

oxygen requirements (Hudak *et al.* 1996; Mondanlou *et al.* 1997; da Costa *et al.* 1999). The dosage of surfactant varies according to the individual product, but there is no evidence that more than two doses result in decreased ventilation requirements or prevent chronic lung disease.

Mechanical ventilation

Different approaches to ventilation have been used to optimise ventilatory support for RDS, whilst minimising lung damage. Pressure-cycled mechanical ventilators are generally used. The results of studies comparing conventional ventilation (CV) with high-frequency oscillatory ventilation (HFOV) have been equivocal. Meta-analysis of eight studies (Henderson-Smart *et al.*, 2002) showed no difference in mortality between CV and HFOV groups. Although there was a trend towards reduction in incidence of chronic lung disease (CLD) in survivors in the HFOV group (6 trials, summary RR 0.73, 95% CI 0.57 to 0.93), this was at the expense of an increased incidence of severe (grades 3 and 4) cerebral intraventricular hae-morrhage and pulmonary air leak. Only two trials reported neurodevelopmental follow-up outcomes; both showed more abnormalities in survivors from the HFOV group (HIFI Study Group 1990; Ogawa *et al.* 1993).

Initiation of mechanical ventilation has been found to be an independent factor in the development of CLD in a case-control study comparing practice at three

American centres, one in New York and two in Boston (van Marter *et al.* 2000). After adjusting for other potential confounding factors, the odds ratios for mechanical ventilation increasing the risk of CLD were 13.4 on day of birth, 9.6 on days 1 to 3, and 6.3 on days 4 to 7. Other factors that contributed towards an increased risk of CLD in the ventilated patients were maximum peak inspiratory pressure >25 cm H_2O and maximum inspired oxygen of 100% on the day of birth, lowest peak inspiratory pressure >20 cm H_2O and maximum partial pressure of carbon dioxide >50 mmHg on days 1 to 3. In view of the potential detrimental effect of ventilation on the premature lung, alternative respiratory strategies such as the use of CPAP, need to be developed and evaluated.

Continuous positive airways pressure

Nasal continuous positive airway pressure (nCPAP) is generally applied by means of soft prongs placed in the anterior nares. It has several roles as a form of ventilatory support in premature neonates. It is used to treat severe apnoeas of prematurity as well as in the management of acute RDS. Nasal continuous positive airways pressure is used in the initial stages of respiratory distress, particularly in Scandinavia, and as temporary support for premature infants in the recovery phase of RDS, usually for a short period immediately after extubation. The benefit of extubating babies to nCPAP rather than into headbox oxygen is that the incidence of re-ventilation is reduced (RR 0.62 (95% CI 0.49 to 0.79), NNT (number needed to treat) 6 (95% CI 4 to 11)). There is also a tendency towards a reduced incidence of oxygen dependence at 28 days in the nCPAP group (RR 0.86 (95% CI 0.67 to 1.10)) (Davis and Henderson-Smart 2002). However, these studies did not use a standardised delivery mechanism for the nCPAP, so further studies to determine optimal mode to administer nCPAP are needed.

Nasal intermittent positive pressure ventilation (NIPPV) is nCPAP delivered via nasal prongs and augmented by ventilator breaths. Three trials comparing extubation to nCPAP or synchronised NIPPV in premature infants all showed a beneficial effect of NIPPV in reducing re-ventilation (RR 0.21 (95% CI 0.1 to 0.45), NNT 3) (Davis *et al.* 2002).

Trials comparing nCPAP with theophylline for the treatment of apnoea of prematurity are awaited.

Postnatal steroids

Chronic lung disease (CLD, bronchopulmonary dysplasia) is a serious cause of morbidity and, rarely, mortality amongst ELBW survivors. The condition is characterised by scarring of the lungs and a prolonged need for oxygen, which persists after the acute effects of surfactant deficiency have passed. The EPICure study (Costeloe *et al.* 2000) that followed infants born less than 26 weeks' gestation prospectively, showed that 76% of the survivors still needed supplemental oxygen at 36 weeks' postmenstrual age, and 51% of survivors at 40 weeks' postmenstrual age.

The development of CLD involves inflammatory processes, so steroids would seem to be a reasonable therapy. They have been shown to be effective in the short term by reducing duration of ventilation when given at 7–10 days' post-natal age. However, this short-term gain is at the expense of potential adverse effects of hypertension, glucose intolerance, adrenal suppression, compromised growth and increased risk of sepsis. Most worryingly, there is concern that brain development may be affected adversely by post-natal steroids (LeFlore *et al.* 2002), causing an increased risk of long-term neurodevelopmental problems.

Further review of glucocorticoids administration for prevention or treatment of CLD have shown no substantial short- or long-term benefit when given either by inhalation or systemically (American Academy of Paediatrics 2002). The routine use of postnatal steroids is therefore not now recommended. It is advised that their use be limited to exceptional clinical circumstances (e.g. an infant on maximal ventilatory and oxygen support) with parental agreement after full discussion of the implications of their use.

Cardiovascular
Patent ductus arteriosus (PDA)

The ductus arteriosus forms a conduit in utero between the pulmonary artery and the descending aorta. Its physiological effect is to allow blood entering the fetal heart from the umbilical veins to bypass the lungs and to carry oxygen and nutrients directly from the placenta to the tissues.

The ductus arteriosus is naturally patent in the majority of preterm infants, especially in the presence of acidosis, hypoxia and severe RDS. Only in a minority, about 20%, does patency of the ductus arteriosus cause symptoms. Common symptoms are tachycardia and tachypnoea and a PDA may cause increased oxygen and ventilatory requirements. Symptomatic PDA tends to be diagnosed earlier than asymptomatic PDA (3.6 days vs. 9.6 days, $p = 0.044$, 95% CI 0.2 to 11.8) (Lee *et al.* 1998). Spontaneous closure following conservative management by fluid restriction and diuretic therapy occurs more often with asymptomatic PDA than symptomatic PDA (58.3% vs. 10.8%, $p < 0.001$, 95% CI 17.9% to 77.1%) (Lee *et al.* 1998).

The adverse effects of a large PDA depend on whether flow is from left-to-right (from the systemic to the pulmonary circulations) or from right-to-left (from the pulmonary to the systemic circulations). This depends on the relative pressures in the pulmonary artery and the systemic circulation. A large PDA allowing systemic to pulmonary flow across it (left-to-right shunting) may cause high output cardiac failure. Flow from left-to-right increases the risk of pulmonary haemorrhage, reduced cerebral and visceral perfusion, which have been implicated in the development of intraventricular haemorrhage and necrotising enterocolitis.

Indomethacin, a cyclo-oxygenase inhibitor, is effective in closing a PDA. When given to premature infants at the time of diagnosis of symptomatic PDA, it resulted in ductal closure in 79% of cases, compared with 35% who received a placebo (Gersony *et al.* 1983). The incidences of retinopathy of prematurity (ROP) and pneumothorax were also reduced in the treatment group, but there was no difference in mortality. More recently, approaches aimed at prophylaxis of PDA by the administration of intravenous indomethacin to high-risk babies have been effective in reducing short-term problems such as intraventricular haemorrhage (Bandstra *et al.* 1988). A review by Fowlie and Davis (2002) showed a reduced incidence of Grade 3 and 4 intraventricular haemorrhage (IVH) (pooled RR 0.66 (95% CI 0.53 to 0.82)). There was no evidence of any impact on mortality, respiratory or long-term outcomes. Indomethacin administration also causes reduced blood flow to various organs, including the kidneys, gut and brain. The investigation of ibuprofen, another cyclo-oxygenase inhibitor, to minimise adverse effects has had promising results (Dani *et al.* 2000; De Carolis *et al.* 2000).

Hypotension

Mean systemic blood pressure (BP) increases with increasing gestation and post-natal age. Although the optimal level for the mean blood pressure is uncertain, clinicians generally aim to maintain a mean BP above the tenth centile for gestation and postnatal age. Various strategies for increasing BP to achieve improved perfusion have been tried. The first step is to correct hypovolaemia. A comparison of saline with albumin for volume expansion found they were equally effective in raising BP, but saline had the advantage of producing less tissue oedema (So *et al.* 1997).

If BP is not maintained adequately following volume expansion (usually as a 10–20 ml/kg bolus), inotropes are started. Low dose dopamine (1–2.5 µg/kg/minute) increases coronary, mesenteric and renal blood flow without affecting BP. Higher doses (6–10 µg/kg/minute) raise BP by increasing cardiac output but also cause peripheral vasoconstriction. Dopamine is more effective than volume expansion in boosting BP to greater than the tenth centile (Gill and Weindling 1993). Dobutamine, a synthetic inotrope, is less effective than dopamine in neonates and requires higher doses to achieve the plasma threshold level required to improve cardiac output, with less change in BP (Martinez *et al.* 1992), but it is most effective when cardiogenic failure is present as it has good chronotropic action. Systematic review of four comparative studies showed that dopamine is more effective than dobutamine in the short-term treatment of hypotension (Subhedar and Shaw 2002).

Hydrocortisone raises BP as effectively as dopamine (Bourchier and Weston 1997), but its potential side effects limit its use to situations when inotropes have failed. Heckmann *et al.* (2002) reported that an infusion of adrenaline at a rate of between 0.05 and 2.6 µg/kg/min increased the mean BP and heart rate without decreasing urine output in very low birthweight infants where hypotension had not responded to a dopamine infusion. A potential adverse effect was an increase in metabolic acidosis, presumably due to its alpha-receptor vasoconstrictive effects. This suggests that adrenaline should probably only be used when other measures have failed (Weindling 2002).

There is no current evidence to demonstrate that treating hypotension has benefits or impact on long-term neurodevelopmental outcome. Generally, clinicians need to direct their efforts at working out strategies to determine the appropriate BP for an individual baby.

Fluids and electrolytes

Preterm infants have up to 86% total body water, much of which is lost after birth especially through the skin and respiratory tract (Sedin 1996). Administration of fluid therapy during the first week of life requires careful adjustment to balance the need to replace the large insensible water losses with the avoidance of fluid overload. Weighing the baby daily is therefore very helpful. High fluid intake is associated with severity of RDS, development of significant PDA (Bell *et al.* 1980), CLD (van Marter *et al.* 1990) and necrotising enterocolitis (Bell *et al.* 1979). A volume sufficient to replace insensible losses and to meet physiological needs and avoid dehydration is recommended (Kavvadia 2000, Bell and Acarregui 2001). A suggested regime is shown in box 11.4.

The best guide to fluid balance is by monitoring of body weight once or twice daily, with similar frequency of serum electrolytes (sodium and potassium) measurement. Hyponatraemia during the first few days in preterm babies is usually due to water excess rather than sodium insufficiency. Sodium supplementation in this situation will delay excretion of extracellular fluid (Hartnoll *et al.* 2000), and may contribute to chronic lung disease (Costarino *et al.* 1992). Abnormally high water losses can lead to hypernatraemia, which should be treated by increases in fluid volume. Later urinary sodium losses due to immature renal tubular function may lead to hyponatraemia, which can be treated with sodium supplementation.

Feeding and nutrition

The introduction of enteral nutrition for ELBW or premature babies is another area of uncertainty. Much of the concern regarding the feeding of premature babies (especially those who are growth restricted) revolves around early feeding or initiation of feeds within the first week of life. Most sick premature infants are

---

Box 11.4   Recommended fluid management guidelines (Liverpool Women's Hospital 2001)

The basic infusion fluid used is 10% dextrose in ml/kg/day. Electrolytes are added as required. A standard starting regime is: sodium 3 mmol/kg/day, potassium 2 mmol/kg/day, calcium 1 mmol/kg/day. The volume is increased daily, unless there is an abnormal weight gain (usually about 20 g per day).

	Fluid dose for babies < 1001g	Fluid dose for babies > 1001g
Day 1	90 ml/kg/day	60 ml/kg/day
Day 2	120 ml/kg/day	75 ml/kg/day
Day 3	150 ml/kg/day	90 ml/kg/day
Day 4	150 ml/kg/day	120 ml/kg/day
Day 5	150 ml/kg/day	150 ml/kg/day

---

catabolic during the first few days after birth and adequate nutrition is essential to provide energy (Steer *et al.* 1992). Enteral feeding during this period may compromise the sick infant for several reasons. Mechanical splinting of the diaphragm impairs respiration and may cause apnoeas or aspiration. The haemodynamic changes associated with feeding may compromise a labile circulation by diverting blood to the gut. During the first days, fluid is therefore usually given parenterally. Optimal amino acid content of parenteral nutrition of 3 g/kg/day and energy intake of 80–90 kcal/kg/day appear to achieve rates of growth comparable to intrauterine weight gain (Heird *et al.* 1992). Prolonged administration of parenteral nutrition has risks. There is an increased risk of nosocomial infection associated with the indwelling central lines. Cholestatic jaundice is not uncommon, but is an association that may be due to lack of enteral feeding rather than parenteral nutrition per se (Rager and Finegold 1975). Osteopenia of prematurity used to be a common problem, but adequate phosphate supplementation in total parenteral nutrition (TPN) solutions has helped reduce this (Lyon *et al.* 1984).

Necrotising enterocolitis

Delayed feeding may lead to gut atrophy due to lack of intestinal stimulation. (Berseth 1990). Exposure of the immature gut to milk has been associated with necrotising enterocolitis (NEC). This is a condition that is almost unique to the preterm infant, rarely affecting the baby at term. It is characterised by inflammation of the gut wall. The gut mucosa becomes vulnerable to bacterial invasion from the lumen and, in the most serious forms of this condition, there is intramural gas and the gut perforates. Although the whole small and large gut may be involved, there is a predilection for areas that have a watershed blood supply, suggesting that gut ischaemia is an important cause. Numerous risk factors have been associated with NEC and feed intolerance. These include: infection, umbilical cannulae, thromboembolism, circulatory compromise and artificial milk feeds more than expressed breast milk (Lucas and Cole 1990).

Several studies have investigated the association between absent end diastolic flow in the umbilical artery and subsequent risk of developing NEC (Malcolm *et al.* 1991; Karsdorp *et al.* 1994; Adiotomre *et al.* 1997). Malcolm *et al.* (1991) reported a small case-control series of 25 pregnancies in which absent or reversed end diastolic flow was identified. Of the 15 morphologically normal offspring, 8 (53%) developed suspected or proven NEC compared with one neonate (6%) from the matched control group. Karsdorp *et al.* (1994) compared the outcome of pregnancies in which Doppler velocity measurements of the umbilical artery were positive (n = 214) with those that had either absent or reverse end diastolic velocities (n = 245). Absent or reverse end diastolic flow did not influence the risk of infants from these pregnancies developing NEC, despite significantly increasing the risk of cerebral haemorrhage, hypoglycaemia and anaemia. Similar findings were reported by Adiotomre *et al.* (1997) in their case-controlled study of 60 infants. In practice the presence of absent end diastolic flow, especially in growth retarded premature infants, prompts a cautious approach to feeding despite the evidence that there may not be an increased risk of NEC.

Kempley *et al.* took Doppler measurements of the superior mesenteric artery in premature babies with in utero growth retardation (IUGR). They demonstrated reduced blood flow velocity compared to those of normal weight premature babies (Kempley *et al.* 1991). In premature babies who developed NEC, however, superior mesenteric artery velocities were higher than in un-fed controls (Kempley and Gamsu 1992). These findings, whilst not straightforward, suggest that inherently abnormal adaptation in the gut circulation of IUGR babies may be another risk factor for NEC. A post-prandial peak mean superior mesenteric artery velocity after feeds has also been shown to correlate well with ability to tolerate early feeds independent of gestational age or birthweight (Fang *et al.* 2001). A 17% rise in superior mesenteric artery velocity at 60 minutes post-feed predicted early feed tolerance (establishment of full enteral feeds by 7 days post-test feed) with a sensitivity of 100% and specificity of 70%.

Good quality large scale feeding studies for ELBW infants are difficult to achieve. The intervention cannot be blinded and important outcomes such as assessment of feed intolerance are difficult to standardise, and they are therefore prone to observer bias. Giving babies small volumes of milk – less than to provide adequate nutrition – is known as minimal enteral nutrition or hypocaloric feeding. There is evidence that minimal enteral nutrition reduces the incidence of NEC and improves feed tolerance (Tyson and Kennedy 2002). The benefits and the risks of early feeding (before four days of life) compared with starting feeds later (after four days of life) are in need of further evaluation. A systematic review revealed two small studies, with 72 subjects, which have looked at this issue (Kennedy *et al.* 2002). Neither reported any clear advantage from 'early' feeding. There were no significant differences in mortality or NEC reported. So, although it seems potentially safe to initiate small amounts of feed within the first week of life in ELBW babies, a larger trial is needed to verify this.

Box 11.5   Suggested feeding approach for the vulnerable infant

- Initiate tube feeds 1ml/kg/2-hourly when stable (no inotropes, stable ventilation)
- Increase increments cautiously: 20 ml/kg/day or 1 ml/kg/hr
- Use expressed breast milk if possible
- Increase feed frequency slowly
- Avoid additives/fortifiers until fully established on feeds

---

Transfusion

Anaemia of prematurity is a common problem encountered during the acute and recovery stages of RDS in premature infants. Very low birthweight babies receive between two and three units of blood before they are discharged from a neonatal unit (Wardle *et al.* 2002).

Acute episodes of bleeding, such as intracranial, abdominal or adrenal haemorrhages may occur in the sickest infants in the first week of life. Pulmonary haemorrhage is usually due to haemorrhagic pulmonary oedema associated with patency of the ductus arteriosus. Transfusions of packed red blood cells may be used for acute blood loss in these circumstances. The rapid turnover of fetal erythrocytes, iatrogenic losses from blood sampling and haemodilution are other risk factors for anaemia. These affect stable premature babies as well as the acutely sick ones. These losses overwhelm the erythropoietic ability of the premature infant. Measures to maintain a normal haematocrit and packed cell volume should include minimising blood sampling in all but the sickest of infants.Transfusions should be reserved for acutely ill babies (e.g. if ventilated or infected) or those with symptomatic anaemia (tachycardia, tachypnoea, increased oxygen requirement or poor weight gain).

Haemoglobin levels alone are a poor indicator of response to transfusion for anaemia. Criteria for transfusion (see Box 11.5) have been formulated from consensus views rather than randomised controlled tinals of transfusion practices

(Whyte and Bifano 2002). Decisions to transfuse should be based on clinical factors in combination with measures of haematocrit or red cell volume rather than haemoglobin alone (Hudson *et al.* 1990).

As there are risks associated with blood transfusion (transmission of infectious agents, alloimmune reactions, extravasation and iron overload), the procedure should be avoided if possible, but monitored closely when required. Blood transfusion also suppresses endogenous erythropoietin production, another reason for trying to reduce its use (Stockmann *et al.* 1977; Lachance *et al.* 1994). Alagappan *et al.* (1998) showed that adherence to guidelines (see Box 11.6) could significantly decrease the number of transfusions given in a neonatal unit to babies less than 1250 g.

Other alternative strategies to blood transfusion that have been explored include iron supplementation (Lundstrom 1977), recombinant erythropoietin (Maier *et al.* 1994, 2002; Ohls *et al.* 1995; Shannon *et al.* 1995) and combinations of the two (Genen and Klenoff 2002). A recent randomised controlled trial reported by Maier *et al.* (2002) compared early versus late weekly administration of recombinant erythropoietin against non-treated controls, in 219 ELBW babies given concurrent oral iron supplements. Thirteen per cent of infants in the early treatment group maintained their haematocrit above 30% compared to 4% of the control group, and thus did not require transfusion. This reduction in transfusion exposure needs to be offset against the cost of erythropoietin and a larger study to assess any cost-benefit would be justified.

Consider transfusion to maintain Hb >7 g/dl if asymptomatic.

All other infants are transfused for significant signs of anaemia if Hb <10 g/dl, such as increasing frequency of apnoeic or bradycardic episodes with no other

---

Box 11.6   Suggested guidelines for transfusion formulated from Shannon *et al.* (1995) and Task Force of the College of American Pathologists Guidelines (Simon *et al.* 1998)

Category	Description	Transfusion Criteria
Severe	RDS/< 5 days old and/or mean arterial pressure (MAP) > 8 cm H_2O, and FiO_2 > 50%; on inotropes or hypoxaemic in FiO_2 100%	Haematocrit (Hct) < 40% or Haemoglobin (Hb) < 14 g/dl
Moderate	MAP 6–8 cm H_2O and/or FiO_2 > 35%, nCPAP, nasal cannula	Hct < 35% or Hb < 12 g/dl
Mild	MAP < 6 cm H_2O and/or FiO_2 25–35% via nCPAP, nasal cannula	Hct < 30% or Hb < 10 g/dl

obvious cause (exclude other causes first). Babies with significant lethargy or poor feeding, particularly with apnoeas may also require consideration for transfusion.

Jaundice in the preterm infant

Jaundice is a common feature in the first few days of life in premature babies. They are vulnerable to the same underlying causes for jaundice as term babies but have additional risk factors (see Box 11.7).

When jaundice is detected it is important to have a logical approach to investigation and treatment so that pathological causes can be discriminated from the majority of physiological reasons.

Box 11.7   Risk factors and causes for jaundice in preterm babies

Prehepatic

Increased red blood cell (RBC) breakdown (shorter fetal RBC lifespan or due to antibodies)

RBC enzyme defects, abnormal RBC shape

trauma and bruising (e.g. breech deliveries/cephalohaematomas)

intracranial haemorrhage

high haematocrit (e.g. IUGR, maternal diabetes)

Hepatic

Slowed glucuronidation due to poor entry to liver

immature enzyme systems

hypothyroidism (transient due to sickness or congenital)

other metabolic disorders (rarely, e.g. neonatal haematochromatosis)

familial or hepatic cell dysfunction due to infection or toxins.

Post-hepatic

Poor drainage of bile due to absent, hypoplastic or obstructed bile canaliculi external obstruction due to stenosis or choledocal cyst.

Enterohepatic circulation

Delayed passage of meconium due to immature gut motility, delayed feeding or absence of enteral feeds, NEC, (rarely malformation, cystic fibrosis (meconium ileus))

Most premature babies will have a combination of the above risk factors. The threshold for treating jaundice associated with prematurity is conventionally lower than term babies. The reasons for this are the potential ease for unbound bilirubin to cross a relatively permeable blood–brain barrier and cause kernicterus. This is especially so in ELBW babies who may also be sick, and therefore have a greater combination of risk factors for hyperbilirubinaemia. Low serum albumin levels in these babies may contribute to the level of free bilirubin in circulation. (Cashore 2000). It is this free or unbound bilirubin that presents the risk of toxicity. Theoretically, measuring this value or albumin binding capacity or bilirubin production rates would be a more accurate way of basing treatment criteria (Bratlid 2001). As none of these methods have been validated in vivo, the threshold for treatment of low birthweight and preterm babies is usually based on measurements of total serum bilirubin alone. The recommended levels for instituting therapy vary according to birthweight (Cashore 2000).

Treatment of significant jaundice in preterm babies is not without potential side effects. Phototherapy is now the universal first-line method of treating jaundice. It has been regarded as a relatively safe non-invasive process for treating unconjugated jaundice in term babies. Premature babies however, may experience increased trans-epidermal water loss (Maayan-Metzger *et al.* 2001; Grunhagen *et al.* 2002) and fluctuations in cerebral and gastrointestinal blood flow depending on the method of delivery of phototherapy (Benders *et al.* 1998; Pezzati *et al.* 2000). Fibre-optic phototherapy potentially reduces these risks but there is insufficient evidence of any benefit over conventional therapy in the overall treatment of jaundice in preterm infants (Pezzati *et al.* 2000; Mills and Tudehope 2001). Recent interest in turquoise light as a safer alternative to the conventional blue light is a new development in this area that requires further evaluation (Ebbesen *et al.* 2003).

Infection

Neonatal infection accounts for much of the early morbidity in premature infants. Managing neonatal infection involves detection, treatment and where possible prevention. The incidence of neonatal infection per se varies between 1–8.1 per 1000 live births in the USA (Klein and Marcy 1995). Early onset infections are usually acquired prenatally and the pathophysiology and implications of this are dealt with elsewhere. Sepsis developing after three days of age is considered to be of late onset. Gram-positive organisms accounted for 70% of late onset septicaemia, and 48% of infections were due to coagulase-negative staphylococci in a 2-year published survey (Stoll *et al.* 2002); in our own unit, 90% of septicaemia is caused by coagulase-negative staphylococci. Other organisms causing late-onset sepsis include: *Staphylococcus aureus, Escherichia coli* and other Gram-negative pathogens and fungi. Mortality is mostly associated with Gram-negative infection (36%) and fungaemia (32%).

The susceptibility of the premature neonate to invasion and thus infection is multifactorial. Exposure results in colonisation of the skin, respiratory tract, gut and mucosal surfaces, including conjunctivae, by any combination of the organisms, potentially followed by invasion. There are many invasive procedures involving handling, with resultant indwelling intravenous catheters and ETTs that may become colonised. This facilitates translocation of these organisms, and possible breach of mucosal surfaces into the bloodstream.

Immature host defences, such as inability to produce antibodies or mount cellular responses to infection, mean that once invasion by an organism has occurred, it spreads rapidly. Premature babies have poor neutrophil function, and reduced chemotactic and phagocytic ability (Kemp and Campbell 1996). The bone marrow only has low stores of immature neutrophils. It is unable to synthesise them rapidly in response to overwhelming peripheral destruction. This compounds neutropenia, which is a poor prognostic sign.

The clinical features of neonatal sepsis are generalised and non-specific (see Box 11.9).

Box 11.8   Clinical features of sepsis in the preterm infant

Temperature lability, either fever or hypothermia

Tachycardia

Respiratory distress (increased work of breathing, increasing O_2 or ventilatory requirements, tachypnoea)

Apnoeas despite patent airway and adequate drug treatment (theophyllines/caffeine)

Feed intolerance/abdominal distension

Lethargy, instability with handling, irritability

Jaundice with or without hepatic or splenic enlargement

Localised lesions – skin abscesses/vesicles/blisters; petechiae

---

Detection of any combination of these signs warrants close monitoring of trends with rapid initiation of investigation and treatment if symptoms persist. Basic investigations suggested for a septic screen are listed in Box 11.8. A differential white cell count, which gives the total neutrophil and immature neutrophil numbers, is more useful and reliable than the total white cell count alone. A high ratio of immature neutrophils to total white cell count has a sensitivity of 90% and specificity of 80% as a marker for early onset sepsis, but its sensitivity is only 29%–58% in late onset sepsis. Thrombocytopenia is also a feature in 50% of cases of sepsis. Haematological scoring systems have been used to help assess which babies are likely to be septic (Rodwell *et al.* 1993). If three or more parameters from a combination of white cell numbers (totals and ratios) and platelet count are abnormal, there is a sensitivity of 96% and specificity of 86% for the presence of sepsis. The C-reactive protein (CRP) is also useful and is a marker that we use in Liverpool, where samples are taken daily. Trends in these haematological and biochemical markers of infection are useful in screening for infection, enabling appropriate samples to be taken and antibiotics to be started before a baby is frankly septicaemic, and for monitoring the response to antibiotic therapy after an infection has been confirmed.

A cytokine assay is a promising test for rapid diagnosis of sepsis. Interleukin (IL)-6 and IL-8 levels were raised in infants with proven bacterial infection in a study investigating the predictive value of cytokines in neonatal infection (Mehr *et al.* 1999). The combination of IL-8 levels with an absolute neutrophil count gave 100% sensitivity and 54% specificity, with a Positive Predictive Value of 68% for infection. The Negative Predictive Value using this combination was 100%, which indicates this would be a useful test for excluding infection. This could potentially help to reduce antibiotic use.

Culture of organisms from normally sterile body fluids remains the gold standard for diagnosing sepsis. Cerebrospinal fluid should be collected in suspected late onset sepsis, as 15%–40% of babies with no growth from blood cultures

---

Box 11.9   Basic Investigations for septic screen in a Preterm Infant

Full blood count with white cell differential and platelet count
CRP
Blood cultures – peripheral and from any indwelling lines
Lumbar puncture – Cerebrospinal Fluid (CSF) for culture, sensitivities, glucose and protein analysis
Urine by supra-pubic aspirate for culture and sensitivities
Other investigations to be considered:
Bacterial or viral antigen detection from urine or CSF
Polymerase chain reaction for detection of Group B streptococcus, herpes simplex virus DNA
Candida – from serum or CSF
Endotracheal aspirates

will have meningitis (Isaacs and Moxon 1999). It is important to detect meningitis, as this will affect the duration of treatment.

The choice of antibiotics should be guided by the spectrum of organisms implicated in infections in each neonatal unit. A standardised approach is recommended to avoid ad hoc use of different antibiotics, encouraging multiple drug resistance (Isaacs and Moxon 1999). Our own practice is to start therapy with first-line antibiotics when sepsis is suspected. If cultures are negative after 48 hours, the antibiotics are stopped. If, however, the infant continues to be septic in spite of adequate blood antibiotic concentrations, we change to second-line therapy. The rationale for this combination of antibiotics is that they cover most nosocomial infections such as coagulase-negative staphylococcus and gram-negative organisms.

Box 11.10   Suggested antibiotic regimes

First-line antibiotics: Benzylpenicillin and gentamicin

Second-line antibiotics: Teicoplanin and ciprofloxacin

Suspected meningitis: Cefotaxime (or other third generation cephalosporin)

It is advisable to remove any indwelling central catheters when there is recurrent sepsis, particularly when the infecting organism is a coagulase-negative staphylococcus, because these organisms produce a slime that surrounds them in the lumen of cannulae and this is relatively resistant to antibiotic penetration.

Other supportive treatments targeting infection have been tried. There have been small studies using neutrophil transfusions that have improved survival in neutropenic septic babies. However, preparation of these transfusions is complex and expensive, and would prohibit generalised use. Another development being studied is colony-stimulating factors and results of trials are awaited (Cairo *et al.* 1996).

Prevention of infection should be a priority for all NICUs. Strategies such as prophylactic intravenous immunoglobulin have been assessed but without any significant clinical benefit (3% reduction in sepsis and a 4 % reduction in any serious infection, but no impact on incidence of NEC, IVH or shortening of hospital stay (Ohlsson and Lacy 2002)). The keystone of any policy to reduce infection is to stress the importance of strict hand-washing for all who enter a neonatal unit, the use of antiseptic hand-rubs before handling any baby and the avoidance by staff of jewellery that interferes with the efficiency of hand-washing.

Predischarge arrangements

Retinopathy of prematurity (ROP)

Babies born at less than 32 weeks' gestation or <1500 g are at risk of developing ROP. Damage to the developing retina by oxygen-derived free radicals has been proposed as the starting point for developing acute ROP. Avoidance of hyperoxia is thus important in limiting ROP. In approximately 11% of babies <28 weeks' gestation, ROP progresses to 'threshold' levels with the formation of scars and vessel overgrowth. Although spontaneous regression may occur, this process may lead to retinal detachment and blindness. There is little consensus about appropriate levels of oxygen for maximising short- or long-term growth and development, whilst minimising harmful effects. In a meta-analysis, restricted compared with liberal oxygen administration significantly reduced the incidence of all forms of ROP in survivors. Cicatricial ROP of any grade was significantly reduced in surviving infants who were exposed to a restricted oxygen regime (RR 0.26, 95% CI 0.11 to 0.58). There was also a significant reduction in the precursor, vascular ROP (any stage), in surviving infants exposed to restricted oxygen (RR 0.34, 95% CI 0.25 to 0.46) (Askie and Henderson-Smart 2001).

Intervention by cryo- or laser-therapy has been shown to be effective (Cryotherapy for Retinopathy of Prematurity Cooperative Group 1988). Screening of high-risk infants, by direct visualisation of the retina to detect these changes, begins at 34 weeks' post-conceptional age. Ophthalmologists apply ablative therapy using cryotherapy or laser photocoagulation to halt the progression of the disease with good results. Strategies to prevent ROP have been investigated. There is no evidence to support reduction of early exposure to light using goggles (Phelps and Watts 2002) to prevent ROP. The use of D-penicillamine as chelation therapy has been suggested. Theoretically it has the potential to mop up oxygen free radicals and disrupt disulphide bonds (such as those found in vascular endothelial growth factor) and may thus reduce ROP disease. Only two randomised controlled trials have so far been conducted, with a trend towards reduction in ROP in the D-penicillamine group (Phelps *et al.* 2002). In view of its potential side effects and the small number in these trials, cautious further study is warranted before the use of D-penicillamine can be recommended.

Neurological screening

Acquired disorders, which affect the developing brain before about 24 weeks' gestation, are either due to abnormalities of neuronal migration (the exact cause of which is unknown) or to intrauterine (so-called 'congenital') infection. Brain damage affecting preterm infants after 24 weeks is usually acquired and is due to periventricular leukomalacia (PVL) and/or periventricular haemorrhage (PVH).

These conditions both affect premature infants born two or more months prematurely but should be considered as separate entities. Although both conditions uniquely affect the brain during its early development, their aetiologies and clinical effects are different. However, both are due in part to disturbances of the cerebral circulation.

The basic pattern of the internal carotid artery and branches of the anterior, middle and posterior cerebral arteries is established by seven weeks' post-conceptional age. The post-embryonic period is characterised by the growth and development of the cerebral hemispheres, which is reflected in the pattern of development of the internal cerebral vessels. Between about 24 and 32 weeks there is a watershed area in the white matter around the lateral cerebral ventricles, which is where PVL develops.

By contrast, PVH is due to bleeding in the germinal matrix and then into the lateral cerebral ventricles with blood tracking into the subarachnoid space. Periventricular haemorrhage is a condition that is unique to the immature brain. Until about 22 weeks, the germinal matrix is densely packed with glioblasts, which take part in the migratory process. The germinal matrix comprises an extensive capillary bed and is reckoned as the source of about 80% of subependymal and IVH (Pape and Wigglesworth 1979). After 30 weeks, PVH becomes increasingly less likely because of regression of this area.

During this critical period of brain development, the periventricular white matter is supplied by two systems of vessels. Meningeal perforating branches pass into the brain parenchyma. The longer branches run towards the ventricles and then send branches back out towards the cortex. Other vessels run towards the ventricles only. As there are no connections between these two arterial systems, the boundary region between them is particularly vulnerable to hypoperfusion, and this is where the lesions of PVL are located.

Three physiological features are relevant to the aetiology of PVH in extremely premature babies: the relative resistance of the preterm brain to hypoxia, the ability to divert blood to essential organs (the diving reflex) and the concept of autoregulation.

Resistance to hypoxia is facilitated by a combination of factors. Fetal blood has a PaO_2 between 20 and 25 mmHg, a pH between 0.1 and 0.15 units below the pH of maternal blood in late gestation and it is about 0.5 °C warmer than the mother is. These factors have the effect of shifting the oxygen dissociation curve to the right, facilitating the release of oxygen from the haemoglobin molecule to the fetal tissues. The high proportion of haemoglobin F and higher haematocrit at earlier gestations ensures that fetal red cell oxygen affinity is greater than that of the maternal blood and has an effect in preserving oxygen delivery to fetal tissues. The net effect of these factors is that fetal arterial blood oxygen content and oxygen saturation are similar to those of the human adult (Delivoria-Papadopoulos and McGowan 1998).

Secondly, the diving reflex, which is well established in the term infant, maintains blood flow to the vital organs; the degree to which it operates in the extremely preterm infant remains uncertain, as is the degree to which it is altered by intrauterine growth restriction.

Thirdly, autoregulation is a factor in the development of PVH. Cerebral blood flow (CBF) is maintained provided BP remains within normal limits. These limits have not, however, been clearly defined in the preterm infant, and are likely to vary with other factors such as the availability of metabolic substrates, e.g. glucose (Pryds 1994) and acidaemia. Cerebral blood flow in the preterm infant seems to be particularly susceptible to hypocarbia, which causes cerebral vasoconstriction, and the condition is associated with the development of PVL (see below).

The term PVH is used to describe the conditions germinal matrix haemorrhage (GMH) or subependymal haemorrhage (SEH), intraventricular haemorrhage (IVH) and intraparenchymal haemorrhage (IPH). It is a disease of prematurity. Periventricular haemorrhage occurs in about 40% of infants below 35 weeks or 1500 g and in only very few babies above 37 weeks. The aetiology of subependymal and IVH is rather different to that of IPH. Infants who have had subependymal and/or IVH also have a much better neurodevelopmental outcome than those damaged by an IPH.

Periventricular haemorrhage arises in the germinal matrix and, in its minor and commoner forms it affects only the germinal matrix or the cerebral ventricles, having such little clinical effect that it is considered benign. When the bleeding involves the adjacent brain parenchyma there may be clinical effects.

A great deal about the timing and clinical associations of PVH has been learnt from cranial ultrasound scanning, the most appropriate imaging modality. Germinal matrix and IVH become more common with increasing immaturity,

---

Box 11.11   Classification of periventricular haemorrhage (based on Papile *et al.* 1978)

Grade	Description
I	subependymal haemorrhage (bleeding confined to germinal matrix)
II	Haemorrhage within the lateral cerebral ventricle
III	As for grade II with distension of the affected ventricle
IV	Intraparenchymal haemorrhage

and have been associated with respiratory distress and its complications (particularly pneumothorax) and asphyxia (Weindling *et al.* 1985b). Bleeding tends to be seen within 48 hours after birth; between 40% and 50% occur within the first 8 postnatal hours (e.g. Ment *et al.* 1994). These findings suggest that maturity of the vascular bed in the germinal matrix may be important in determining whether bleeding occurs here.

Clinical features

Small haemorrhages may be clinically undetected and are only observed by cranial ultrasound scan. Larger bleeds may be accompanied by circulatory collapse, with hypotension and a fall in haematocrit. The complications of PVH depend on the size of the haemorrhage, and whether there is associated white matter injury. When there is haemorrhagic infarction, an affected infant may be comatose, suffer from seizures (notoriously difficult to detect and varied in manifestation in the premature neonate), or the bleeding may be entirely unnoticed even by the most vigilant and experienced clinical staff. Mostly infants are asymptomatic.

In the medium term, the main complication of PVH is post-haemorrhagic hydrocephaly, particularly when there is haemorrhagic infarction of the brain parenchyma. The treatment of this has been the subject of a randomised trial that looked at the effectiveness of ventricular taps compared with the use of diuretic therapy. The outcome was that there was no clear advantage to ventricular tapping (Ventriculomegaly Trial Group 1990; review by Whitelaw 2002). There has also been interest in fibrinolytic therapy (reviewed by Whitelaw *et al.* 1996). However, when the "clot-busting" drug, streptokinase, was introduced into the ventricular system, and the effects were compared with conservative management of post-haemorrhagic ventricular dilatation, the numbers of deaths and babies with shunt dependence were identical in both groups (Whitelaw *et al.* 1992, 1996; Hudgins *et al.* 1994).

The incidence of post-haemorrhagic hydrocephaly has, however, declined markedly over the last five years or so, probably because of the increased use of antenatal steroids.

Periventricular leukomalacia

Periventricular leukomalacia was first fully described by Banker and Larroche (1962), although Virchow described a similar condition in 1867. Periventricular leukomalacia typically affects infants before 34 weeks' gestation. Although it may affect a baby at term, this is unusual, and the peak timing of this condition means that it occurs at a time of white matter development before active myelination (Back *et al.* 2001).

Estimates of the prevalence of PVL vary. A general figure (the median of 13 studies between 1983 and 1992 reviewed by de Vries and Levene 1995) is that it affects approximately 8% of infants below 32 weeks' gestation, and such infants comprise about 0.7% of all babies born.

The following description of histopathological changes is based on Kinney and Back (1998) and Back *et al.* (2001). Between three and eight hours after injury starts, there is coagulation necrosis of all cells followed by proliferation of astrocytes and capillary hyperplasia. Between the next three and ten days, microglia start to infiltrate the damaged area, followed by reactive hypertrophic astrocytes and there is accumulation of lipid-laden cells. As the damaged area becomes organised, reactive gliosis occurs. Then, over the next few weeks, there is cavitation and/or gliosis.

The understanding of PVL has advanced considerably with the development of cranial ultrasound scanning using a high-resolution 7.5 MHz scanhead. This is the best of the imaging modalities during the weeks after birth. Ultrasound scans have shown how the condition evolves after the causative injury. Firstly, echodense areas appear around the ventricles. Then, between two and four weeks later, cavities, known as cysts, appear; the average time before cysts or cavities appear on ultrasound is three weeks (e.g. Weindling *et al.* 1985a; Trounce *et al.* 1986). Because the condition invariably represents white matter damage, it is much more serious than PVH.

The distributions of the lesions are mainly in the periventricular watershed area, strongly suggesting that hypoxia and ischaemia are important in their pathogenesis. Three other factors are also implicated. The first relates to haemodynamics and the observation that the lesions of PVL are in an area of the developing brain that is particularly vulnerable to ischaemia. An association with hypocarbia has been described (Calvert *et al.* 1987; Greisen *et al.* 1987). Hypocarbia leads to vasoconstriction and hence hypoperfusion of the vulnerable periventricular region.

Another observation, linked to this first one, is that an increased risk of cerebral palsy (probably due to PVL) has been noted in monochorionic twins. The likely cause is altered intrauterine haemodynamics. It is argued that, in a significant proportion of singletons, spastic cerebral palsy may be due to the death of a monochorionic co-twin (Pharoah and Cooke 1996, 1997). The mechanism is probably through the disruption of the supply of blood and oxygen to the surviving fetus, causing damage to vulnerable areas of the brain, for example in the watershed areas.

Secondly, an association with chorioamnionitis, observed by Spinillo *et al.* (1995) amongst others, has become established, although a single causative organism has not been identified (Romero *et al.* 1991). There is a persuasive argument (summarised by Dammann and Leviton 1997) that the action of inflammation-related cytokines link chorioamnionitis with PVL. A rabbit model demonstrated that intrauterine infection can cause fetal brain white matter lesions (Yoon *et al.* 1997), and the same group found raised IL-6 concentrations in umbilical cord plasma in infants who had PVL-associated lesions on early cranial ultrasound scan (Yoon *et al.* 1996).

Verma *et al.* (1997) recorded that clinical chorioamnionitis doubled the chance of an abnormal cranial ultrasound scan during the neonatal period (OR 2.03, 95% CI 1.24–3.30). A recent meta-analysis found that clinical chorioamnionitis and preterm delivery was significantly associated with both cerebral palsy (RR 1.9%, 95% CI 1.4–2.5) and cystic PVL (RR 3.0, 95% CI 2.2–4.0) (Wu and Colford 2000). Since intrauterine infection causes premature labour (Goldenberg *et al.* 2000), it is possible that the brain damage is a consequence of the infection, and that the time of birth (prematurity) affects the pattern of injury, rather than being its cause. There is also a suggestion that delivery by Caesarean section might be helpful; Baud *et al.* (1998) reported that in 99 infants, 16 of whom developed cystic PVL, the risk of developing PVL was reduced significantly in those delivered by Caesarean section (OR 0.15, 95% CI 0.04 to 0.57).

A third point is that neonatal cerebral white matter is particularly vulnerable to injury before about 34 weeks' gestation. Cell culture has shown that the early differentiating oligodendrocyte is more susceptible to injury by oxygen-derived free radicals than the mature cell, possibly because of poorly developed anti-oxidant systems at this stage of development (Kinney and Back 1998; Volpe 1998). The observation that there is coagulation necrosis suggests that glutamate toxicity may play a part in perinatal white matter injury and the evidence has been summarised by Kinney and Back (1998).

There are no clinical manifestations associated with PVL during the immediate neonatal period. Because the sites of periventricular infarction lie in the path of the motor tracts, the motor disability due to PVL is usually manifested as spasticity (stiffness) affecting the legs more than the arms. This condition is known as spastic diplegia. Sigmund Freud appropriately called it 'spasticity of prematurity'. Clinical signs are not usually manifest before a baby is about eight months old or later. When the lesions are widespread, all limbs may be affected (spastic quadriplegia). Because PVL affects the periventricular white matter, usually bilaterally although not necessarily evenly, it is likely that it is caused by a generalised brain injury and, depending on the extent of the damage, there may also be associated cognitive loss.

In summary, PVL is the result of injury to the white matter around the lateral cerebral ventricles. Infection, both as antenatal maternal infection, such as chorioamnionitis, and postnatal infection, hypocapnia and hypoperfusion are implicated in its aetiology. There is debate about whether the condition originates before or after birth; it is likely that the disease represents the consequence of a process, which often begins before birth but which is manifest afterwards. Although cavities in the brain parenchyma ('cystic lesions') are clearly seen on ultrasound scans during the days and weeks just after birth, it is surprisingly difficult to make reliable predictions about outcome. In one intervention study where entry depended on the presence of signs of serious brain damage on an ultrasound brain scan, cerebral palsy was only accurately predicted in 54% infants (Weindling *et al.* 1996). There are two possible reasons for this. One is that it is difficult to identify the precise anatomical location of the lesions. The other is that the damaging process occurs relatively early in the brain's development, and neuronal plasticity may compensate. Although it might have been hoped that a decrease in the incidence of this condition would be seen with the widespread use of antenatal steroids, this has not yet been demonstrated to be the case.

Discharge arrangements

Most preterm babies not requiring supplemental oxygen at 36 weeks' post-conceptional age are ready for discharge within a week or so of their expected due date. The main criteria for discharge are that the baby should be able to maintain his/her temperature in a cot at room temperature, be fully orally fed and be gaining weight adequately in air or a low concentration of added oxygen. Acceptable oxygen saturation levels to enable infants to go home in air vary between individual NICUs. The Liverpool Women's Hospital NICU devised a range of oxygen saturation values in healthy preterm infants as a standard to which babies are compared to ascertain need for supplementary oxygen (Ng *et al.* 1998). It is the policy that infants who are stable in minimal nasal cannula oxygen and are fully fed have overnight oxygen saturation studies to evaluate the optimal oxygen flow required to maintain saturations within that predefined range. Arrangement of installation of oxygen concentrators is made through the infant's GP.

Before discharge, all parents of preterm infants should have basic resuscitation training and advice regarding prevention of cot death by laying the baby on his/her back.

It is usual for low birthweight or preterm babies to be given folic acid, iron and vitamin supplements for the first few months after discharge.

Summary

The postnatal progress of premature infants in today's NICUs involves anticipation and prevention of long-term morbidity as much as interventional and supportive treatments. Provision of respiratory support in the initial stages is being refined to avoid damage to vulnerable developing organs. The importance of developing a sound scientific basis for therapies cannot be over-emphasised. The danger of hyperoxia was only recognised after thousands of babies were blinded. Then, when the administration of oxygen was restricted, others were damaged by hypoxia (Cross 1973) and screening for ROP and effective therapy was only introduced after randomised controlled trials. Other apparently promising therapies such as postnatal steroids appeared to have a role in achieving short-term targets such as reduced duration of ventilation, but there are now indications that the dosage used may be responsible for serious long-term neurodevelopmental morbidity.

The peri-viable neonate

The most recent and comprehensive study of viability of extremely premature infants in Britain was a prospective observational study of all births from 20 to 25 weeks' gestation during a 9 month period in 1995 (Costeloe *et al.* 2000). There were a couple of surprising findings. One was that an unexpectedly high proportion (80%) of these extremely premature babies failed to survive long enough to be admitted for neonatal intensive care. Of 4004 births, only 811 survived to be admitted to an intensive care unit. Three hundred and fourteen (39%) of these infants survived to be discharged from hospital and 308 survived to 30 months (Wood *et al.* 2000). There were no survivors at 21 weeks' gestation, but survival to discharge increased progressively with increasing maturity: 9% at 22 weeks, 20% at 23 weeks, 34% at 24 weeks, 52% at 25 weeks (summarised in Table 11.1). In the UK today, survival at 28 weeks is better than 90%.

The outcome for babies born small, whether because of prematurity or intrauterine growth restriction, is poor. The second surprising finding of this EPICure study was the high occurrence of disability among survivors assessed when they were two and a half years old; about half had some disability, and, of these, about half were severely disabled (Wood *et al.* 2000). Add to this the information from Hack *et al.* (2002) that fewer very low birthweight young adults graduate from high school than those who are of normal birthweight (74% vs. 83% p = 0.04) and that the mean IQ at 20 years of age of these small babies is 5 points below that of normal birthweight controls (87 vs. 92). Cole (2000) suggested that such studies indicate two paths for future research and public policy. One is research aimed at reducing the frequency of extremely premature birth. The other is to increase access by parents and parents-to-be to information about outcome.

There are no limits in the UK below which resuscitation is not undertaken. Clinical practice is to discuss the range of likely outcomes with parents and decisions about whether or not resuscitation of a baby at the margins of viability should be undertaken are made in partnership with them. Such discussions need

Table 11.1. Survival and disability outcomes amongst preterm infants between 22 and 25 weeks gestation

Gestation	22 weeks	23 weeks	24 weeks	25 weeks
Live births	138	241	382	424
Died in labour ward	116 (84%)	110 (46%)	84 (22%)	67 (16%)
Died in neonatal unit	20 (14%)	105 (44%)	198 (52%)	171 (40%)
Survived to 2.5 years	2 (1%)	25 (10%)	108 (28%)	183 (43%)
No disability	1	11	45	98
Severe disability	1	8	24	40

to be skilled and the counsellor needs to have a sound knowledge of the possibilities and their implications; it is therefore helpful to involve a senior paediatrician. In Britain, the interests of the child are considered paramount, and parents need to be able to recognise that their own interests are secondary to those of their child, even one who has not yet been delivered.

The way in which a doctor presents information regarding likely outcome is very important. The prospect of having a very immature baby is an enormously difficult time for parents, most of whom will have had no previous experience of a baby born extremely prematurely. McCormick (1999) suggested that parents' views are more likely to be based on their own preconceptions and beliefs than on an understanding of the statistical probability of outcome. Counselling should therefore be by the most experienced person available; it is often best done by a consultant obstetrician together with a consultant paediatrician. In Liverpool, we show parents charts of current outcomes both by birthweight and gestation (since in most cases the estimated fetal weight is known and gestation is certain) (Figure 11.3a and 11.3b).

The UK Royal College of Paediatrics and Child Health has recognised that intensive care may not be instituted (or that it may be withdrawn) if the prognosis is hopeless. If the decision is then taken not to resuscitate but the baby at the margins of viability is born alive, there is no legal obligation to undertake resuscitation. The baby must, however, be treated in a dignified manner and kept comfortable, even if intensive care is not instituted. This means offering the baby to the parents to hold if they wish, keeping the baby warm and placing the baby in a cot. The expectation is that the baby in this situation will not survive, but parents should be warned that death might not occur immediately.

Long-term follow-up

51% of babies in the EPICure study (born <26 weeks' gestation) were still in supplemental oxygen at the time of the expected date of delivery (Costeloe *et al.*

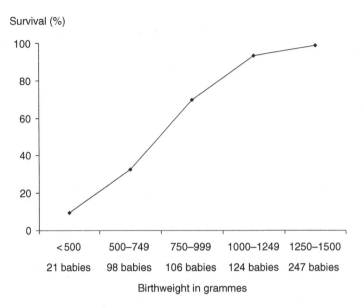

Figure 11.3a   Survival of preterm babies by birthweight.

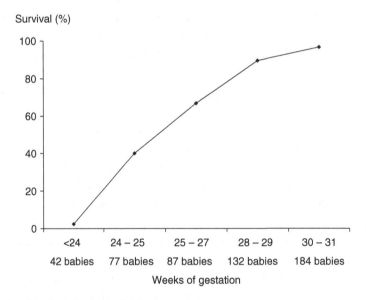

Figure 11.3b   Survival of preterm babies by gestation.

2000). Most of them would have been discharged home with domiciliary oxygen. Our practice is for these families to be supported by a specialist nurse and for the children who receive home oxygen to be followed at a specialist clinic. Preterm infants born in Britain also have regular ophthalmological surveillance until it is clear that they are no longer at risk of developing ROP (see above). All very premature infants also have formal hearing screening.

Apart from the special cases described above, even babies born extremely prematurely are not followed up routinely in hospital. Most paediatricians will see such children until they are reasonably certain that development is normal. In practice, this may be when the child is walking and talking appropriately, or regular hospital follow-up may end sooner. Community paediatric services have responsibility for ensuring that babies who were born prematurely are promptly offered appropriate treatment if they develop disability and all children are surveyed regularly by their health visitor.

REFERENCES

American Academy of Pediatrics Committee on Fetus and Newborn. (2002) Postnatal corticosteroids to treat or prevent chronic lung disease in preterm infants *Pediatrics* **109**, 330–8.

Adiotomre, P. N., Johnstone, F. D. and Laing, I. A. (1997) Effect of absent end diastolic flow velocity in the fetal umbilical artery on subsequent outcome. *Arch. Dis. Child. Fetal Neonatal Ed.* **76**, F35–8.

Ainsworth, S. B., Beresford, M. W., Milligan, D. W. *et al.* (2000). Pumactant and poractant alfa for treatment of respiratory distress syndrome in neonates born at 25–29 weeks' gestation: a randomised trial. *Lancet* **355**(9213), 1387–92.

Alagappan, A., Shattuck, K. E. and Malloy, M. H. (1998) Impact of transfusion guidelines on neonatal transfusions. *J. Perinatol.* **18**, 92–7.

Askie, L. M. and Henderson-Smart, D. J. (2001) Restricted versus liberal oxygen exposure for preventing morbidity and mortality in preterm or low birthweight infants. *Cochrane Database Syst. Rev.* **4**, CD001077.

Bandstra, E. S., Montalvo, B. M., Goldberg, R. N. *et al.* (1988) Prophylactic indomethacin for prevention of intraventricular haemorrhage in premature infants. *Pediatrics* **82**, 533–42.

Back, S. A., Luo, N. L., Borenstein, N. S. *et al.* (2001) Late oligodendrocyte progenitors coincide with the developmental window of vulnerability for human perinatal white matter injury. *J. Neurosci.* **21**(4), 1302–12.

Banker, B. and Larroche, J. (1962) Periventricular leukomalacia of infancy: a form of neonatal anoxic encephalopathy. *Arch. Neurol.* **7**, 386–410.

Baud, O., Ville, Y., Zupan, V. *et al.* (1998) Are neonatal brain lesions due to intrauterine infection related to mode of delivery? *BJOG* **105**, 121–4.

Bell, E. F., Warburton, D., Stonestreet, B. S. and Oh, W. (1979) High volume fluid intake predisposes premature infants to necrotising enterocolitis. *Lancet* **ii**, 90.

  (1980) Effect of fluid administration on the development of symptomatic patent ductus arteriosus and congestive heart failure in premature infants. *N. Engl. J. Med.* **302**, 598–604.

Bell, E. F. and Acarregui, M.J. (2001) Restricted versus liberal water intake for preventing morbidity and mortality in preterm infants. *Cochrane Database Syst. Rev.* **3**, CD000503.

Benders, M.J., van Bel, F. and van de Bor, M. (1998) The effect of phototherapy on cerebral blood flow velocity in preterm infants. *Acta Paediatr.* (**7**), 786–91.

Berseth, C. L. (1990) Neonatal small intestinal motility: the motor responses to feeding in term and preterm infants. *J. Pediatr.* **117**, 777–82.

Berseth, C. L., Kenny, J.D., and Durand, R. (1986) Longitudinal development in pediatric residents of attitudes towards neonatal resuscitation. *American J. Dis. Child.* **140** (8): 766–9.

Bourchier, D. and Weston, P.J. (1997) Randomised trial of dopamine compared with hydrocortisone for the treatment of hypotensive very low birthweight infants. *Arch. Dis. Child. Fetal Neonatal Ed.* **76**, F174–8.

Bratlid, D. (2001) Criteria for treatment of neonatal jaundice. *J. Perinatol.* **21** suppl 1, S88–92.

Cairo, M. S., Seth, T. and Fanaroff, A. (1996) A double-blinded, randomized placebo controlled pilot study of RhGM-CSF in low birthweight neonates. *Paediatr. Res.* **39**, 294A.

Calvert, S. A., Hoskins, E. M., Fong, K. W. and Forsyth, S. C. (1987) Etiological factors associated with the development of periventricular leukomalacia. *Acta Paediatr. Scand.* **76**, 254–9.

Cashore, W.J. (2000) Bilirubin and jaundice in the micropremie. *Clin. Perinatol.* **27**(1), 171–9, vii.

Cole, F. S. (2000) Extremely preterm birth – Defining the limits of hope. *N. Engl. J. Med.* **343**, 429–30.

Costarino, A. T., Gruskay, J. A., Corcoran, L., Polin, R. A. and Baumgart, S. (1992) Sodium restriction versus daily maintenance replacement in very low birthweight premature neonates: a randomised, blind therapeutic trial. *J. Pediatr.* **120**, 99–106.

Costeloe, K., Hennessy, E., Gibson, A. T., Marlow, N. and Wilkinson, A. R. (2000) The EPICure study: outcomes to discharge from hospital for infants born at the threshold of viability. *Pediatrics* **106**, 659–71.

Cross, K. W. (1973) Cost of preventing retrolental fibroplasia? *Lancet* **ii**, 954–6.

Crowley, P. (1995) Antenatal corticosteroid therapy: a meta-analysis of the randomized trials 1972–1994. *Am. J. Obstet. Gynecol.* **173**, 322–35.

Crowley P. (1999) Prophylactic corticosteroids for preterm delivery. In *The Cochrane Library* Issue 2. Oxford: Update Software.

Cryotherapy for Retinopathy of Prematurity Cooperative Group. (1988) Multicenter trial of cryotherapy for retinopathy of prematurity: preliminary results. *Pediatrics* **81**, 697–706.

Dammann, O. and Leviton, A. (1997) Maternal intrauterine infection, cytokines, and brain damage in the preterm newborn. *Pediatr. Res.* **42**, 1–8.

Dani, C., Bertini, G., Reali, M. F. *et al.* (2000) Prophylaxis of patent ductus arteriosus with ibuprofen in preterm infants. *Acta Paediatr.* **89**, 1369–74.

da Costa, D. E., Pai, Mg. and Al Khusabiby, S. M. (1999) Comparative trial of artificial and natural surfactants in the treatment of respiratory distress syndrome of prematurity: experiences in a developing country. *Pediatr. Pulmonol.* **27**(5), 303–4.

Davis, P. G. and Henderson-Smart, D. J. (2002) Prophylactic post-extubation nasal CPAP in preterm infants. (Cochrane Review) In *The Cochrane Library*, Issue 4. Oxford: Update Software.

Davis, P. G., Lemyre, B. and De Paoli, A. G. (2002) Nasal intermittent positive pressure ventilation (NIPPV) versus nasal continuous positive airway pressure (NCPAP) for preterm neonates after extubation (Cochrane Review). In *The Cochrane Library*, Issue 2. Oxford: Update Software.

De Carolis, M. P., Romagnoli, C., Polimeni, V. *et al.* (2000) Prophylactic ibuprofen therapy of patent ductus arteriosus in preterm infants. *Eur. J. Pediatr.* **159**, 364–8.

Delivoria-Papadopoulos, M. and McGowan, J. E. (1998) Oxygen transport and delivery. In R. A. Polin and W. W. Fox *Fetal and Neonatal Physiology*. eds., W. B. Saunders Co, pp. 1105–17.

de Vries, L. and Levene, M. I. (1995) Cerebral ischaemic lesions. In M. I. Levene, R. J. Lilford, M. J. Bennet and J. Punt eds., *Fetal and Neonatal Neurology and Neurosurgery*. Edinburg: Churchill Livingstone, pp. 367–860.

Ebbesen, F., Agati, G. and Pratesi, R. (2003) Phototherapy with turquoise versus blue light. *Arch. Dis. Child. Fetal Neonatal Ed.* **88**(5), F430–1.

Fang, S., Kempley, S. T. and Gamsu, H. R. (2001) Prediction of early tolerance to enteral feeding in preterm infants by measurement of superior mesenteric artery blood flow velocity. *Arch. Dis. Child. Fetal Neonatal Ed.* **85**, F42–5.

Finer, N. N., Rich, W., Craft, A. and Henderson, C. (2001) Comparison of methods of bag and mask ventilation for neonatal resuscitation. *Resuscitation* **49** (3), 299–305.

Fowlie, P. W. and Davis, P. G. (2002) Prophylactic intravenous indomethacin for preventing mortality and morbidity in preterm infants (Cochrane Review). In *The Cochrane Library*, Issue 4. Oxford: Update Software.

Genen, L. H. and Klenoff, H. (2002) Iron supplementation for erythropoietin-treated preterm infants (Protocol for a Cochrane Review). In *The Cochrane Library*, Issue 4. Oxford: Update Software.

Gersony, W. M., Peckham, G. J., Ellison, R. C., Mettinen, O. S. and Nadas, A. S. (1983) Effects of indomethacin in premature infants with patent ductus arteriosus: results of a national collaborative study. *J. Pediatr.* **102**, 895–906.

Gill, A. B. and Weindling, A. M. (1993) Randomised controlled trial of plasma protein fraction versus dopamine in hypotensive very low birthweight infants. *Arch. Dis. Child.* **69**, 284–7.

Goldenberg, R. L., Hauth, J. C. and Andrews, W. W. (2000) Intrauterine infection and preterm delivery. *N. Engl. J. Med.* **342**, 1500–7.

Greisen, G., Munck, H. and Lou, H. (1987) Severe hypocarbia in preterm infants and neuro-developmental deficit. *Acta Paediatr. Scand.* **76**, 401–4.

Grunhagen, D. J., de Boer, M. G., de Beaufort, A. J. and Walther, F. J. (2002). Transepidermal water loss during halogen spotlight phototherapy in preterm infants. *Pediatr. Res.* **51**(3), 402–5.

Hack, M., Flannery, D. J., Schluchter, M. *et al.* (2002) Outcomes in young adulthood for very low birthweight babies. *N. Engl. J. Med.* **346** (3), 149–57.

Hammarlund, K. and Sedin, G. (1979) Transepidermal water loss in newborn infants. III Relation to gestational age. *Acta Paediatr. Scand.* **68**, 795–801.

Hartnoll, G., Betremieux, P. and Modi, N. (2000) Randomised controlled trial of postnatal sodium supplementation on body composition in 25 to 30 week infants. *Arch. Dis. Child. Fetal Neonatal Ed.* **82**, F24–8.

Heckmann, M., Trotter, A., Pohlandt, F. and Lindner, W. (2002) Epinephrine treatment of hypotension in very low birthweight infants. *Acta Paediatr.* **91**, 566–70.

Heird, W. (1992) Parenteral feeding. In J. C. Sinclair, and M. B. Bracken, eds., *Effective Care of the Newborn*. Oxford: Oxford University Press, pp. 141–160.

Henderson-Smart, D. J., Bhuta, T., Cools, F. and Offringa, M. (2002) Elective high frequency oscillatory ventilation versus conventional ventilation for acute pulmonary dysfunction in preterm infants (Cochrane Review). In *The Cochrane Library*, Issue 4. Oxford: Update Software.

HIFI Study Group. (1990) High frequency oscillatory ventilation compared with conventional mechanical ventilation in the treatment of respiratory failure in preterm infants: neurodevelopmental status at 16 to 24 months of post-term age *J. Pediatr.* **117**, 939–46.

Hudak, M. L., Farrell, E. E., Rosenberg, A. A. *et al.* (1996) A multi-centre randomized masked comparison trial of natural versus synthetic surfactant for the treatment of respiratory distress syndrome. *J. Pediatr.* **128**, 396–406.

Hudgins, R. J., Boydston, W. R., Hudgins, P. A. and Adler, S. R. (1994) Treatment of intraventricular hemorrhage in the premature infant with urokinase. A preliminary study. *Pediatr Neurosurg.* **20**, 190–7.

Hudson, I., Cooke, A., Holland, B. *et al.* (1990) Red cell volume and cardiac output in anaemic preterm infants. *Arch. Dis. Child.* **65**, 672–5.

Isaacs, D. and Moxon, E. R. (1999) (eds) Handbook of Neonatal Infections, a Practical Guide. London: W. B. Saunders.

Jobe, A. H., Kramer, B. W., Moss, T. J., Newnham, J. P. and Ikegami, M. (2002) Decreased indicators of lung injury with continuous positive expiratory pressure in preterm lambs *Pediatr. Res.* **52**, 387–92.

Jonsson, B., Katz-Salamon, M., Faxelius, G., Broberger, U. and Lagercrantz, H. (1997) Neonatal care of very-low-birthweight infants in special-care units and neonatal intensive-care units in Stockholm. Early nasal continuous positive airway pressure versus mechanical ventilation: gains and losses. *Acta Paediatr. Suppl.* **419**, 4–10.

Karsdorp, V. H., van Vugt, J. M., van Geijn, H. P. *et al.* (1994) Clinical significance of absent or reversed end diastolic velocity waveforms in umbilical artery. *Lancet* **344**, 1664–8.

Kattwinkel, J., Niermeyer, S., Nadkarni, V. *et al.* (1999) ILCOR advisory statement: resuscitation of the newly born infant: an advisory statement from pediatric working group of the International Liason Committee on Resuscitation. *Circulation* **99**, 1927–38.

Kavvadia, V., Greenough, A., Dimitrou, G. and Hooper, R. (2000) Randomised trial of fluid restriction in ventilated very low birthweight infants. *Arch. Dis. Child. Fetal Neonatal Ed.* **83**, F91–6.

Kemp, A. S. and Campbell, D. E. (1996) The neonatal immune system. *Semin. Neonatol.* **1**, 67–75.

Kempley, S. and Gamsu, H. R. (1992) Superior mesenteric artery blood flow velocity in necrotising enterocolitis. *Arch. Dis. Child.* **67**, 793–6.

Kempley, S. T., Gamsu, H. R., Vyas, S. and Nicolaides, K. (1991) Effects of intrauterine growth retardation on postnatal visceral and cerebral blood flow velocity. *Arch. Dis. Child.* **66**, 1115–18.

Kennedy, K. A., Tyson, J. E. and Chamnanvanikij, S. (2002). Early versus delayed initiation of progressive enteral feedings for parenterally fed low birthweight or preterm infants (Cochrane Review). In *The Cochrane Library*, Issue 4. Oxford: Update Software.

Kinney, H. C. and Back, S. A. (1998) Human oligodendroglial development: relationship to periventricular leukomalacia. *Semin. Pediatr. Neurol.* **5**, 180–9.

Klein, J. O. and Marcy, S. M.(1995) Bacterial sepsis and meningitis In J. S. Remington and J. O. Klein, eds., *Infectious Diseases of the Fetus and Newborn Infant*, 4th edn. Philadelphia: W. B. Saunders, pp. 835–90.

Lachance, C., Chessex, P., Fouron, J. C., Widness, J. A. and Bard, H. (1994) Myocardial, erythropoietic, and metabolic adaptations to anaemia of prematurity. *J. Pediatr.* **125**, 278–82.

Lee, C. S., Hwang, B., Lu, J. H., Soong, W. J. and Chen, S. J. (1998) Symptomatic patent ductus arteriosus in very low birthweight infants. *Zhonghua Yi Xue Za Zhi (Taipei)* **61**, 93–8.

LeFlore, J. L., Salhab, W. A., Broyles, R. S. and Engle, W. D. (2002) Association of antenatal and postnatal dexamethasone exposure with outcomes in extremely low birthweight neonates. *Pediatrics* **110**, 275–9.

Liverpool Women's Hospital. (2001) Neonatal Intensive Care Unit, Fluid and Electrolyte Administration Guidelines (unpublished).

Lucas, A. and Cole, J. (1990) Breastfeeding and necrotising enterocolitis. *Lancet* **336**, 1519–23.

Lundstrom, U. (1977) At what age does iron supplementation become necessary in low-birth-weight infants. *J. Pediatr.* **91**, 878–83.

Lundstom, K. E., Pryds, O and Greisen, G. (1995) Oxygen at birth and prolonged cerebral vasoconstriction in preterm infants. *Arch. Dis. Child.* **73**, F81–6.

Lyon, A. J., McIntosh, N., Wheeler, K. and Brooke, O. G. (1984) Hypercalcaemia in extremely low birthweight infants. *Arch. Dis. Child.* **59**, 1141–4.

Maayan-Metzger, A., Yosipovitch, G., Hadad, E., and Sirota, L. (2001) Transepidermal water loss and skin hydration in preterm infants during phototherapy. *Am. J. Perinatol.* **18**(7), 393–6.

McCormick, M. C. (1999) Conceptualizing child health status: observations from studies of very premature infants. *Perspect. Biol. Med.* **42**, 372–86.

Mackintosh, M. (2003) CESDI. Project 27/28: An enquiry into quality of care and its effect on the survival of babies born at 27–28 weeks. London:The Stationary Office.

Maier, R. F., Obladen, M., Scigalla, P. *et al.* European Multicenter Erythropoietin Beta Study Group. (1994) The effect of epoetin beta (recombinant human erythropoietin) on the need for transfusion in very-low-birthweight infants. *N. Engl. J. Med.* **330**(17), 1173–8.

Maier, R. F., Obladen, M., Muller-Hansen, I. *et al.*; European Multicenter Erythropoietin Beta Study Group. (2002) Early treatment with erythropoietin beta ameliorates anemia and reduces transfusion requirements in infants with birthweights below 1000 g. *J. Pediatr.* **141**, 8–15.

Malcolm, G., Ellwood, D., Devonald, K., Beilby, R. and Henderson-Smart, D. (1991) Absent or reversed end diastolic flow velocity in the umbilical artery and necrotising enterocolitis. *Arch. Dis. Child.* **66**, 805–7.

Martinez, A. M., Padbury, J. F. and Thio, S. (1992) Dobutamine pharmacokinetics and cardio-vascular responses in critically ill neonates. *Pediatrics* **89**, 47–51.

Mehr, S. S., Vervaart, P., Henschke, P., Doyle, L. W. and Rice G. E. (1999) The predictive value of interleukin-6 (IL-6) and interleukin-8 (IL-8) in infants with bacterial sepsis (abstract) *Proceedings of the Perinatal Society of Australia and New Zealand 3rd Annual Congress.*

Ment, L. R., Oh, W., Ehrenkranz, R. A. *et al.* (1994) Low-dose indomethacin therapy and extension of intraventricular hemorrhage: a multicenter randomized trial. *J. Pediatr.* **124**, 951–5.

Mills, J. F., Tudehope, D. (2001) Fibreoptic phototherapy for neonatal jaundice. *Cochrane Database Syst. Rev.* 1, CD002060.

Mondanlou, H., Beharry, K., Padilla, G. and Norris, K. (1997) Comparative efficacy of Exosurf and Survanta surfactants on early clinical course of respiratory distress syndrome and complications of prematurity. *J. Perinatol.* **17**, 455–60.

Morley, C. (1999) Personal Practice: Continuous distending pressure. *Arch. Dis. Child. Fetal Neonatal Ed.* **81**, F152–6.

Niermeyer, S., Kattwinkel, J., Van Reempts, P. *et al.* (2000) International Guidelines for Resuscitation: An excerpt from the Guidelines 2000 for Cardiopulmonary Resuscitation and Emergency Cardiovascular Care: International Consensus on Science. Contributors and reviewers for the Neonatal Resuscitation Guidelines *Pediatrics* **106**(3), E29.

Nijima, S., Shortland, D. B., Levene, M. I. *et al.* (1988) Transient hyperoxia and cerebral blood flow velocity in infants born prematurely and at full term. *Arch. Dis. Child.* **63**, 1126–30.

Ng, A., Subhedar, N., Primhak, R. A. and Shaw, N. J. (1998) Arterial oxygen saturation profiles in healthy preterm infants. *Arch. Dis. Child Fetal Neonatal Ed.* **79**, F64–6.

O'Donnell, A. I., Gray, P. H. and Rogers, and Y. M. (1998) Mortality and neurodevelopmental outcome for infants receiving adrenaline in neonatal resuscitation. *Journal of Paediatrics and Child Health* **34**(6), 551–6.

Ogawa, Y., Miyasaka, K., Kawano, T. *et al.* (1993) A multi-centre randomised trial of high frequency oscillatory ventilation as compared with conventional mechanical ventilation in preterm infants with respiratory failure. *Early Hum. Dev.* **32**, 1–10.

Ohls, R. K., Osborne, K. A. and Christensen, R. D. (1995) Efficacy and cost analysis of treating very low birthweight infants with erythropoietin during their first two weeks of life: a randomized, placebo controlled trial. *J. Pediatr.* **126**, 421–6.

Ohlsson, A. and Lacy, J. B. (2002) Intravenous immunoglobulin for preventing infection in preterm and/or low-birth-weight infants (Cochrane Review). In *The Cochrane Library*, Issue 4. Oxford: Update Software.

Pape, K. E. and Wigglesworth, J. S. (1979) Haemorrhage, ischaemia and the perinatal brain. *Clinics in Developmental Medicine* Nos 69/70. London: Spastics International Medical Publications. William Heinemann.

Papile, L. A., Burstein, J., Burstein, R. and Koffler, H. (1978) Incidence and evolution of subependymal and intraventricular haemorrhage: a study of infants with birthweights less than 1,500 gm. *J. Pediatr.* **92**, 529–34.

Pezzati, M., Biagiotti, R., Vangi, V. *et al.* (2000) Changes in mesenteric blood flow response to feeding: conventional versus fiber-optic phototherapy. *Pediatrics* **105**(2), 350–3.

Pharoah, P. O. and Cooke, T. (1996) Cerebral palsy and multiple births. *Arch. Dis. Child. Fetal Neonatal Ed.* **75**, F174–7.

(1997) A hypothesis for the aetiology of spastic cerebral palsy–the vanishing twin. *Dev. Med. Child Neurol.* **39**, 292–6.

Phelps, D. L. and Watts, J. L. (2002) Early light reduction for preventing retinopathy of prematurity in very low birthweight infants (Cochrane Review). In *the Cochrane Library*, Issue 4. Oxford: Update Software.

Phelps, D. L., Lakatos, L. and Watts, J. L. (2002) D-Penicillamine for the preventing retinopathy of prematurity in preterm infants (Cochrane Review) In *The Cochrane Library*, Issue 4. Oxford: Update Software.

Pryds, O. (1994) Low neonatal cerebral oxygen delivery is associated with brain injury in preterm infants. *Acta Paediatr.* **83**, 1233–6.

Rager, R. and Finegold, M. J. (1975) Cholestasis in immature infants: is parenteral alimentation responsible? *J. Pediatr.* **86** (2), 264–9.

Ramji, S., Ahuja, S., Thirupuram, S. *et al.* (1993) Resuscitation of asphyxiated newborn infants with room air or 100% oxygen. *Pediatr. Res.* **34**, 809–12.

Resuscitation Council UK. (2001) Algorithm for neonatal life support. In *Resuscitation at Birth; The Newborn Life Support Provider Course Manual* (ISBN 1 903823 011), p. 64.

Rodwell, R. L., Taylor, K. M., Tudehope, D. I. and Gray, P. H. (1993) Haematologic scoring system in the early diagnosis of sepsis in neutropenic newborns. *Pediatr. Infect. Dis. J.* **12**, 372–6.

Romero, R., Ghidini, A., Mazor, M. and Behnke, E. (1991) Microbial invasion of the amniotic cavity in premature rupture of membranes. *Clin Obstet. Gynecol.* **34**, 769–78.

Saugstad, O. D., Rootwelt, T. and Aalen, O. (1998) Resuscitation of asphyxiated newborn infants with room air or oxygen: an international controlled trial: the Resair 2 study. *Pediatrics* **102**(1), E1.

Sedin, G. (1996) Fluid management in the extremely preterm infant. In T. N. Hansen and N. McIntosh, eds., *Current Topics in Neonatology*. London: W. B. Saunders, pp. 50–66.

Shannon, K. M., Keith, J. F. 3rd, Mentzer, W. C. *et al.* (1995) Recombinant human erythropoietin stimulates erythropoiesis and reduces erythrocyte transfusions in very low birthweight preterm infants. *Pediatrics* **95**, 1–8.

Simon, T. L., Alverson, D. C., AuBuchon, J. *et al.* (1998) Practice parameter for the use of red blood cell transfusions: developed by the Red Blood Cell Administration Practice Guideline Development Task Force of the College of American Pathologists. *Arch. Pathol. Lab. Med.* **122**, 130–8.

Sims, D. G., Heal, C. A. and Bartle, S. M. (1994) Use of adrenaline and atropine in neonatal resuscitation. *Arch. Dis. Child. Fetal Neonatal Ed.* **70** (1): F3–9.

Sinclair, J. C. (2002) Servo-control for maintaining abdominal skin temperature at 36C in low birthweight infants (Cochrane Review). In *The Cochrane Library*, Issue 4. Oxford: Update Software.

So, K. W., Fok, T. F., Ng, P. C., Wong, W. W. and Cheung, K. L. (1997) Randomised controlled trial of colloid or crystalloid in hypotensive preterm infants. *Arch. Dis. Child.* **76**, F43–6.

Soll, R. F., Blanco, F. (2003) Natural surfactant versus synthetic surfactant for neonatal respiratory distress syndrome (Cochrane Review). In *The Cochrane Library*, Issue 4. Chichester, UK: John Wiley & Sons, Ltd. CD000144.

Soll, R. F. and McQueen, M. C. (1992) In J. C. Sinclair and M. B. Bracken, eds., *Effective Care of the Newborn Infant*. Oxford: Oxford University Press, 325–58.

Spinillo, A., Capuzzo, E., Stronati, M. *et al.* (1995) Effect of preterm premature rupture of membranes on neurodevelopmental outcome: follow up at two years of age. *BJOG* **102**, 882–7.

Stanley, F. J. and Alberman, E. D.(1978) Infants of very low birthweight. 1 Factors affecting survival. *Dev. Med. Child Neurol.* (**20**), 300–12.

Steer, P. A., Lucas, A. and Sinclair, J. (1992) Feeding the low birthweight infant In J. C. Sinclair and M. B. Bracken, eds., *Effective Care of the Newborn*. Oxford: Oxford University Press, pp 94–140.

Stockman, J. A., Garcia, J. F. and Oski, F. A. (1977) The anaemia of prematurity. Factors governing the erythropoietin response. *N. Engl. J. Med.* **296**, 647–50.

Stoll, B. J., Hansen, N., Fanaroff, A. A. *et al.* (2002) Late-onset sepsis in very low birthweight neonates: the experience of the NICHD Neonatal Research Network. *Pediatrics* **110**, 285–91.

Subhedar, N. V. and Shaw, N. J. (2002) Dopamine versus dobutamine for hypotensive preterm infants (Cochrane Review). In *The Cochrane Library*, Issue 4. Oxford: Update Software.

Subramaniam, P., Henderson-Smart, D. J. and Davis, P. G. (2000) Prophylactic nasal continuous positive airways pressure for preventing morbidity and mortality in very preterm infants (Cochrane Review). In *The Cochrane Library*, Issue 4. Oxford: Update Software.

Tan, A., Schulze, A. and Davis, P. G. (2002) Air versus oxygen for resuscitation of infants at birth (Protocol for a Cochrane review) In *The Cochrane Library*, Issue 4. Oxford: Update Software.

Thompson, M. and Kempley, S. (1999) Proceedings of Debate: Early prophylactic versus rescue administration of surfactant. Royal London Hospital Ventilation Workshop, July 1999 (unpublished).

Trounce, J. Q., Rutter, N. and Levene, M. I. (1986) Periventricular leukomalacia and intraventricular haemorrhage in the preterm neonate. *Arch. Dis. Child.* **61**, 1196–202.

Tyson, J. E. and Kennedy, K. A. (2002) Minimal enteral nutrition for promoting feeding tolerance and preventing morbidity in parenterally fed infants (Cochrane Review). In *The Cochrane Library*, Issue 4. Oxford: Update Software.

van Marter, L. J., Leviton, A., Allred, E. N., Pagano, M. and Kuban, K. C. (1990) Hydration in the first days of life and the risk of bronchopulmonary dysplasia in low birthweight infants. *J. Pediatr.* **116**, 942–9.

Van Marter, L. J., Allred, E. N., Pagano, M. *et al.* (2000) Do clinical markers of barotrauma and oxygen toxicity explain interhospital variation in rates of chronic lung disease? The Neonatology Committee for the Developmental Network. *Pediatrics* **105**, 1194–201.

Vento, M., Asensi, M., Sastre, J. *et al.* (2001) Resuscitation with room air instead of 100% oxygen prevents oxidative stress in moderately asphyxiated term neonates. *Pediatrics* **107**, 642–7.

Ventriculomegaly Trial Group. (1990) Randomised trial of early tapping in neonatal post-haemorrhagic ventricular dilatation. *Arch. Dis. Child.* **65**, 3–10.

Verma, U., Tejani, N., Klein, S. *et al.* (1997) Obstetric antecedents of intraventricular hemorrhage and periventricular leukomalacia in the low-birth-weight neonate. *Am. J. Obstet. Gynecol.* **176**, 275–81.

Volpe, J. J. (1998) Neurologic outcome of prematurity. *Arch. Neurol.* **55**, 297–300.

Wardle, S. P., Garr, R., Yoxall, C. W. and Weindling, A. M. (2002) A pilot randomised controlled trial of peripheral fractional oxygen extraction to guide blood transfusions in preterm infants. *Arch. Dis. Child. Fetal Neonatal Ed.* **86**, F22–7.

Weindling, A. M. (2002) Epinephrine treatment in hypotensive newborns. *Acta Paediatr.* **91**, 500–2.

Weindling, A. M., Wilkinson, A. R., Cook, J. *et al.* (1985b) Perinatal events which precede periventricular haemorrhage and leukomalacia in the newborn. *BJOG* **92**, 1218–23.

Weindling, A. M., Rochefort, M. J., Calvert, S. A., Fok, T. F. and Wilkinson, A. (1985a) Development of cerebral palsy after ultrasonographic detection of periventricular cysts in the newborn. *Dev. Med. Child. Neurol.* **27**, 800–6.

Weindling, A. M., Hallam, P., Gregg, J. *et al.* (1996) A randomized controlled trial of early physiotherapy for high-risk infants. *Acta Paediatr.* **85**, 1107–11.

Whitelaw, A. (2002) Repeated lumbar or ventricular punctures in newborns with intraventricular hemorrhage (Cochrane Review). In *The Cochrane Library*, Issue 4. Oxford: Update Software.

Whitelaw, A., Rivers, R., Creighton, L. and Gaffney, P. (1992) Low dose intraventricular fibrinolytic therapy to prevent posthaemorrhagic hydrocephalus. *Arch. Dis. Child.* **67**, F12–4.

Whitelaw, A., Saliba, E., Fellman, V. *et al.* (1996) Phase 1 study of intraventricular recombinant tissue plasminogen activator for treatment of posthaemorrhagic hydrocephalus. *Arch. Dis. Child. Fetal Neonatal Ed.* **74**, F20–6.

Whyte, R. K. and Bifano, E. M. (2002) Early erythrocyte transfusion in very-low-birth-weight infants (Protocol for a Cochrane Review). In *The Cochrane Library*, Issue 4. Oxford: Update Software.

Wood, N. S., Marlow, N., Costeloe, K., Gibson, A. T. and Wilkinson, A. R. (2000) Neurologic and developmental disability after extremely preterm birth. *N. Engl. J. Med.* **343**, 378–84.

Wyckoff, M. H., Perlman, J. and Niermeyer, S. (2001) Medications during resuscitation – what is the evidence? *Semin. Neonatol.* **6** (3), 251–9.

Wu, Y. W. and Colford, J. M. (2000) Chorioamnionitis as a risk factor for cerebral palsy. A meta-analysis. *JAMA* **284**, 1417–24.

Yoon, B. H., Romero, R., Yang, S. H. *et al.* (1996) Interleukin-6 concentrations in umbilical cord plasma are elevated in neonates with white matter lesions associated with periventricular leukomalacia. *Am. J. Obstet. Gynecol.* **174**, 1433–40.

Yoon, B. H., Chong, C. J., Romero, R. *et al.* (1997) Experimentally induced intrauterine infection causes fetal brain white matter lesions in rabbits. *Am. J. Obstet. Gynecol.* **177**, 797–802.

Yost, C. C. and Soll, R. F. (2002) Early versus delayed selective surfactant treatment for neonatal respiratory distress syndrome (Cochrane Review). In *The Cochrane Library*, Issue 4. Oxford: Update Software.

12

Organisation of high risk obstetric and neonatal services

Karl Murphy[1] and Sara Twaddle[2]

[1]St Mary's Hospital, London
[2]Scottish Intercollegiate Guideline Network, Edinburgh

Service requirements

Background: the need for change

The current provision of perinatal services in the UK is under intense scrutiny and many fundamental and far-reaching changes are in the pipeline. The impetus for these changes has come largely from the neonatal specialties, which are experiencing difficulties providing comprehensive care for very preterm and sick term infants. This chapter will review the provision of perinatal services, together with potential and proposed changes in service provision. The London region will be used as an example of service provision, but the issues discussed are relevant to the majority of regions in the UK.

Up to 10% of all newborns need admission to a neonatal unit, and 2%–3% need intensive care. In the UK we are generating large numbers of inappropriate transfers of complex cases between units, often out of specialist centres, before and after birth because of inadequate capacity in our neonatal units (Parmanum *et al.* 2000). The fact that our neonatal intensive care is not centralised and we have a large number of relatively small neonatal units providing some intensive care is a key issue here. These transfers cause great misery and distress to families at a time of crisis, and waste a great deal of medical and midwifery staff time. Moreover, siblings of multiple pregnancies may receive care in different neonatal units in up to one third of cases. Another problem is that intensive care cots are blocked by infants who should be nursed in high-dependency or even special care because of a lack of specialist nursing staff. London has a particular problem with recruitment and retention of specialist nursing staff. Although there is no direct evidence that the high numbers of long distance transfers are responsible for poor clinical outcomes, a recent study supports the gathering view that UK neonatal intensive care survival outcomes are less impressive than those for other countries (International Neonatal Network 1997). In fact there is evidence available to show that well planned transport of babies improves outcome (CESDI 2001a; Clinical Standards Advisory Group 1996).

Preterm Labour Managing Risk in Clinical Practice, eds. Jane Norman and Ian Greer. Published by Cambridge University Press. © Cambridge University Press 2005.

Litigation costs may also be contributing to the perceived need for change in the provision of perinatal services. For example, in 2002 there were £5.25 billion worth of outstanding claims against the NHS to be settled over a 10-year period. In 2001, this outstanding amount represented about 8% of the total NHS budget. While one in five claims relates to obstetrics, the cost of these claims is 80% of all medicolegal claims (CESDI 2001b). Clearer standards and guidelines with respect to lines of responsibility and care of high-risk pregnancies may help to curb this costly, exponential growth in litigation. The 'Bristol Inquiry' report provided us with useful guidance on the organisation of neonatal surgical services, guidance that is very relevant to neonatal intensive care – also a highly technical specialty with the constant risk of iatrogenic complications. The report recommended that specialist care be concentrated in a limited number of centres where staff had the prerequisite skills and experience (Bristol Royal Infirmary Inquiry 2001) There is evidence that increasing size of neonatal units is associated with improved clinical outcomes (International Neonatal Network 1993; Shann, 1994) but much of it is contradictory, and the current arguments in favour of increasing centralisation have grown stronger as a result of the chronic problems with staffing and service provision. Certainly, there are data which suggest that larger units use resources more efficiently than smaller ones (NHS Executive, Fordham *et al.* 1992; Northern Neonatal Network 1993; Young 1994; Mother and Child Initiative 2000).

Review Groups

In response to the problem the London Regional Specialised Commissioning Group (LRSCG) and the Thames Regional Perinatal Group (TRPG) undertook a review of neonatal intensive care and high-dependency care and published a discussion document entitled 'Modernising Neonatal Intensive Care in London and the Implications for Related Services' in 2001. More recently, the Department of Health has formed an External Advisory Group for Neonatal Intensive Care with multidisciplinary and lay membership to advise on the organisation of neonatal services

The LRSCG/TRPG discussion document accepts the standards provided by the British Association of Perinatal Medicine (BAPM) standards (BAPM 2001). The BAPM and Neonatal Nurses Association (NNA) have reclassified the existing categories of neonatal care. Briefly, they describe three levels of neonatal care: a *Level 3 neonatal unit* will provide the full range of services. It cares for the sickest babies, requires the presence of a competent doctor on-site, and may or may not provide specialist neonatal services such as paediatric surgery or cardiology on site. A *Level 2 unit* will provide only short-term intensive care (mechanical ventilation for 24 hours or less), and high-dependency care (now to include continuous positive airways pressure category). A *Level 1 unit* will provide special care only and will not be expected to provide any intensive or high-dependency care, and may or may not have resident medical staff. Full details on the standards for each level of care are available from the BAPM Publications website (BAPM 2001).

Service infrastructure

Perinatal intensive care requires the close collaboration of obstetricians, midwives, neonatologists and anaesthetists, in addition to all of the appropriate equipment and facilities. Where the appropriate facilities are not available there must be procedural mechanisms in place to ensure the patient still has equity of access to treatment. Based on the recommendations of the Bristol Inquiry the LRSCG/TRPG review group considered that a central principle of any proposed reorganisation of the perinatal services was that care should be provided as close as possible to the place of residence, but that ease of access should never take precedence over quality and safety.

The LRSCG/TRPG document sets out a vision for the future of perinatal services in which all hospitals providing maternity and neonatal care collaborate to deliver integrated services through the development of Managed Clinical networks. The networks would provide an overarching framework and, where possible, obstetric and neonatal networks would be coterminous. It was estimated for example that London would need 5 to 9 networks each serving 12–20 000 births. It is proposed that the neonatal networks should be managed by a steering committee, which would be administered from the lead centre and, ideally, chaired by a clinical director. Each network would have one hospital that is a major perinatal centre. This centre would include both a specialist obstetric department providing materno-fetal medicine services in combination with a Level 3 Neonatal Intensive Care Unit. The perinatal centre would act as the lead hospital for the network. Most of the other hospitals in the network would provide neonatal high-dependency care and some short-term neonatal intensive care (Level 2), while some would offer only special and normal care (Level 1). It is recommended by TRPG that Level 3 units should have 8–12 intensive care cots, and Level 2 at least 4 such cots. However, all hospitals providing any maternity or neonatal care would be expected to make arrangements with the appropriate perinatal centre for the training and maintenance of skills in neonatal resuscitation and stabilisation of babies (Expert Maternity Group 1993).

The target would be that 95% of all neonatal work for the defined population would be provided within the network. To achieve this target the review group estimated that for London the average bed occupancy would need to be less than 70%. On the thorny issue of numbers of neonatal intensive care cots required, data are available to suggest that something like 1.2 cots per 1000 births would suffice, but obviously this would need to be flexible in accordance with local needs

(Northern Neonatal Network 1993; Burton *et al.* 1995). Additional funding will obviously be required for expansion of the existing Level 3 units. To facilitate the provision of services within a single network, the LRSCG/TRPG suggested the following guidelines:

- Medical and nursing staff from the perinatal centre would need to be available at all times to give advice to the other units in the network.
- All pregnant women expected to deliver before a gestational age of 29 weeks or with an estimated fetal weight of less than 1 kg should be transferred to the perinatal centre antenatally.
- All babies with a birth weight less than 1 kg or needing mechanical ventilation for longer than 24 hours should be transferred to the perinatal centre postnatally.
- All babies weighing less than 1.5 kg or with a gestational age of less than 33 weeks should be transferred out from a Level 1 unit.
- The perinatal centre must provide on-going contact with the staff from the referring centre together with early return of babies to the base unit.

Maternity services

The proposed changes in neonatal services will inevitably have a major impact on the maternity services. About 20% of women develop a problem in pregnancy that requires the services of a specialist in materno-fetal medicine. Severe maternal morbidity can be expected in about 1.2% of all births (Waterstone *et al.* 2001) The number of hospitals providing neonatal intensive care will be reduced in the medium to long term, and high-risk women will need to be transferred to perinatal centres so that they can receive obstetric/medical and neonatal care in the same centre. High-risk women should not be delivered in maternity hospitals separate from acute hospital facilities (Confidential Enquiries into Maternal Deaths in the UK 2002). Changing public expectations will be a key aspect of achieving acceptance of the reforms. There are data to show that patients are prepared to travel for care if they believe it will benefit them (Greenberg *et al.* 1988)

The LRSCG/TRPG review group provided guidelines for the provision of maternity services within the context of the perinatal centres. They are based on the 1998 BAPM recommendations (BAPM 1998), and include the following:

- At the perinatal centre at least one obstetrician (preferably more) should have a major interest in perinatal obstetrics and devote the majority of their working week to organising and running the service.
- There should be a multidisciplinary team including a physician with an interest in obstetric medicine, obstetric anaesthetists and specialist midwives all of whom would participate in the on-call rota so that the service functions appropriately out of hours.

- There should be consultant level obstetric cover for labour ward at all times and for 40 hours per week the covering consultant should have no other fixed commitment.
- A fully trained obstetric anaesthetist should be available at all times and a dedicated consultant session should be available per 500 deliveries.
- The higher dependency level of patients in perinatal centres should be reflected in the level of midwifery staffing. The Royal College of Obstetricians and Gynaecologists (RCOG) now recommend 50 full time equivalents per 1000 deliveries (Whittle *et al.* 1994)

With respect to facilities and equipment at the perinatal centre the guidelines include the following:

- There should be a recovery area, a high dependency unit and at least one dedicated obstetric theatre, on the same floor as the delivery suite, per 3000 deliveries.
- Obstetric ultrasound equipment must comply with RCOG/Royal College of Radiologists (RCR) guidelines.
- There should be one fetal monitor per 500 deliveries.
- There should be 24-hour availability of haematological, biochemical and micro-biological support.
- An epidural service should be available 24 hours per day.
- Services for genetic counselling should be available on site.

The use of complicated invasive diagnostic procedures such as cordocentesis or fetal blood transfusion will become the preserve of the perinatal centres but clearly high-risk obstetricians will need to be given sessional commitments in the perinatal centres if their base unit becomes Level 1 or 2. Funding for obstetric services must then be reviewed and it is essential in future that it follows the high-risk patient.

Transport services

A co-ordinated transport service would organise retrievals and returns to the base hospital, and provide consultation services and education for outlying practitioners. There are data to show that transportation of neonates to Level 3 units improves outcomes (Delaney-Black *et al.* 1989; Chiu *et al.* 1993), although shortcomings in the provision of the transport service have been documented (Medical Devices Agency 1995). Currently, antenatal and postnatal transfers are arranged with the London Ambulance Service, but in future postnatal transfers would need an independent, dedicated transport service to transfer babies within and between networks. There would need to be clear protocols applicable throughout the network for antenatal transfers, resuscitation, stabilisation, postnatal transfers and for prompt return. Senior medical staff would need to be available to assess suitability of patients for in utero and postnatal transfer, and, ultimately, it would be desirable for the retrieval team to be present at the delivery and conduct the stabilisation and transfer. The mother should always be accommodated in the perinatal centre under these circumstances.

Adult intensive care facilities

Many babies needing intensive care are born to mothers who have conditions such as severe pre-eclampsia and who themselves require intensive care, and any unit offering Level 3 neonatal care must be able to provide high level care for sick mothers as well. Regardless of the original diagnosis, the quality of the intensive care may determine the outcome (Confidential Enquiries into Maternal Deaths in the UK 2002).

The recent Department of Health (DOH) publication 'Comprehensive Critical Care' sets out an ambitious modernisation programme that is far reaching and has important implications for trusts providing this type of care (Department of Health 2000). Again, care is reclassified according to the severity of illness and the level of care that individual patients need. A doctor with specialist training in intensive care medicine should lead every critical care service and, in the longer term, all consultants in intensive care medicine should possess the Royal College specialist competencies. Trust-wide critical care delivery groups need to be formed with an executive director taking the lead. Regional offices and NHS trusts will need to form networks so that providers and commissioners work together to cover specific geographical areas. In general terms, hospitals admitting emergencies should normally have all levels of care available. As will be the case for the new perinatal centres, the modernised adult critical care service should ensure that transfers occur within the network as much as possible.

Staffing requirements

The intention for the proposed new structures would be to have 24 hour consultant on-site cover for all Level 3 neonatal units. The move towards shorter working hours will adversely affect continuity of care provided by the junior staff, and it is anticipated that the slack will be picked up by increased numbers of consultants. At the very least the attending neonatologist will need to hold certificate of completion of specialist training (CCST) qualifications. In order to allow for study leave, annual leave and sick leave, the review group calculated that seven whole time equivalent consultant neonatal staff would be needed to provide a safe service. Current trainees should be made aware of the increased opportunities for jobs and for career development.

Nursing recruitment and retention are serious problems for the NHS and national initiatives are urgently needed to make nursing and midwifery careers more attractive (Buchan 2002). A lack of trained staff may lead to care that is unsafe and it must be remembered that units need to allow for sick leave, annual leave and study leave. The BAPM/NNA recommend that for neonatal intensive care there should be a staff to patient ratio of 1:1, for high dependency it should be 2:1, and for special care it should be 4:1 (BAPM/NNA 1992).

Affordable accommodation is an urgent requirement for improving recruitment and retention in the London area. In addition, the traditional nursing role needs to change and adapt to meet the new requirements of the NHS Plan. For example, the extended clinical role should be encouraged, and competency based grading is helpful in recognising new nursing skills. Neonatal transfers could be co-ordinated by specialist nurses, so that a team of nurse practitioners with specialised training in the transport of babies would be a future requirement.

Specialist neonatal services

Although not all networks would be expected to provide specialist neonatal services such as paediatric surgery and cardiology, it is mandatory that all would have formal arrangements in place with specialist centres to allow patients appropriate access. Obviously, networks providing specialist neonatal services to neighbouring networks will need to have a capacity that reflects this.

A Level 3 Neonatal Intensive Care Unit needs input from paediatric specialists and during the reconfiguration every effort should be made to bring these services together in the first place. Trusts could consider joint senior staff appointments or clearly defined service agreements so that specialists would be free to visit and advise freely in neighbouring networks. If a specialist centre were not a perinatal centre it would need to demonstrate that it has enough competent staff to provide the service at all times. The specialist centre may of course be a member of more than one network.

Effects on postgraduate training and academic infrastructure

Training, research and development remain the responsibility of Level 3 units. However, many of these units are struggling to achieve the throughput which makes this possible. The development of fewer, larger units (perinatal centres) should facilitate training, research and development. Funding bodies will need to recognise this need as well.

Proposals for subspecialty training in neonatal medicine have been drawn up by the Royal College of Paediatrics and Child Health specialist advisory committee for neonatal medicine (RCPCH 2001). All consultants must have done one year of higher training on a Level 3 neonatal unit. All future consultant appointments to a Level 3 unit must have their CCST in neonatal medicine plus have spent at least two years training in a Level 3 unit. The new perinatal centres should enhance the quality of training for both neonatal paediatricians and obstetricians, presenting increased opportunities for integrated experience. The postgraduate deaneries will need to take on board the particular problems of consultant recruitment in London.

It is important that the perinatal research base is protected both during and after the reconfiguration. Close links between university and clinical departments should ensure its protection without detriment to clinical services because of vested interests. It is desirable that there is an active perinatal research programme in place in the perinatal centre. The networks would be responsible also for collating joint obstetric and paediatric data on staffing levels, clinical activity and outcomes to facilitate benchmarking, and clinical governance (including risk management, audit and continuing professional development). The networks would also be responsible for publishing annual reports according to BAPM standards (BAPM 1997). Information Technology resources would be shared within the network facilitating the use of common protocols and the adequate dissemination of patient information and literature.

The way forward

Implementation of the changes will require a programme of training and reorganisation over many years. The DOH External Advisory Group for Neonatal Intensive Care is planning the increased centralisation of the services. In the meantime, there are the immediate problems of excessive numbers of long-distance transfers and inadequate capacity at the referring centres for returns.

The networks should be identified now and the staff within each network would then be responsible for integrating their services with the aim of reducing the number of transfers outside the network. An integrated transport system would be a priority. National and regional strategies are needed to sort out consultant and nursing recruitment and retention problems and deployment issues relating to the reconfiguration. Once the perinatal centres have adequate capacity and are staffed properly then a resident senior shift in neonatology could be considered. All of these issues will need full consultation, an end to open competition between trusts, protection of existing contracts and full explanation to prospective patients. There will be a need for common agreed protocols and information technology strategies.

The advantages of the changes would be a reduction in the rates of long-distance transfers, a reduction in the split transfers of multiple births and more equity of access to specialist obstetric and neonatal services. It is anticipated that the changes will provide the relevant healthcare workers with improved job satisfaction, which in turn will lead to better recruitment and retention rates in the hard pressed specialties. Finally, it is to be *hoped* that the changes will result in improved clinical outcomes.

The economics of service provision

Introduction

This section introduces the basic concepts of economic evaluation, before discussing the relevance of such an approach to the provision of high-risk obstetric and neonatal services. Evidence relating to the cost effectiveness of different forms of care for women with preterm labour, and other high-risk pregnancies, is then discussed. The section concludes by identifying areas where further work is required.

Economic evaluation

In areas where resources such as hospital beds, obstetricians and midwives are scarce, the use of such resources for one group means that they are not available for other groups. For example, if a midwife undertakes a domiciliary visit then s/he is not available to see a number of women in an antenatal clinic. This is the concept of opportunity cost.

Economic evaluation is the way in which the economic implications of alternative courses of action are reviewed. It is about making explicit the trade-off involved and has been defined as *'the comparative analysis of alternative courses of action in terms of both their costs and consequences'* (Drummond *et al.* 1987). An important prerequisite to economic evaluation is evidence of clinical effectiveness; an ineffective clinical service can never be cost effective. The results of an economic evaluation provide information about the efficiency, or cost effectiveness, of one alternative compared with another.

Economic evaluation can address two distinct types of questions. The first relates to what is the best way of doing something, such as 'what is the best way of managing preterm labour?' and is about technical efficiency. The second type of question is whether something is worth doing, such as 'should second trimester scans be provided for all pregnant women?' and relates to allocative efficiency.

There are three main types of economic evaluation as shown in Table 12.1. Cost effectiveness analysis and cost utility analysis are used to answer technical efficiency questions and provide information on either the way of obtaining a unit of outcome at minimum cost, or the maximum amount of outcome that can be obtained for a given cost. Cost benefit analysis is used to answer allocative efficiency questions and provides information on the net benefit (benefits minus costs) of each programme.

Economic evaluation involves a number of distinct stages as follows: *Stage 1: define study question, including perspective to be adopted and alternatives under review.* It is important that the perspective of any evaluation is made clear; an evaluation from the perspective of the health service may give very different results from one from the perspective of the woman experiencing preterm labour.

Table 12.1. Types of economic evaluation

Type of evaluation	Cost analysis	Outcomes included	Uses
Cost effectiveness analysis	Expressed in £	Natural units (e.g. cases of preterm labour averted, life years gained)	To compare programmes with an effect on the same outcome, such as bed rest or tocolysis for preterm labour
Cost utility analysis	Expressed in £	Quality adjusted life years (QALYs), a measure encompassing both quality and quantity of life gained	To compare programmes with different health effects, such as bed rest for preterm labour with drug therapy for multiple sclerosis
Cost benefit analysis	Expressed in £	Expressed in £	To compare programmes in terms of their worth to society, such as choosing between antenatal care programmes or road building projects

Source: further information can be obtained in Palmer *et al.* (1999)

It is also vital that the alternatives under review are stated clearly to enable those reading the evaluation to identify whether these are useful from their perspective. It is not possible to undertake an economic evaluation without an alternative.

Stage 2: identify, measure and value all costs and outcomes required to answer the question posed. The perspective of an evaluation will determine to a large degree the costs and outcomes included in the evaluation, but there is also an issue of timing. In preterm labour, costs and outcomes may refer to the immediate intranatal period, or may include costs and outcomes of long-term sequelae.

Stage 3: take account of differential timing of costs and outcomes. Not all costs and outcomes occur within the first year; this is particularly true when long-term sequelae are included. There is therefore a need to ensure that account is taken of this in the analysis.

Stage 4: present the findings in such a way as they are relevant to decision makers. In many respects this is the most difficult component of an economic evaluation, requiring presentation of information for decision makers in a user friendly format.

Although economic evaluation is not new, it has been infrequently applied to alternative means of managing complications of pregnancy. The next section discusses why this may be the case.

Why are we interested in the economics of preterm delivery?

Interest in the economic evaluation of health care has arisen due to a number of factors, all of which place increasing pressure on scarce health service expenditure. These factors include technological advance, which in itself may be costly but may also increase the number of people potentially benefiting from medical care, increasing life expectancy and consumer pressure. As a result there is increasing interest in ways in which scarce healthcare resources can be allocated efficiently.

Interest in economic evaluation is also heightened when there is significant expenditure on a service, although this may reflect misunderstandings about the role of economic evaluation and its requirement for evidence of clinical effectiveness of the alternatives being compared.

Obstetrics, particularly the management of high-risk pregnancies, and neonatology would appear to be ideal candidates for economic evaluation because of the increasing use of technology, alongside high levels of consumer pressure. Additionally, the existence of the Cochrane Pregnancy and Childbirth database (now at the Cochrane Library http://www.nelh.nhs.uk/cochrane.asp) provides information about the effectiveness of interventions in an easily accessible form, allowing secondary economic evaluations to be performed.

There is also significant activity and expenditure associated with hospital services for preterm labour, although much of the literature in this area comes from America. A study by Scott *et al.* (1997) found that, in California, 33% of all admissions prior to delivery were for preterm labour. Nicholson *et al.* 2000 used a cross-sectional study of hospital discharges for pregnancy and delivery in Maryland to assess the relationship between patient characteristics and costs of preterm labour. From this, they estimated the total costs to the USA of more than $820 million for 1994 and concluded that *'physicians must better understand the cost consequences of preterm labour to assess the costs effectiveness of new screening strategies and clinical management of preterm labour'*.

In Scotland, preterm births accounted for 7.3% of all live births in 2000/1 (Information & Statistics Division 2002). Applying the California estimate to Scottish admissions prior to delivery would suggest that approximately 13 000 admissions per annum relate to preterm labour. During 1998/9 there were 8205 episodes of care in neonatal units in Scotland, 3262 (40%) of which were for preterm infants (Information & Statistics Division 2001). Early detection of preterm labour and preventive action to avoid preterm delivery therefore have the potential to make large health gains and free up resources for other groups. More recent data show that the cost to NHSScotland of care in neonatal units is in excess of £35 million per annum (Information & Statistics Division 2003).

A recent review of the economic consequences of preterm birth and low birth-weight (Petrou 2003) describes how the costs associated with such babies are substantial even after the initial hospital stay. Such costs place a burden not just on health services, but also on education services, local authorities, the voluntary sector and very significantly on families and carers.

Economic analysis of obstetric services has, however, not attracted high priority in research terms, with the possible exceptions of neonatal intensive care and prenatal screening, with a bibliography of economic evaluations listing only 34 studies under the heading up to 1992. A crude Medline search found only 102 citations using the terms economic evaluation, cost benefit analysis, cost effectiveness and obstetrics between 1966 and October 2002.

One possible explanation for the lack of published research into the economics of obstetric services is that there are inherent difficulties in undertaking such evaluations. This was first raised in 1968 when Levin argued that, although difficult, economic evaluation should not be abandoned in maternal programmes as it serves to stimulate awareness of the lack of effectiveness data (Levin 1968). The main source of difficulty stems from the fact that obstetrics differs from virtually all other medical areas in that there are two patients involved in receiving care, the mother and the baby. Actions that affect the mother may therefore directly, or indirectly, affect the baby and vice versa and the effects may operate in different directions from each other. This additional confusion has tended to limit the role of economic evaluations to areas of technical efficiency.

There are, however, other aspects to the 'difference' of obstetrics, compared to other branches of medicine. In particular, maternity services have become more 'consumer orientated' than other services, with emphasis on satisfaction and choice. This emphasis on choice is unusual in medicine; although alternative forms of care do exist in other areas, such as between day surgery and inpatient surgery, the choice of care setting is rarely made in consultation with the patient, but according to clinical need and availability of services. This does not mean, however, that clinical need is ignored in the pursuit of choice for women and it is unlikely that mothers would choose services that disadvantage their babies. It is an important distinction, however, between obstetrics and other healthcare services and may be a contributory factor to the dearth of studies in the area.

Cost effectiveness of different strategies for managing preterm labour

Although detection and management of preterm labour is an area of interest and has attracted considerable attention particularly in the US literature, because of the potential impact on neonatal costs, there is very little high quality economics literature available. A small number of economic evaluations were identified; these are cost effectiveness analyses with cases of adverse outcome prevented as the measure of outcome. They address the different ways of managing preterm labour, but do not address whether treatment of preterm labour is more cost effective to society than treating other pregnancy complications. In addition to these economic evaluations, there is some limited literature that reports the effect on costs and the effect on outcomes of alternative programmes of care, without formally presenting these as an economic evaluation. These have been included when they provide useful information.

Detection of preterm labour

Effective management of preterm labour requires early intervention to allow targeting of treatments with the aim of reducing morbidity and health service costs. Morrison *et al.* (1989) undertook a small randomised trial and cost analysis of ambulatory uterine monitoring compared with self-palpation in women at risk of preterm labour. They found that ambulatory monitoring significantly reduced neonatal intensive care days and improved the proportion of babies born at term. This was associated with lower total costs to the health service, but costs per woman were not significantly lower. The authors conclude, therefore, that the results point to ambulatory uterine monitoring being cost effective.

Kosasa *et al.* (1990) undertook a prospective study of ambulatory uterine monitoring in 79 women at high risk of preterm labour. They found significant reductions in the cost associated with preterm labour and early delivery associated with its use, compared with 192 women admitted with preterm labour, who received inpatient tocolysis.

Management of preterm labour

Korenbrot *et al.* (1984) retrospectively compared the costs of using tocolytic agents at different gestations to the expected costs associated with no gestational delay. They found that the increased costs of prenatal medical care were offset by decreased costs of neonatal medical care when treatment was given before 34 weeks of gestation, whereas there was no saving after 34 weeks.

Two modelling studies have been published in the last five years using information from a variety of sources to predict the relative cost effectiveness of different management strategies for preterm labour. In both cases these were cost effectiveness analyses using cases of respiratory distress syndrome prevented as the outcome of interest.

Myers *et al.* (1997) used a Markov model to compare tocolysis and corticosteroids, amniocentesis and fetal lung maturity testing and treatment based on test results, with no treatment in women with preterm labour and intact membranes in a tertiary care centre. They found that testing for fetal lung maturity was cost effective only under certain circumstances and was sensitive to the probability and costs associated with respiratory distress syndrome. For their own unit fetal lung maturity testing was only cost effective between 34 and 36 weeks' gestation.

Mozurkewich *et al.* (2000) used decision analytic techniques to compare nine alternative strategies for assessment and treatments of threatened preterm labour in gravid women with intact membranes. They found that fetal fibronectin testing or cervical length assessment with corticosteroid therapy were associated with lower costs and similar outcomes to a policy of treating all women with threatened preterm labour, avoiding unnecessary hospitalisation and tocolytic treatment for women not at risk of preterm labour.

Home based care

Increasing costs of hospital care and a recognition of the value of community based care in obstetrics has led to increasing interest in the effect of different locations of care on the management of preterm labour and other high-risk pregnancies. Studies have been undertaken in the areas of home based care and daycare, although there is a dearth of high quality evidence for the cost effectiveness of such programmes.

Harrison (2001) compared cohorts of women with preterm labour before and after the introduction of a home based care system for high risk pregnancies in Canada. They showed that a home based service, offering nursing and support services for women with an established diagnosis of preterm labour, had significantly better birth outcomes than the previous hospital based service, but with no significant difference in costs. This new service is therefore cost effective, as it offers better outcomes for the same cost. This study also found no significant differences in either birth outcomes or costs for women with hypertension in pregnancy.

Conclusion

Economic evaluation is the means by which the economic implications of alternatives courses of action are compared. Despite high levels of morbidity and resource use for both mothers and their babies associated with preterm labour, there is a dearth of studies that address the most cost effective way of managing this common condition. There is a need, therefore, for more research in this area to assist decision makers in identifying the best allocation of their scarce resources.

Counselling issues

Introduction

For a parent the experience of preterm labour and delivery may be a life-changing event. When it occurs unexpectedly the perinatal team may have only a small window of opportunity in which to deal with some very complex issues. These include: preparing the parents for the birth of a preterm infant; discussing strategies of therapeutic intervention to delay labour; deciding whether elective delivery is in the fetal interest; choosing the route of delivery; transfer of the mother antenatally or the baby postnatally to another unit; and discussing appropriate levels of intervention in the neonatal unit for a given gestational age. Couples may have little idea about the long-term implications of the birth of an extremely premature infant, and the perinatal team will be responsible for educating them to the point that they are able to participate in decision making. On the other hand the preterm birth may be elective, as for example in severe pre-eclampsia, and the couple may have had more time to come to terms with the likely course of events. Such couples are likely to have more realistic expectations as to what is medically possible and about the future prospects for their infant. However, where maternal health is compromised they may experience some degree of guilt that they sacrificed their baby in their own interest.

Recommendations for the management of fetuses and newborn at gestational ages of 22–26 weeks are available from the BAPM Publications website (BAPM 2000). These deal with some of the most complex clinical scenarios when the fetus or neonate is at the threshold of viability (Table 12.2). Very preterm infants have an increased risk of survival with long-term damage and this raises serious ethical dilemmas about professional and parental obligations in the face of great uncertainty.

Principles of counselling

Counselling should be honest and accurate and decisions should be based on the ethical principles of beneficience, nonmaleficence, justice, futility, autonomy, quality of life and best interests and legal rights of the infant. The counsellor, obstetrician or neonatologist, needs to build a close working relationship with the couple in so far as this is possible. He or she should always try to gain insight into the parents' views during the discussions. Parents will bring a unique perspective to the meeting based on their own knowledge and experience. Each will have their own fears, some realistic, some imaginary, and it will be the job of the counsellor to address these and to put them into proper perspective. The counsellor should never impose his or her own moral or religious views on the patient, and when there is a problem should be prepared to offer the patient a second opinion. The doctor should always try to share difficult decisions with the whole team of healthcare workers. The burden of complex decisions should not be placed on the parents – it is the responsibility of a multidisciplinary team including obstetricians, paediatricians, midwives and nurses and associated healthcare workers.

Parents making difficult decisions should always be encouraged to seek help from other family members or close friends, or other support networks or religious bodies of relevance to them. Prior to the birth counselling should take into account

Table 12.2. Guidelines relating to the Birth of Extremely Immature Babies
(22–26 weeks' gestation)

The following points are emphasised in the guidelines:
- Good communication with the parents
- Management decisions should not be influenced by the child's gender, religion or demography
- When the Doctors' beliefs interfere with proper counselling they have a duty to involve a colleague
- Involvement of the most experienced clinician available is mandatory
- The perinatal team needs up-to-date national and local statistics on mortality and morbidity
- Advance authorisation for the non-resuscitation of very preterm neonates are not binding on the perinatal team
- Recording management plans in the casenotes is important
- The outcome for babies less than 24 weeks' gestation is very poor
- Intrauterine transfer becomes an option only after 22 weeks' gestation
- Cardiac resuscitation is rarely appropriate before 25 weeks' gestation
- Caesarean section before 25 weeks' gestation is rarely appropriate
- The desirability of full or limited post-mortem examination should be emphasised by a senior neonatologist
- Developmental follow-up for very preterm infants should be for 2–5 years

Source: based on Thames Regional Perinatal Group Guidelines (2000) and the British
Association of Perinatal Medicine Memorandum (July 2000) (unpublished data).

the fact that the mother's wishes are paramount (see Chapter 13 for a discussion of
the legal issues). Immediately after the birth, however, the situation changes and
decisions will invariably be based on what is considered to be in the infant's best
interest. Decisions should not be influenced by the child's gender, or by religious
or demographic factors. Parents and families may bring personal, cultural and
religious beliefs into their relationship with their doctors that have the potential to
conflict with medical perceptions of good care. In a very small number of cases it
may be necessary to involve the courts.

Close collaboration between obstetricians and neonatologists is crucial in the
decision making process, particularly when the decisions are complex and time is
short. Decision making will be most effective when there has been prior agreement
between the obstetrician and the neonatologist about how things will be handled.
Written protocols and guidelines should be available in each unit to facilitate this
process. Interestingly, the obstetrician's view is regarded as very important by parents
who are required to make critical decisions at the margins of viability (Munro *et al.*

2001). Advanced planning is particularly important in complex fetal medicine cases, and a comprehensive plan for the birth and aftercare should be drawn up well in advance of the anticipated delivery date and documented clearly in the case notes.

Preliminary discussions

The obstetrician is usually the first person to break the news to the patient that preterm birth is a possibility. Who should be there at the time? A major teaching round on the labour ward may not be the most appropriate setting in which to conduct the session. Prior arrangements should be made with the couple where possible so that they can prepare their questions and both attend. The consultant obstetrician could then see the couple in a relatively private setting, perhaps with the on-call registrar and a senior midwife from the labour ward. The obstetrician would then cover all the relevant issues such as the use of tocolysis, possibility of in utero transfer, mode of delivery, and provide an overview of the baby's chances of survival. The couple should be given plenty of time to assimilate the information and ask questions. Following this meeting the parents should be encouraged to meet with the neonatal team. They would then provide the couple with survival and morbidity data from their own unit and from national sources such as *The EPICure Study*, taking into account the specific circumstances of the case (Costeloe *et al.* 2000). Morbidity data should include the incidence and severity of disability among survivors up to at least two years of age. Parents must be made aware that long-term follow-up will be required (two to five years). The planned development of perinatal centres should facilitate the provision of reliable information, as the perinatal centres will be responsible for collating data and publishing annual reports for each unit within the network (LRSCG/TRPG 2001). A guided visit to the neonatal unit would be appropriate for the prospective parents at this stage.

Labour and delivery

The mode of delivery can present particular difficulties when the gestational age is at the threshold of viability. Caesarean delivery, which in very preterm pregnancies often requires a classical uterine incision, may reduce fetal risks in some circumstances but it increases maternal risk both in the index pregnancy and in subsequent ones. There is a consensus now that Caesarean section before 25 weeks' gestation confers little benefit in terms of survival (Kitchen *et al.* 1985) even for breech presentation (Wolf *et al.* 1999). The prognosis is similarly poor when the estimated fetal weight is below 500 g. A second opinion is advisable if the parents disagree strongly. For breech infants with an estimated fetal weight of 1.5 kg and above delivery by caesarean is usually recommended. These issues need to be discussed sensitively with the parents who may be disappointed that their 'right' to labour and deliver normally has been taken away relatively early in pregnancy.

Although the decision about the route of delivery is primarily an obstetric one, the neonatal team should be encouraged to contribute as well.

When fetal monitoring in labour is deemed inappropriate the carers must be particularly sensitive to the parents wishes. It may be agreed that intermittent auscultation of the fetal heart is desirable so that the parents would be aware if and when fetal demise were to occur. Some parents may request continuous monitoring in previable situations and then it should be done discreetly and prior agreement should be recorded that action would not be taken in the presence of fetal heart irregularities. The information may sometimes be helpful for the paediatricians when deciding about resuscitation and prognosis after birth.

In utero and postnatal transfers

Last minute transfers from the booking unit can be traumatic for prospective parents and every effort should be made to deal with these events sensitively. Parents may have developed a strong bond of trust with the perinatal team at the base hospital and may be shocked to discover that in their hour of need they are being moved on. Clearly, there is a need to minimise this type of transfer particularly from the tertiary units. The proposed new perinatal centres (see Chapter 11) will help but in future women will need to be told at their booking visit about the neonatal facilities available at their unit and the likelihood of transfer to perinatal centres in these situations. Obviously couples are reassured when they are being transferred to another centre that they perceive as offering better or more specialist care. Sadly, at the present time this is not always the case.

Resuscitation of the infant and withdrawal of support

Delivery of a very preterm infant should be regarded as a major emergency and the most senior neonatologist available should be present in the delivery room. There must be an agreed protocol for the calculation of gestational age in the unit so as to allow staff to recognise the emergency and respond appropriately. In the case of an unexpected very preterm delivery the paediatrician may initiate resuscitation and provisional intensive care until a full assessment clarifies the position. Clinical examination may reveal a more mature fetus than expected leading to continuation of treatment. This might be applied even in cases where the parents have given advanced authorisation for non-resuscitation. Parents should be made aware that advanced authorisations are not binding. When parents do not agree with the doctors' advice on whether to withhold or withdraw care, treatment should be continued until agreement is reached or until a change in the baby's condition clarifies the situation. The hospital ethics committee may offer helpful advice in particularly complex situations. A case would only be referred to the courts when all the normal procedures have failed, and when the perinatal team consider it is in the best interests of the infant. When a decision is made not to resuscitate then all of the original discussions and subsequent actions must be documented carefully in the casenotes. Most neonatologists will not actively resuscitate infants below 23 weeks' gestation (Sanders *et al.* 1995; Munro *et al.* 2001).

The decision to withdraw life support from very preterm infants is particularly emotional and fraught. The staff must provide basic comfort care, including the appropriate use of opiates, for infants who are being allowed to die. The parents should be encouraged to remain closely involved and obviously should receive the best possible support to help them through this traumatic experience (RCPCH 1997). After death the senior paediatrician should spend time with the parents and discuss the benefits of post-mortem examination. If the parents decline a post-mortem a limited examination involving the use of X-rays, magnetic resonance imaging and needle biopsy with histology and karyotyping will often be acceptable. Again the most senior clinician should counsel the couple, discuss organ donation if relevant, and request the post-mortem (Rankin *et al.* 2002). Learning from the Alder Hey Inquiry it is mandatory that parents now receive more detailed information, written and oral, about the post-mortem (The Royal Liverpool Children's Hospital Inquiry Report 2001). Formal, written consent must be obtained and pathologists need to be aware of the constraints in the use of tissue imposed by that consent (CESDI 2001c). Despite a lack of scientific evidence that psychological support after perinatal loss is beneficial it is considered good practice to offer bereavement counselling after the follow-up medical visit (Chambers and Chan 2000; Jennings 2002). Communication with the patient's general practitioner and, when there is a long interval until death, with the obstetric team, is paramount. Afterwards, it is recommended by BAPM that a full summary of the perinatal and postnatal events should be written and circulated to all members of the healthcare team, and copied to the parents.

REFERENCES

Bristol Royal Infirmary Inquiry. (2001) *Learning From Bristol: the public inquiry into children's heart surgery at the Bristol Royal Infirmary 1984–1995.* Available at www.bristol inquiry.org.uk.

British Association of Perinatal Medicine and Neonatal Nurses Association (BAPM/NNA). (1992) Report of the working group. Categories of babies requiring neonatal care. *Arch. Dis. Child.* **67**, 868–9.

British Association of Perinatal Medicine (BAPM). (1997) *A minimum dataset to support annual reports from neonatal intensive care units: report of a working group.* London: BAPM.

(1998) *Obstetric Standards for the provision of Perinatal Care.* Joint committee RCOG/ RCPCH. Available at www.bapm-london.org.

(2000) *Fetuses and Newborn Infants at the Threshold of Viability: A Framework for Practice*. Available at www.bapm-london.org/publications.

(2001) *Standards for hospitals providing Neonatal Intensive and High Dependency Care (Second Edition) and Categories of Babies requiring Neonatal Care*. Available at www.bapm-london.org.

Buchan, J. (2002) Global nursing shortages- are often a symptom of wider health system or societal ailments. *BMJ* **324**, 751–2.

Burton, P., Draper, E., Fenton, A. and Field, D. (1995) Neonatal intensive care cots: estimating the requirements in Trent, UK. *J. Epid. Comm. Health* **49**, 617–28.

Chambers, H. M., and Chan, F. Y. (2000) Support for women/families after perinatal death. *Cochrane Database Syst. Rev.* **2**, CD000452.

Chiu, H. S. H., Vogt, J. F., Chan, L. S. and Rother, C. E. (1993) Regionalisation of infant transports: the Southern California experience and its implications. I: Referral pattern. *J. Perinatol.* **13**, 288–96.

Clinical Standards Advisory Group. (1996) *Access and availability of neonatal intensive care*. Second Report, London: HMSO.

Confidential Enquiries into Maternal Deaths in the UK. (2002) *Why Mothers Die 1997–1999*. London: HMSO.

Confidential Enquiries of Stillbirths and Deaths in Infancy (CESDI) (2001a) *CESDI 8th Annual Report. Survival rates of babies born between 27 and 28 weeks' gestation in England, Wales and Northern Ireland 1988–2000*. Maternal & Child Health Consortium, p. 83–100.

(2001b) *CESDI 8th Annual Report. Changing Practice-a view from the clinical negligence scheme for trusts*. Maternal & Child Health Research Consortium, p. 101–7. Available at www.cesdi.org.uk.

(2001c) *CESDI 8th Annual Report. Update on issues surrounding the post-mortem*. Maternal and Child Health Research Consortium, p. 63–71.

Costeloe, K., Hennessy, E., Gibson, A. T., Marlow, N. and Wilkinson, A. R. (2000) The EPICure study: outcomes to discharge from hospital for infants born at the threshold of viability. *Pediatrics* **106**, 659–71.

Delaney-Black, V., Lubchenco, L. O., Butterfield, J. *et al.* (1989) Outcome of VLBW infants: are populations of neonates inherently different after antenatal versus neonatal referral? *Am. J. Obstet. Gynecol.* **160**, 545–52.

Department of Health. (2000) *Comprehensive Critical Care: A review of adult critical care services*. London: Department of Health. Also available at www.doh.gov.uk/nhsexec/compcritcare.htm

Drummond, M., Stoddart, G. and Torrance, G. (1987) *Methods for the Economic Evaluation of Health care Programmes*. Oxford: Oxford University Press.

Expert Maternity Group. (1993) *Changing Childbirth – Report of the Expert Maternity Group*. London: HMSO.

Fordham, R., Field, D., Hodges, S. *et al.* (1992) Cost of neonatal care across a regional health authority. *J. Pub. Health Med.* **14**, 127–30.

Greenberg, E. R., Dain, B., Freeman, D., Yates, J. and Korson, R. (1988) Referral of lung cancer patients to university hospital cancer centres. *Cancer* **62**, 1647–52.

Harrison, M. J., Kushner, K. E., Benzies, K. *et al.* (2001) In home nursing care for women with high risk pregnancies: outcomes and cost. *Obstet. Gynecol.* **97**, 982–7.

Information & Statistics Division. (2001) *Scottish Health Statistics 2000* Edinburgh. Available at http://www.isdscotland.org.

(2002) *Scottish Health Statistics 2001* Edinburgh. Available at http://www.isdscotland.org.

(2003) *Scottish Health Statistics* 2002. Edinburgh. Available at http://www.isdscotland.org.

International Neonatal Network. (1993) The Crib Score: a tool for assessing initial neonatal risk and comparing performances of NICUs. *Lancet* **342**, 193–8.

(1997) Scottish neonatal consultants, nurses Collaborative Study Group. Risk adjusted and population based studies of the outcome for high risk infants in Scotland and Australia. *Arch. Dis. Child. Fetal Neonatal Ed.* **82**, 118–23.

Jennings, P. (2002) Should paediatric units have bereavement support posts? *Arch. Dis. Child.* **87**, 40–2.

Kitchen, W., Ford, G. W., Doyle, L. W. *et al.* (1985) Caesarean section or vaginal delivery at 24 to 28 weeks' gestation: comparison of survival and neonatal and two-year morbidity. *Obstet. Gynecol.* **66**,149–57.

Korenbrot, C. C., Aalto, L. H. and Laros, R. K. (1984) The cost effectiveness of stopping preterm labour with beta-adrenergic treatment. *N. Engl. J. Med.* **310**, 691–6.

Kosasa, T. S., Abou-Sayf, F. K., Li-Ma, G. and Hale, R. W. (1990) Evaluation of the cost effectiveness of home monitoring of uterine contractions. *Obstet. Gynecol.* **76**, 71S–75S.

Levin, A. L. (1968) Cost effectiveness in maternal and child health. *N. Engl. J. Med.* **278**, 1041–7.

London Regional Specialist Commissioning Group/Thames Regional Perinatal Group (LRSCG/TRPG). (2001) *Modernising Neonatal Intensive Care in London and the Implications for Related Services.* Discussion document LRSCG/TRPG.

Medical Devices Agency. (1995) Transport of neonates in ambulances (TINA). Medical Devices Agency, London

Morrison, J. C., Martin, J. N., Martin, R. W. *et al.* (1989) Cost effectiveness of ambulatory uterine activity monitoring. *Int. J. Gynecol. Obstet.* **28**, 127–32.

Mozurkewich, E. L., Naglie, G., Krahn, M. D. and Hayashi, R. H. (2000) Predicting preterm birth: a cost effectiveness analysis. *Am. J. Obstet. Gynecol.* **182**, 1589–98.

Munro, M., Yu, V. Y., Partridge, J. C. and Martinez, A. M. (2001) Antenatal counselling, resuscitation practices and attitudes among Australian neonatologists towards life support in extreme prematurity. *Aust. N. Z. J. Obstet. Gynaecol.* **41**, 275–80.

Myers, E. R., Alvarez, J. G., Richardson, D. K. and Ludmir, J. (1997) Cost effectiveness of fetal lung maturity testing in preterm labor. *Obstet. Gynecol.* **90**, 824–9.

NHS Executive, Mother and Child Initiative. (2000) *UK Neonatal Staffing Study-Final Report. A prospective evaluation of risk-adjusted outcomes of neonatal intensive care in relation to volume, staffing and workload in UK neonatal intensive care units.* BAPM Publication available at www.bapm-london.org.

Nicholson, W. K., Frick, K. D. and Powe, N. R. (2000) Economic burden of hospitalizations for preterm labour in the United States. *Obstet. Gynecol.* **96**, 95–101.

Northern Neonatal Network. (1993) Requirements for neonatal cots. *Arch. Dis. Child.* **68**, 544–9.

Palmer, S., Byford, S. and Raftery, J. (1999) Types of economic evaluation. *BMJ* **318**, 1349.

Parmanum, J., Field, D., Rennie, J. and Steer, P. (2000) National census of availability of neonatal intensive care. *BMJ* **321**, 727–9.

Petrou, S. (2003) Economic consequences of preterm birth and low birthweight. *BJOG* **110** (*suppl* 20), 17–23.

Rankin, J., Wright, C. and Lind, T. (2002) Cross sectional survey of parents' experience and views of the post-mortem findings. *BMJ* **324**, 816–18.

Royal College of Paediatrics and Child Health (RCPCH). (1997) Withholding or Withdrawing Life Saving Treatment in Children- A Framework for Practice. Pub Royal College of Paediatrics and Child Health.

Specialist Advisory Committee for Neonatal Medicine. (2001) sub-specialty training in neonatal medicine v. 2.2, available at http://www.rcpch.ac.uk/publications/education_and_training_documents/HST/subspecialty_training_in_neonatal_medicine_oct_2001.pdf

Sanders, M. R., Donohue, P. K., Oberdorf, M. A., Rosenkrantz, T. S. and Allen, M. C. (1995) Perceptions of the limit of viability: neonatologists' attitudes toward extremely preterm infants. *J. Perinatol.* **15**, 494–502.

Scott, C. L., Chavez, G. F., Atrash, H. K. *et al.* (1997) Hospitalizations for severe complications of pregnancy, 1987–1992. *Obstet. Gynecol.* **90**, 225–9.

Shann, F. A. (1994) Review of the report 'The Care of Critically Ill Children'. In *A Critical Appraisal of the Care of Critically Ill Children*. York: NHS Centre for Reviews and Dissemination.

The Royal Liverpool Children's Hospital Inquiry Report (Alder Hey). (2001) London: The Stationary Office.

Waterstone, N., Bewley, S. and Wolfe, C. (2001) Incidence and predictors of severe obstetric morbidity: case control study. *BMJ* **322**, 1089–94.

Whittle, M., Cavenagh, A. G. M., Halliday, H. L. *et al.* (1994) *Minimum Standards of Care in Labour*, pp. 1–28. London: RCOG.

Wolf, H., Schaap, A. H., Bruinse, H. W. *et al.* (1999) Vaginal delivery compared with caesarean section in early preterm breech delivery: a comparison of long term outcome. *BJOG* **106**, 486–91.

Young, G. L. (1994) The place of birth. In G. Chamberlain and N. Patel, eds., *The Future of the Maternity Services*, London: RCOG.

13

The management of pregnancy and labour

Sheila A. M. McLean and Sarah Elliston

University of Glasgow

Introduction

Medicine's increased capacities make intervention at all stages of pregnancy and labour both more common and more successful. The capacity to see the developing fetus in the womb and the skills of healthcare professionals around the moment of birth, when coupled with the sophistication of their knowledge about fetal development, genetics and safe delivery, also enhance the professionals' perceived responsibility to the child-to-be as well as to the mother.

Generally speaking this is likely to be both uncontroversial and welcome. Most pregnant women (and their partners) are likely to view the progress in prenatal screening and managed childbirth as being a definite bonus, increasing their reproductive liberties and maximising the safety of pregnancy and childbirth. Undoubtedly, in the vast majority of cases this will be the experience of women and their partners. However, this is not to say that the modern management of pregnancy is entirely uncontroversial, and – perhaps unfortunately – it is necessary to consider such controversy in this chapter. These controversies are often intimately linked to the primary focus of this chapter; namely issues surrounding consent and negligence.

Consent

It is widely accepted that – except in limited circumstances – consent is a prerequisite of both an ethical and a legal intervention. In an emergency situation where consent cannot be sought because of the patient's lack of consciousness, treatment may proceed without the patient's consent. However, even here, care must be taken to do no more than is immediately necessary until the patient is able to consider treatment decisions for herself. Making decisions for patients with incapacity outside an emergency situation is considered later. However, in the normal case the individual has the right to make decisions, based on appropriate information, about whether or not to agree to any intervention, irrespective of its expected medical value. Indeed,

Preterm Labour Managing Risk in Clinical Practice, eds. Jane Norman and Ian Greer. Published by Cambridge University Press. © Cambridge University Press 2005.

the individual can legally refuse treatment even when it is life preserving (*B v. An NHS Hospital Trust* (2002)). The modern law of consent is said to reflect the statement made in an elderly US case that:

Every human being of adult years and sound mind has a right to determine what shall be done with his own body … (*Schloendorff v. Society of New York Hospital* (1914)).

Any treatment given to a patient without his or her consent, indeed, any 'touching' of a patient without consent, is an assault on the patient, and could result in the responsible doctor or other medical professional being sued by the patient, or even prosecuted for assault in sufficiently serious cases. Criminal prosecutions of members of the medical profession for assault on their patients are rare, but see *Hussain v. Houston* (1995). In practice, of course, people's capacity to agree to or reject medical care is dependent on a number of factors, which can broadly be summarised as information and capacity or competence.

For a consent to be legally valid it is generally agreed to require the provision of information. Thus, the law requires that an individual should receive a certain amount of information before anyone may undertake any medical intervention, however benign or well-motivated. Before considering how much information is necessary, it is worth at this point noting that – because of the information disclosure requirement – healthcare providers should be careful not to become too enthusiastic about the notion of 'implied' consent. It is sometimes said that consent to treatment can be evidenced by the patient's apparent willingness to undergo the treatment. For example, the patient who holds out his or her arm for an injection is sometimes said to be providing implied consent by so doing. Manifestly, if information is the key to the validity of consent, this may be a dubious presumption to make. The patient may indeed be *compliant*, but this is not the same as being *informed*, and consent without information (unless it has been explicitly refused) can seldom – if ever – satisfy the requirements of a valid consent.

So what does the law require a patient to be told? For some, the only genuinely valid consent follows the provision of the fullest possible information. This, however, is not what is required by law. It is necessary that patients are informed in broad terms of the nature and purpose of the treatment. Failure to do so may result in an action for assault, or trespass to the person, if treatment is given. This could be the case regardless of an objectively beneficial outcome of treatment, since legal validity is concerned with consented to physical intervention rather than the consequences of the intervention (although this will be relevant to the level of any award if litigation ensues). Patients must also be given adequate information about material risks associated with a procedure, the expected benefits of the intervention, and any alternative treatments that may be available.

Warning of risks should also include the risks of not proceeding with proposed treatment. Failure to provide adequate information may lead to an action in negligence (*Chatterton v. Gerson* (1981)).

The difficulty lies in determining what is regarded as adequate information and what risks need to be discussed with the patient in the specific circumstances of the case. In the routine medical intervention,[1] UK law adopts what has been referred to as a 'professional standard'; that is, one where judgement as to whether or not sufficient information has been provided is effectively based on a standard set by a 'responsible body of medical opinion'.[2] Thus, judges have been criticised as passing the content of a *legal* duty to doctors. (See, for example, Lord Scarman's judgement in *Sidaway v. Board of Governors, Bethlem and Royal Maudsley Hospital* (1985); McLean, (1989). See also the later discussion on negligence, p. 000.) That aside, the law requires that patients are told in broad terms of the risks associated with a particular intervention; not every piece of information known to the doctor (*Chatterton v. Gerson* (1981)). The doctor's decision about what to tell will, if challenged, be subject to the negligence test outlined above (known as the '*Bolam Test*'). The *Bolam* test will be discussed in more detail in the section on negligence, below. However, reliance upon what information the doctor of ordinary skill would disclose to establish the proper standard of information disclosure has proved controversial, since it places priority on what medical practitioners usually tell patients, rather than on what the patient wishes to know. It should, however, be noted that professional guidelines issued by the General Medical Council suggest that full disclosure should be made (General Medical Council, 1999).

Therefore, even if reliance is placed on the standard of what the doctor of ordinary skill would disclose, the level of disclosure that would be expected today is likely to be significantly higher than would have been expected when the House of Lords decided the case of *Sidaway v. Board of Governors, Bethlem and Royal Maudsley Hospital* (1985). *Pearce v. United Bristol Healthcare NHS Trust* (1998) is an interesting recent case from England. This case suggests that the courts may be becoming more sympathetic to the view that doctors should disclose information to patients about significant risks that would be expected to affect the decision of a reasonable person whether or not to proceed with treatment, thereby focusing more upon patient expectation than professional practice. *Pearce* also considered the case of *Bolitho v.*

---

[1] Different rules apply where the intervention is experimental, but there is insufficient space to consider this here. However, for those wishing to follow this up, the case of *Halushka v. University of Saskatchewan* (1965) may be instructive. See also Mason *et al.* (2002): para. 19.4.

[2] This standard is taken from the case of *Bolam v. Friern Hospital Management Committee* (1957). It was subsequently endorsed (in large part) by the majority in *Sidaway v. Board of Governors, Bethlem and Royal Maudsley Hospital* (1985), and was expressly said to equate to the law in Scotland in the case of *Moyes v. Lothian Health Board* (1990).

City and Hackney Health Authority (1997), which indicated that expert evidence should be subjected to scrutiny by the courts in order to establish that the opinion expressed is logical and credible, and applied it to information disclosure. Although the judgement in *Bolitho* was explicitly stated to be concerned with diagnosis and treatment, rather than with information disclosure, it now therefore seems likely that it will be extended to this situation. In the case of *Smith v. Tunbridge Wells Health Authority* (1994), failure to warn of risks, despite expert evidence supporting this approach, was held to be negligent, since it was neither reasonable nor responsible. (See also *Newell and Newell v. Goldenberg* (1995) and *Lybert v. Warrington Health Authority* (1996).)

Where the patient is a conscious adult, then, the doctor's duty is to ensure that she is informed of the benefits, risks and alternatives to the proposed treatment, but not to provide every detail. If the patient asks direct questions it might be assumed that the law would require that the doctor answer them fully. Although case law had previously suggested that this was not in fact the case (*Blyth v. Bloomsbury Health Authority* (1993)), the professional guidance already mentioned makes it clear that doctors must be honest in these circumstances.

Once the necessary information has been disclosed, it is of course for the patient to decide what to do with it. Treatment can, as has been said, be accepted or rejected, and the doctor who attempted to enforce treatment would by and large be guilty of assaulting a patient. The provision of information is designed to facilitate the patient's autonomy, not to provide a reassurance to the clinician as to his or her legal position, although it may well also achieve that.

However, it is in the use to which information is put that conflict can arise. When a patient receives information, coupled with the optimal clinical recommendation, and then chooses to do something that appears irrational, even risky, it is tempting to seek a resolution by recourse to some other principles. Thus, increasingly in obstetrics, a conflict has been identified between the wishes of the pregnant woman and those of her professional carers. This, in fact, is one of the major controversies to which we referred above, and can arise both in the management of pregnancy and the management of labour.

The Management of pregnancy

The modern pregnancy is managed effectively by, amongst other things, the availability of extensive screening, which is now offered to all pregnant women in the United Kingdom. As the British Medical Association (BMA) noted in 1998:

Prenatal screening might be by family history, serum screening, molecular tests, or ultrasound. Ultrasound scanning is currently offered routinely to all pregnant women in the UK and, although it is undertaken to monitor the development of the fetus, it can also detect both major and minor defects. (British Medical Association 1998: 38)

However, one concern expressed both by the BMA and by other commentators, is that the very fact that such screening is routine may place pressure on women to accept it. Failure to do so might be seen as irresponsible; yet some may prefer not to receive certain information or be unsure about the implications of accepting the tests (British Medical Association 1998. See also Marteau, 1995). Thus it is important that '[any] decision about whether to opt for prenatal screening or genetic testing must be based on good quality, objective information'. (British Medical Association 1998: 38). In other words, the fact that screening is routine does not obviate the need for the provision of appropriate information; the law still requires this. Equally, women should be free to decline such screening for any reason that is reasonable *to them*. It should also be remembered that the results of prenatal screening are not necessarily a bonus, even if they are seen as enhancing reproductive choice. Indeed, they can 'present parents with dilemmas which, with hindsight, they might prefer to have avoided'. (British Medical Association 1998: 50).

Nonetheless, once information is known, it cannot be unlearned. For this reason, as well as for the enhancement of autonomy, it is vital that screening is presented as an actual choice rather than merely as a routine event that every woman is expected to accept. Of course the availability of screening is something that requires to be disclosed in the first place. The BMA reports, for example, that some ethnic groups are not offered screening because of the assumption that they would not be interested in it (British Medical Association 1998: 51). Equally, the BMA notes that:

In the past, some health professionals restricted access to prenatal diagnosis to those individuals who planned to terminate an affected pregnancy. Although this approach is now widely regarded as paternalistic and unacceptable, a 1993 survey of obstetricians found that one-third still generally required an undertaking to terminate an affected pregnancy before proceeding with prenatal diagnosis. (British Medical Association 1998: 52)

This, the BMA goes on to say, it regards as 'unacceptable'. What these last examples show, however, is the true value of the process of information disclosure. Firstly, it cannot be assumed that people, because they belong to a particular culture or religion, are homogeneous in the choices they will make; nor can it be right to pressurise people into making particular decisions before or after the provision of information, since the information-giving process is designed to facilitate a free choice on their part, not a coerced one. As Robertson and Shulman have said:

Developments in obstetrics, genetics, fetal medicine and infectious diseases will continue to provide knowledge and technologies that will enable many disabled births to be prevented. While most women will welcome this knowledge and gladly act on it, others will not. The ethical, legal, and policy aspects of this situation require a careful balancing of the offspring's welfare and the pregnant woman's interest in liberty and bodily integrity. (Robertson and Shulman 1987: 32)

Arguably, however, there is no legal balance to be struck, although there may be an ethical one. Although the law is clear that the embryo/fetus has no standing (*Paton v British Pregnancy Advisory Service* (1979)) the ethical position is less clear. Both the *Report on the Review of the Guidance on the Research Use of Foetuses and Foetal Material* (Polkinghorne Report 1989) and the *Committee of Inquiry into Human Fertilisation and Embryology* (Warnock Report 1984) concluded that the embryo of the human species is worthy of some respect from an ethical perspective. However, neither recommended that this should become a legal reality.

Of course, in the management of a pregnancy the decisions made by the woman will often, if not invariably, have an effect on the developing embryo or fetus, and it is for this reason that they may become subject to challenge. Developments in fetal medicine have enabled doctors to envisage themselves as having not one patient – the woman – but rather two patients – the woman and the embryo/fetus. Or at least they may feel themselves to have responsibilities to the embryo or fetus in addition to those that they owe to the women. (See, for example, the discussion in Mattingly (1992). Ways of considering the relationship between women and the fetus are explored at length in Seymour (2000), particularly Chapters 1, 8 and 9.) This dilemma has in part been created by medical advance, but it is also accentuated by it. Knowledge about fetus unfriendly behaviour (such as the ingestion of drugs, or even smoking or drinking caffeine) inclines doctors to warn women about these risks, quite naturally. Also naturally, most women will heed such warnings and minimise the controllable risks to the developing embryo/fetus.

However, not all women will be prepared to make lifestyle changes in order to do this, for reasons that may be unknown or unintelligible to third parties. In strict law, this should be irrelevant. It has been made very clear that the right to make a decision '. . . exists notwithstanding that the reasons for making the choice are rational, irrational, unknown or even non-existent' (*Re T (adult) (refusal of medical treatment)* (1992) at p. 653). One possible exception to this general rule was mooted by Lord Donaldson, however, when he said:

An adult patient who . . . suffers from no mental incapacity has an absolute right to choose whether to consent to medical treatment, to refuse it or to choose one rather than another of the treatments being offered. The only possible qualification is a case in which the choice may lead to the death of a viable foetus. (*Re T (adult) (refusal of medical treatment)* (1992) at pp. 652–3).

It is unclear on what authority such a statement was made and subsequent cases have not directly endorsed it. Whatever status a fetus may have emotionally, it is clear that it has no legal status whatsoever. Although once born alive a child can sue for damage sustained prenatally, or even pre-conception, and can inherit under a will, it has no rights before birth. Any rights that accrue do so after the fact of live birth and are therefore attributable to a person in being, not a person in waiting. As McCullough and Chervenak say:

> ... the fetus cannot be thought to possess subjective interests. Because of the immaturity of its central nervous system, the fetus has no values and beliefs that form the basis of such interests. It obviously follows from this that the fetus cannot possess deliberative interests, since these, in turn, are based on subjective interests and reflection on subjective interests. The latter is a task no fetus can accomplish. Hence, there can be no autonomy-based obligations to the fetus. Hence, also, there can be no meaningful talk of fetal rights, the fetus's right to life in particular, in the sense that the fetus itself generates rights. (McCullough and Chervenak 1994:102)

Thus, the proposal that a person with rights (the pregnant woman) should have these rights reduced or removed in the interests of something that has no legal rights (the fetus) is surely wrong in law, even if the fetus is deemed viable (however that is assessed).

The consequences of deciding otherwise can perhaps best be illustrated by the US case of Angela Carder. Mrs Carder had suffered from leukaemia as a child. This went into remission, she married and became pregnant. Sadly, however, in the course of her pregnancy the leukaemia returned aggressively and it was clear that she was terminally ill. With her agreement, her care was managed in such a way as to maximise the length of the pregnancy, so as hopefully to allow for the delivery of a preterm but viable child. In the event, at about twenty six and a half weeks of pregnancy, her condition was such that her attending physicians decided that a Caesarean section was required to salvage the fetus.

This, Mrs Carder refused. Although legally irrelevant, she was supported in her decision by her husband and her parents. From the hospital's perspective, how-ever, what they had was a possibly viable fetus and a woman who was dying. For it, the concern was the potential of the fetus to become a child. The hospital therefore summoned a judge to the premises and a hearing took place, without Mrs Carder present and without clarification of her views (on the grounds that she was now too ill to be asked questions; a conclusion that was itself open to challenge). The judge agreed to the surgery being performed and his decision was supported on appeal. The child survived for about two hours and Mrs Carder for about two days. This classic, and tragic, example of the difficulties associated with seeing the fetus as a separate patient with equal (even in this case apparently superior) rights led the American commentator George Annas to say:

> They treated a live woman as though she were already dead, forced her to undergo an abortion, and then justified their brutal and unprincipled opinion on the basis that she was almost dead and her fetus's interests in life outweighed any interest she might have in her own life and health. (Annas 1988: 25).

The case was, however, appealed by Angela Carder's parents who fronted a vigorous media campaign. This appeal was supported by, amongst others, the American College of Obstetricians and Gynaecologists and the American Medical Association and the decision was ultimately overturned, albeit too late for Angela Carder (*In re AC* (1990)). It is, however, widely considered to be the turning point in a move away from court ordered medical treatment of pregnant women. (Gallagher 1987)

This case demonstrates clearly why there is such controversy about the treatment of the fetus as a person with rights, and it is not alone (see, for example, *Jefferson v. Griffin Spalding County Hospital* (1981); *In re Madyyun* (1986); *Taft v. Taft* (1983)). The Angela Carder case also demonstrates why it is that pregnant women should have their choices respected even if they appear to be 'wrong'. Attributing rights to the fetus (pre or post viability) could ultimately result not just in the kind of decision taken in Angela Carder's case, but also in all fertile and sexually active women being required to behave at all times as if they were pregnant in order to avoid being accused of damaging the fetus. This is because there are a whole host of fairly ordinary choices and behaviours that might impact negatively on the fetus, such as the ingestion of substances like caffeine. Behaviour harmful to the fetus, however, may be more anti-social – even unlawful – but yet again, the USA can provide clear examples of the consequences of attempting to intervene in these decisions because of the existence of a pregnancy. Women have reportedly been incarcerated during their pregnancies in order to ensure that they behaved 'properly'. In the case of Pamela Rae Stewart, a woman was charged under child protection laws for harm caused to her child as a result of her drug abuse during the pregnancy. The consequence of these actions, however, was as often as not to discourage women from seeking prenatal care, particularly as the women targeted were disproportionately poor and from ethnic minorities. (See Kolder *et al* (1987); Solomon (1991).) Even crediting the authorities with the best of intentions, the policy was rights reducing and counterproductive.

In the UK also, however, attempts to safeguard the fetus by modulating maternal behaviour have been made. In *Re F (in utero)* (1988), a local authority attempted to make a fetus a ward of court to protect it from the behaviour of its mother. This application was refused, however, on the basis that 'until the child was actually born, there would be an inherent incompatibility between any projected exercise of the wardship jurisdiction and the rights and welfare of the mother'. (Mason *et al.* 2002: para. 5.57). Nevertheless, in *Re D (a minor) v. Berkshire County Council* (1987) a local authority was held to be competent to make a care order in respect of a child who had been born suffering from drug dependency. In doing so, the court felt able to take into account conditions existing during pregnancy, as well as those existing after birth, in order establish whether it could be said that there had been continuing impairment of the child's proper development. Mason *et al.* (2002) suggest that this was very much a case decided on its own facts, so it should be treated with some caution as a precedent. Nevertheless, they point out that the decision means that 'the remedy is there should it be needed in serious cases'. (Mason *et al.* 2002: para. 5.58).

It is clear, therefore, that a pregnant woman in the UK ostensibly has the right to live her life as she chooses throughout the course of her pregnancy, although in exceptional cases this may be taken into account in deciding whether her child is at risk when it is born. Thus, even if fully informed of the risks to which she might put a fetus, she may effectively do with that information as she pleases during pregnancy.

As in the Angela Carder case, another area of interest arises when the mother's behaviour is not in itself problematic, but rather some medical intervention on the fetus would enhance its well-being or ensure its safety. In most cases it is likely that any such intervention will be agreed to by the pregnant woman who will generally see her interests as lying in having the healthiest possible child. However, again, there may be some women who will refuse to cooperate. In the UK, this refusal, even if it is to only minimally invasive intervention, must also be respected. In such cases, given that any intervention will inevitably involve the body of the woman, effectively the woman is being asked to agree to treatment of her own body, albeit for the benefit of the fetus. Her right to refuse treatment is exactly the same as it would be were she not pregnant. Indeed, were the law to step in and require women to submit to such interventions on behalf of a legal non-person, as argued earlier it would be open to the most strenuous objections, particularly since the law does not ordinarily force women (or anyone else) to agree to interventions, even when they could save an existing person. While there has been no case on precisely this point in Britain, it seems unlikely in the extreme that British courts would take a different position to that taken in America. (See *McFall v. Shimp* (1978).)

Problems in the course of pregnancy are exacerbated at the stage at which the birth process commences and throughout it. The image of the fetus as a separate patient is at its most acute when it is waiting to be born and become a live child with the full panoply of legal rights. Again, most women will be only too willing to accept medical advice about the management of birth, but some may not be. For the attending healthcare professionals, the failure of a woman to act at this stage in the interests of the fetus is doubtless more frustrating – even distressing – than any failure to do so earlier in the pregnancy. Perhaps for this reason, healthcare professionals have been willing to ask the law to reinforce their professional opinion about the welfare of the child to be, and have asked for the authority of the court to override a woman's decision in a number of cases. These can be dealt with relatively briefly.

The management of labour and birth

The case of Angela Carder has already been referred to, but there are UK cases in which similar (if less dramatic) events have occurred and the attitude of the law in these cases is instructive. The first of these cases was that of *Re S* (1992). In this case, the woman refused a Caesarean section on religious grounds. The best medical advice was that neither she nor the fetus would survive unless the surgery was carried out, and this information was made clear to the pregnant woman. Despite this, she continued to refuse the operation and her doctors sought the authority of the court to proceed in the face of her refusal. Because of the urgency of the case, the hearing lasted only a short period of time and – as was the case with Angela Carder – the woman was unrepresented. In the event, the judge authorised the surgery to go ahead, based – at least in some measure – on the interests of the fetus in being born alive. Extensive reference was made to the welfare of the fetus (*Re S* (1992) at p. 70).

Although this case is not now taken as having any legal authority, it remains worthy of some consideration, as it highlights clearly a series of assumptions which, it has been suggested, underpin the problems associated with what has come to be called maternal/fetal conflict. (For further discussion, see, for example, Chapter 3 in McLean (1999) and also Mair (1996).) A number of features emerge, perhaps most importantly that the woman was making a decision based on religious conviction (which is generally respected by law). This was extensively discussed in the case of *Re T (adult) (refusal of medical treatment)* (1992). See also the Canadian case of *Malette v. Shulman* (1990). It is also worthy of note that the European Convention on Human Rights, now incorporated into UK law by the Human Rights Act 1998, expressly refers to the right to freedom of thought, conscience and religion in Article 9. There was also no suggestion in *Re S* (1992) that the woman was not competent to make a decision. (The issue of competence will be discussed later (p. 000).) In other words, despite what appears to be a clear legal position, the judge was prepared to force major surgery on an unwilling woman in large measure because of the alleged interests of the fetus. This is reminiscent of the words of Lord Donaldson in *Re T (adult) (refusal of medical treatment)* (1992), referred to above. As an interesting footnote, it is worth noting that – in the absence of any UK precedent on this matter – the judge relied on the case of Angela Carder as authority for permitting the surgery, seemingly unaware that the case had already been overturned.

This case, unsurprisingly perhaps, was widely criticised and essentially ignored by the courts. This was shown some years later in the case of *Re MB* (1997), in which the court affirmed that:

The fetus up to the moment of birth does not have any separate interests capable of being taken into account when a court has to consider an application for a declaration in respect of a caesarean section operation. The court does not have the jurisdiction to declare that such medical intervention is lawful to protect the interests of the unborn child even at the point of birth. (Per Butler-Sloss, *Re MB* (1997) at p. 227).

This case laid down guidelines, which it was anticipated would be followed in the future. Broadly, they were that everyone is presumed to be competent to make medical decisions unless the contrary can be proved and a competent woman can make her own decisions even if this results in her own death or that of the fetus. Indeed, in a case already discussed, *Re F (in utero)* (1988), the court had indicated that any change to this position would need to come from Parliament. Finally, the case of *St George's Healthcare NHS Trust v. S* was heard in 1998. In this case, an apparently competent woman was eventually sectioned under the Mental Health legislation following her refusal of a Caesarean section, a route of which the Court of Appeal expressly disapproved. The court did, however, recognise the kinds of pressures under which healthcare professionals work in these circumstances; indeed, the pressure under which the courts are working. As Judge, LJ said:

When a human life is at stake the pressure to provide an affirmative answer authorising unwanted medical intervention is very powerful. Nevertheless, the autonomy of each individual requires continuing protections even, perhaps particularly, when the motive for interfering with it is readily understandable, and indeed to many would appear commendable. (*St George's Healthcare NHS Trust v. S* (1998) at p. 688).

Thus, it would appear, UK law is now relatively settled. A competent person may refuse medical treatment, even if that person is a pregnant woman. This is entirely in line with the jurisprudence of the European Court of Human Rights in its interpretation of the Convention on Human Rights to which the UK is now bound by statute. (See, for example, the case of *X v Austria* (1980).)

Competence

However, what if the person lacks competence? As has already been noted, the presumption in law is that people are competent unless the contrary can be proved. The fact of pregnancy – even the fact of being in labour – does not reduce that presumption. Indeed, even in cases where a person is suffering from a diagnosed mental illness, it cannot simply be presumed that they are incompetent for all purposes. This was clearly demonstrated in the case of *Re C (adult: refusal of treatment)* (1994). In this case, C was suffering from paranoid schizophrenia. His doctors asked the court to authorise the amputation of a gangrenous foot in the interests of preserving C's life and in the face of his refusal to submit to surgery.

The court refused to do so, and, indeed, forbade the doctors to amputate in the future should C lapse into incompetence. In the court's view, C was able to meet the tests required to establish competence; namely that he could understand the nature, purpose and effects of the treatment, believe the information and use it to arrive at a choice.

These tests form the basis of the common law on competence and have relevance also in obstetric cases. In the case of *Tameside and Glossop Acute Services Trust v. CH* (1996) a woman was held to be incapable of understanding that if she continued to refuse intervention the fetus would die, an outcome that she expressly did not wish. In *Norfolk and Norwich Healthcare (NHS) Trust v. W* (1996) a woman presented at hospital in labour, but refused to accept that she was in fact pregnant. Although a psychiatrist indicated that she was not mentally ill, there was some difficulty in deciding whether or not she could meet the tests for competence. In this case the court found her not to be competent and authorised surgery to go ahead if necessary.

Again, these cases reflect the common law position in respect of consent and, if anything, reinforce the view that women should not be treated differently because they are pregnant. The same outcome could have been anticipated in *any* case where the individual was not competent, but manifestly in need of medical treatment, although Mason *et al.* do point to the somewhat unusual conclusion in *Tameside* that a Caesarean section could be treatment of a mental disorder for the purposes of the Mental Health Act 1983. (Mason *et al.* 2002: para. 10.65).

Some pregnant women, therefore, will not be competent to make decisions and the courts will then have the authority to reach decisions on their behalf. However, these decisions should by and large reflect the best interests of the woman; not the purported best interests of the fetus. Of course, it might be assumed that the woman's best interests are served by the birth of a healthy child, rather than the death of the fetus, and so this point might seem to be little more than academic. The authority of the law to intervene in such cases is, however, not always clear. At the time of writing, in England and Wales, no statutory power exists to make decisions for those who are incapacitated (although clearly statutes exist giving certain powers over those falling within the remit of the Mental Health legislation). Historically, the authority of the courts was to be found in the *parens patriae* jurisdiction, traditionally vested in the High Court. However, perhaps unintentionally, this jurisdiction, which historically allowed the Monarch to take care of citizens who were unable to take care of themselves, disappeared from English law following the passing of the Mental Health Act 1959. For an interesting and brief account of this jurisdiction see Mason *et al.* (2002: paras. 10.31–10.34). As they note:

The net result was that no-one, not even a court, can now consent to or refuse medical treatment on behalf of an incapable adult which does not fall within the provisions of the mental health legislation. (Mason *et al.* 2002: para. 5.64).

Despite recommendations from the Law Commission dating back nearly a decade (Law Commission 1995), no legislation has hitherto been in place in England and Wales to remedy this situation, and their courts were therefore required to be creative in such circumstances. Where failure to provide treatment would result in serious risk to the incompetent individual, of course, the doctrine of necessity may be used to authorise the treatment to go ahead, and in some obstetric situations this may well be a valuable doctrine. However, it must be borne in mind that necessity has a precise meaning in law and cannot be used as a convenient catch-all provision to justify enforcing treatment even on incapacitated adults. The use of necessity as a justification for intervention, say on an unconscious adult, is limited by the fact that '[t]he treatment undertaken . . . must not be more extensive than is required by the exigencies of the situation . . .' (Mason *et al.* 2002: paras 10.12–10.15. See also the Canadian cases of *Marshall v. Curry* (1933) and *Murray v. McMurchy* (1949). In the UK see *Devi v. West Midland Regional Health Authority* (1981)). If the treatment cannot be given under the doctrine of necessity, the courts must then fall back on the device of issuing a declaration that treatment will not be unlawful if it is given in the best interests of the incompetent person (*Re F (mental patient: sterilisation)* (1990)). The meaning of best interests is one that falls to be determined on the facts of the case, although it appears that the courts are moving away from a narrow medical outcome approach to one that takes into account the patient's overall best interests. This approach mandates taking into account any known wishes, feelings and values of the patient (see for example *Re MB* (1997) and *Re A (mental patient: sterilisation)* (2000)). Not all cases involving incompetent adults need come before the courts but the dividing line between those that do and those that do not is unclear.

The position is clearly unsatisfactory and at the time of writing the issue of providing treatment to incompetent adults in England and Wales is in the process of major reform. A Draft Mental Capacity Bill has been published and is making its way through the Parliamentary process.[3] Broadly, it is proposed that there will be a general authority for those caring for adults with incapacity, including healthcare practitioners, to make decisions and act on behalf of the adult. Treatment could be provided if the practitioner reasonably believed that the adult lacked capacity with

---

[3] Draft Mental Incapacity Bill, presented to Parliament by the Secretary of the Department of Constitutional Affairs, June 2003. It is available at the website of the Department of Constitutional Affairs, along with other information about the proposed reforms. http://www.dca.gov.uk/menincap/legis.htm. During its passage through Parliament, the Bill has undergone a name change.

regard to the particular treatment, it was reasonable for the practitioner to treat the adult and the practitioner considered the treatment to be in the best interests of the adult. This decision could only be reached after working through a statutory checklist of matters to be considered and consulting with others interested in the welfare of the adult. As the legislation may be subject to amendment during its passage through Parliament, it will not be considered further here.

In Scotland, on the other hand, although the doctrine of necessity continues to have a role to play, following the recommendations of the Scottish Law Commission (Scottish Law Commission 1995), the Adults with Incapacity (Scotland) Act 2000 is now in place. This legislation gives statutory authority to medical and nursing practitioners to treat adults who are deemed to be incapable of making decisions for themselves (section 47 (1)). The medical practitioner primarily responsible for the medical treatment of the patient must certify that s/he is incapable of acting; making decisions; communicating decisions; understanding decisions; or retaining the memory of decisions, ' . . . by reason of mental disorder or of inability to communicate because of physical disability' (section 1(6)). The term 'mental disorder' was intended to have the same meaning as section 1 of the Mental Health (Scotland) Act 1984, and so is defined as:

mental illness (including personality disorder) or mental handicap however caused or manifested; but an adult shall not be treated as suffering from mental disorder by reason only of promiscuity or other immoral conduct, sexual deviancy, dependence on alcohol or drugs, or acting as no prudent person would act.

Any intervention must be for the benefit of the adult, rather than the more common test of being 'in the adult's best interests'. This term was deliberately chosen, as the Scottish Executive accepted the Scottish Law Commission's (SLC) view that the concept of best interests was derived from child-care law and was, therefore, inappropriate for adults whose wishes ought to be respected even if they run counter to what might be regarded as their 'best interests'. In addition, the SLC had said, 'by itself, "best interests" is a vague principle which would require to be supplemented by other factors' (Scottish Executive 1999: para. 2.41).

The outcome of the rejection of the 'best interests' approach is that the adult patient's past wishes must be taken into account in determining whether medical treatment should be given. Accordingly, if a form of treatment had been refused when a patient was competent, unless there is good reason to believe s/he would have changed his/her mind in the circumstances that have arisen, treatment cannot be provided simply because s/he is now incompetent. There are a number of principles to be taken into account, such as the intervention needing to be the minimum necessary and the least restrictive of the freedom of the adult. There are also provisions for a range of people close to the adult to be consulted and a Code of Practice for people giving medical treatment under the Act.[4]

However, it has been accepted that there may still be circumstances where there is insufficient time to follow the certification procedures required under the Act; for example, where delay might endanger the person's life or lead to serious deterioration in his/her condition. In such circumstances it has been stated that doctors may provide treatment immediately as a matter of good practice and under existing law, since the Act was an addition to, rather than a substitute for, the ability to treat emergencies at common law (Scottish Executive 2002: paras. 2.2–2.6). There may also be circumstances where the patient is believed to lack capacity to make a treatment decision but this is not due to mental disorder or inability to communicate because of physical disability. In these circumstances too, the Act may be inapplicable and reliance may have to be placed on the principle of necessity. However, it was noted that the Act was introduced because of uncertainties in the law about the definition of emergency, urgent and routine procedures and doctors are advised to use the authority of the Adults with Incapacity (Scotland) Act 2000 wherever it is reasonable and practicable to do so.

One further group requires attention before leaving the topic of capacity; namely children and young people. Pregnancy is no respecter of age, and the continued high incidence of teenage pregnancies means that doctors will often be confronted by young people desirous of making their own decisions even following full disclosure of information. In this group, competence is a complex issue, and one that again varies between the UK jurisdictions. Space does not permit a detailed discussion here, but a wealth of commentaries exists in this area should the reader wish to follow up this issue. (See, for example, Elliston (1996) and British Medical Association (2001).)

Briefly, the position is as follows. In England and Wales, following the case of *Gillick v. West Norfolk and Wisbech Area Health Authority* (1985) it was made clear that, although doctors should try to convince young people to seek the agreement of their parents to medical interventions, the mature or '*Gillick* competent' child can authorise medical treatment on his/her own behalf. (See also *Re P (a minor)* (1986).) However, more controversial is the situation when the young person's decision is to reject rather than accept treatment. It might be assumed that if a person under the age of majority is able in law to accept medical treatment, the corollary logically would be that they also have the right to refuse it. However, a number of recent judgements have demonstrated this simple equation to be flawed.

In the case of *Re R* (1992) a 15-year-old girl, whose capacity was described as fluctuating, refused treatment during her lucid intervals. Lord Donaldson likened

---

[4] Detailed guidance on the workings of the Act, including a Code of Practice in respect of Part 5 of the Act (Scottish Executive 2002), is available at the Scottish Executive Justice department website: www.scotland.gov.uk/justice/incapacity

the provision of consent to a key opening a door. In the case of the minor, there was, he argued, more than one key-holder: the minor him or her self, those with parental authority and ultimately the court. In his view, consent obtained from either of these parties was sufficient to authorise treatment to go ahead. Thus, if the child consents and the parents do not, the child's consent is sufficient. Unfortunately, perhaps, for the young person, the converse is also true in this analogy; that is, if the child refuses treatment and the parents agree to it, their consent is sufficient to override the refusal by the young person, even if s/he is otherwise '*Gillick* competent'.

Lord Donaldson took this analogy to a different level in the case of *Re W (a minor) (medical treatment)* (1992). This case has added interest in that it concerned a young person of 16 years of age, who was therefore covered by the terms of the Family Law Reform Act 1969, s 8(1) of which gives the young person between the ages of 16 and 18 the specific authority to consent to medical treatment on his/her own behalf. However, s8(3) of the Act says:

Nothing in this section shall be construed as making ineffective any consent which would have been effective if this section had not been enacted.

The impact of this subsection led the court to agree that parental consent could override the refusal of the young person. Thus, the legal authority to refuse treatment is not the other side of the coin which permits young persons to consent to treatment on their own behalf, despite the apparent logic of the assumption that it is. Many commentators regard this decision with concern (for example, Elliston 1996) although others would suggest that '[a] level of comprehension sufficient to justify a refusal of treatment certainly includes one to accept treatment but the reverse does not hold . . .' (Mason *et al.* 2002: para. 10.47).

In Scotland the law seems to take an approach that is different and, arguably for the young person, infinitely preferable. It had always been assumed, even before the *Gillick* case, that children under the age of 16 had the power to consent to a number of things, including certain medical interventions, on their own behalf once they reached a certain level of maturity. This assumption was clarified by the terms of the Age of Legal Capacity (Scotland) Act 1991. Section 2(4) of the Act reads as follows:

A person under the age of sixteen years shall have legal capacity to consent on his own behalf to any surgical, medical or dental procedure or treatment where, in the opinion of a qualified medical practitioner attending him, he is capable of understanding the nature and possible consequences of the procedure or treatment.

Although not explicit in the terms of the Act, it is widely assumed that this extensive right would also include the right to refuse medical treatment. This conclusion is reinforced by the companion legislation, the Children (Scotland) Act 1995. Section 15(5) of this Act makes it clear that a third party (parent) can only act as a child's legal representative for so long as the child is incapable of acting on his/her own behalf. Thus, if the child acquires capacity (under the terms of the 1991 Act) the parent or guardian loses the right to act on his/her behalf, presumably irrespective of what his/her decision is. For the sake of completeness it is also worth noting that section 1(1)(b) of the 1991 Act expressly permits anyone over the age of 16 to enter into any legal transaction, which is defined in section 9 as 'the giving by a person of any consent having legal effect'. Unlike their counterparts in England and Wales, then, those aged 16 and over in Scotland may be fully entitled to accept or refuse, medical treatment, although since there have been no cases in the superior courts on this point, the law may not be regarded as being settled. (See also British Medical Association (2001).)

Whether young people are able to give a legally binding consent to or refusal of treatment or not, professional guidance emphasises the need to involve them in decision making as much as possible. (See, for example, Department of Health (2001a), (2001b); British Medical Association (2001).)

Liability for negligence in obstetric care

As has been seen, failure to provide sufficient information before seeking consent to treat is one extremely important subset of clinical negligence. However, there are issues specific to negligence in treatment – as opposed to the provision of information – which require separate consideration. Specifically, it is necessary to discuss actions raised in negligence in more detail. (For a useful account of negligence in obstetric care see Chapter 4 in Harpwood (1996). For a more recent review of medical negligence see Chapter 9 in Mason *et al.* (2002).)

The essence of negligence in law is that there must be a duty of care owed by A to B, that duty must be breached and the harm caused to B must arise as a consequence of A's breach of duty. (The leading case from which this doctrine is derived is that of *Donoghue or McAlister v. Stevenson* (1932).) Thus, not all adverse outcomes or incidents will form the basis of an action for compensation. For example, although a healthcare professional who offers to care for a pregnant woman undoubtedly owes her a duty of care, the extent and scope of that duty will need to be clear before liability will be imposed. An interesting and important issue to consider is the extent to which a duty of care is owed to the fetus or to the child the fetus will become. In any negligence case, the link between the alleged breach and the harm claimed (legally known as the link in causation) may also not be easy to establish. Finally, in obstetric cases there may be some argument about whether or not a harm has actually occurred.

Duty of care, standard of care and breach of duty

The first issue to consider is what the nature of the duty of care is and how it can be shown to have been breached. It should be obvious that, in a field such as health care, sometimes things will go wrong and patients will be harmed as a result. These may be pure accidents, where no amount of preparation or precaution could have prevented the harm occurring. Others could perhaps have been avoided but the measures that would have had to be undertaken to avoid the harm would have been out all proportion to the likelihood of harm occurring, or its severity. The law recognises that it is not appropriate to hold individuals or organisations liable for all harm caused by their actions in all circumstances, since in that case liability would be unlimited and this could effectively prevent any normal conduct of business or even social life. There are rare examples where the so-called doctrine of strict liability operates; that is, people are held liable for the consequences of their actions, irrespective of any degree of personal fault on their part. However, in the main, liability for harm rests upon some degree of culpability in the form of deliberate wrongful actions or, as is being considered here, negligence. Where negligence is concerned, since there is no intention to harm, there is an additional requirement that there be some kind of relationship between the alleged wrongdoer and the person harmed.

The need for this relationship is because potentially many of our actions or our failures to act could harm other people. The law, however, sets a limit upon those to whom we may be liable in respect of negligent actions by utilising the notion of the duty of care. The scope of the duty is set by the 'neighbour' principle expounded by Lord Atkin in the leading negligence case of *Donoghue or McAlister v. Stevenson* (1932) (at p. 44). He stated that we owe a duty of care to our 'neighbours' who in law are:

> ... persons who are so closely and directly affected by my act that I ought to reasonably have them in contemplation when I am directing my mind to the acts or omissions which are called in question.

In the healthcare context, establishing that a health carer owed a duty of care to a patient he or she is responsible for is generally straightforward, since it is implicit in the professional relationship that reasonable care will be taken.

Much more difficult for patients, however, is establishing whether there has been a breach of the duty of care. What must be established is whether the health carer has fallen below the standard expected of him/her in this situation. The law does not therefore require the health carer to achieve the highest attainable standard. Rather, to escape liability, it requires that a minimum standard is met. This minimum is the standard of care.

In most negligence cases, the test that is used to decide what the standard of care actually is in a given situation will be the test of the hypothetical reasonable person in that situation. This person used to be referred to as the man on the Clapham omnibus, more recently expressed as the commuter on the London Underground (*McFarlane v. Tayside Health Board* (1999), per Lord Steyn). The difficulty in professional negligence cases is that the average person, whatever their means of transport, does not have the kind of skills that the professional is expected to exercise. Judging the professional by what the hypothetical reasonable person might be expected to do, therefore, would not be a sufficient standard against which to test the professional.

It is for this reason that the professional negligence standard in medicine was expressed in what has come to be known as the *Bolam* test:

The test is the standard of the ordinary skilled man exercising and professing to have that special skill. A man need not possess the highest expert skill at the risk of being found negligent. It is a well-established law that it is sufficient if he exercises the ordinary skill of an ordinary man exercising that particular art...A doctor is not guilty of negligence if he has acted in accordance with a practice accepted as proper by a responsible body of medical men skilled in that particular art. (Per McNair J in *Bolam v. Friern Hospital Management Committee* (1957) at pp. 121–122).

This test followed an earlier Scottish decision *Hunter v. Hanley* (1955), which is the case still preferred in Scotland. There is a slight difference in the wording of the standard of care in these two cases. However, it has been held in both jurisdictions that the standard of care in Scotland and in England and Wales is part of the same law and the standards are equivalent. (See *Moyes v. Lothian Health Board* (1990) and *Maynard v. West Midlands Regional Health Authority* (1985).) The same general approach is also taken to dealing with other healthcare professions. (See for example *Corley v. North West Herefordshire HA* (1997), a case involving midwives.)

The *Bolam* test, therefore, relies upon evidence being led to establish whether other professionals in the same field of practice believe it was appropriate to treat the patient in the way that the defendant did. It might be thought that this test is just common sense. Judges are clearly not experts in health care and would expect to receive guidance on what is possible, and what is done, in professional practice in order to consider the reasonableness of the defendant's actions. However, reliance on expert evidence is also at the heart of criticism of the professional standard, in that the accusation may be made that professionals are in effect able to set their own standards. This would be the case if what they do, or say they would do, is uncritically accepted by judges as being what it is *appropriate* to do. Commentators on medical law (such as Teff (1998)) have remarked on the discrepancy between the proportion of successful cases brought in general negligence cases and the much lower success of medical negligence cases. Many reasons can be suggested for this, such as unrealistic expectations of patients and their lawyers in commencing actions with no hope of success; difficulties in establishing causation; and the complexity of medical cases compared with other types of negligence cases. Nevertheless, there has been some suspicion that the courts have been insufficiently rigorous in exercising their own judgement on whether the practices adopted or endorsed by the medical profession are acceptable (Teff 1998). In other words, even though expert evidence should *inform* the decision it should not *determine* whether professional practice is acceptable. This assessment should remain the prerogative of the courts.

In this respect, perhaps the most significant English case since *Bolam* is that of *Bolitho v. City and Hackney Health Authority* (1997). *Bolitho* was unusual, since it involved a failure to attend a patient, so treatment was not given. Expert evidence was led that if treatment, in the form of intubation, had been given then the child patient's life would have been saved. Since the doctor had not attended, the case largely hinged upon causation, an issue that will be looked at later in this discussion. However, for the moment, it is enough to note that the defence case was that, even if the doctor had attended, she would not have intubated, so that her failure to attend was irrelevant to the harm suffered by the child. It was further contended that failure to intubate would have been an appropriate response. Expert evidence on the defendant's behalf supported the view that a reasonable doctor might not have intubated. The parents' contention was that this was illogical, given the relative simplicity of the intervention and the severity of the consequences it would have averted. The House of Lords dismissed the parents' case but importantly Lord Browne-Wilkinson held that:

> ... in cases involving, as they often do, the weighing of risks against benefits, the judge before accepting a body of opinion as being responsible, reasonable or respectable will need to be satisfied that, in forming their views, the experts have directed their minds to the question of comparative risks and benefits and have reached a defensible conclusion on the matter. (*Bolitho v. City and Hackney Health Authority* (1997) at p. 9)

This was immediately qualified by the warning that it would 'seldom be right for a judge to reach the conclusion that views genuinely held by a competent medical expert are unreasonable'. Nevertheless, it may signal a more critical approach by the courts to expert evidence in medical negligence cases, although commentators vary in the extent to which they consider this will be borne out in future cases. (For example, see Brazier and Miola (2000) compared with Maclean (2002).)

It is worth noting here that even where it is admitted, or the courts hold, that there has been a mistake by the professional, this does not prove there has been negligence. The case of *Whitehouse v. Jordan* (1981) concerned the management of a delivery where it was alleged that forceps were used for too long and with excessive force, although this evidence was contested. The child was born with brain damage resulting from asphyxia. According to Lord Fraser:

> The true position is that an error of judgement may, or may not, be negligent: it depends on the nature of the error. If it is one that would not have been made by a reasonably competent professional man professing to have the standard and type of skill that the defendant holds himself out as having, and acting with ordinary care, then it is negligence. If, on the other hand, it is an error that such a man, acting with ordinary care, might have made, then it is not negligence. (*Whitehouse v. Jordan* (1981) at p. 281).

As in all negligence cases, the burden of proving that the defendant fell below the required standard of care is on the person bringing the action; namely the patient, or in the event of the patient's death, his/her next of kin or dependants. Claimants must establish on the balance of probabilities (which means that it is more likely than not) that their version of events is correct and that the health carer was in breach of the duty of care he or she owed them. If a case goes to trial, there will be evidence representing both sides. If the court finds the evidence to be credible, and that it is given by sufficiently qualified experts, the court cannot choose between them (*Maynard v. West Midlands Regional Health Authority* (1985)). In such cases, the claimant will have failed to establish that 'no doctor of ordinary skill' would have treated him/her in this way if acting with ordinary care. It is also not appropriate simply to compare the numbers of practitioners who would act as the defendant did with those who would not. A relatively small number of specialists can form a responsible body of medical opinion, provided that they are sufficiently qualified in the area of practice under consideration (*DeFreitas v. O'Brien* (1995) and *Gordon v. Wilson* (1992)). *Bolitho* does not alter this. All that *Bolitho* does is to emphasise the fact that the court is entitled to conclude that professional practice is negligent. Following usual professional practice may not therefore guarantee escape from liability for negligence, although it is likely to remain highly persuasive.

The converse is also true: the fact that a doctor has not conformed to usual practice in treating a patient is not in itself evidence of negligence (*Hunter v. Hanley* (1955) at p. 217). Again, this may be regarded as a matter of common sense, since failure to allow for deviations from usual practice would mean that there could be no innovations in medical care. After all, every technique now in use was a departure from standard practice once; indeed research and innovation are the lifeblood of medical advance. It is not possible to discuss research in this chapter. However, even in an everyday treatment situation it may not be easy to establish that there was a normal and usual practice, since there may be many treatment options available, any of which could be adopted by a practitioner exercising a reasonable professional judgement.

This is also relevant in the context of what duty of responsibility practitioners have to keep abreast of developments in practice. It has been held that it is not possible for a practitioner to read every article published in his/her field of practice, nor would it necessarily be reasonable to expect practitioners to implement a new technique as soon as it is publicised (*Crawford v. Board of Governors, Charing Cross Hospital* (1953)). There are sound reasons for this approach, since the increasing opportunities for publication may lead to problems of information overload. Equally, it is difficult on occasion to evaluate the quality of information on offer. Even when techniques are published in reputable and peer reviewed journals they may subsequently prove to be harmful. Nevertheless, this is not a licence to practitioners to continue with outmoded techniques; again the critical assessment will relate to the reasonableness of the practitioner continuing to offer the form of treatment given.

It should also be remembered that health carers must consider each case individually, so that, although they may ordinarily use a certain technique, they must be prepared to vary their technique in particular circumstances depending on what they find. (See, for example, *Devaney v. Greater Glasgow Health Board* (1987).) This caution must be borne in mind even when dealing with evidence-based guidelines, since there may be circumstances where slavishly following them would result in harm to the individual. However, as with any departure from recommended and standard practice the reason for doing so should be clearly justifiable.

While the burden of proof always remains on the patient to prove his/her case, in some cases the doctrine of *res ipsa loquitur* may apply. For a detailed discussion of this doctrine see Reid (1999). This doctrine allows negligence to be inferred from the facts of what happened. Thus, the court may conclude that, in the absence of an adequate explanation of how what occurred could have happened without negligence, the claimant has established negligence. This doctrine would be parti-cularly useful where the patient was unable to establish exactly what did happen but the facts of the case strongly suggest that something went wrong that should not have done. However, the use of this doctrine in medical cases is rare since courts are reluctant to infer negligence except in the most obvious cases, such as where swabs have been left in a patient during surgery (*Mahon v. Osborne* (1939); see also *Cassidy v. Ministry of Health* (1951)).

A final and interesting question is the standard of care to be expected of the newly qualified or junior practitioner. The issue arose in the case of *Wilsher v. Essex Area Health Authority* (1986). Here a baby had been born prematurely and it was discovered that the baby had retrolental fibroplasia. The parents alleged that a junior doctor had taken a measurement of oxygen from a vein rather than an artery and consequently that too much oxygen had been given to the child. It was argued on behalf of the Health Authority that a lower standard of care should apply, since hospital staff can only gain experience by working with patients and it would be unfair to expect juniors to provide the same level of treatment as a more senior or experienced member of staff. This argument was rejected on the grounds that '[doctors] are not the only people who gain their experience not only from lectures or from watching other people perform, but from tackling live customers or clients'. (*Wilsher v. Essex Area Health Authority* (1986) per Lord Mustill). To allow a lower standard of care would mean that patients could never know what level of treatment to expect as this could be endlessly variable depending on the precise qualifications of the individual professional. If people are offering treatment then they are expected to be sufficiently well trained and supervised to do so. While junior members of staff may not be morally or personally at fault if they are not able to meet their obligations, lack of adequate training or supervision is still likely to lead to liability of senior staff or the employing organisation for failing to have appropriate systems in place.

Causation

Claimants also have the burden of proving that it is more likely than not that their injuries were caused by the negligence complained of. This can often be a significant hurdle in itself and may prove impossible to overcome. The difficulty is often acute where a child is diagnosed with problems soon after birth. A notable case is that of *Wilsher v. Essex Area Health Authority* (1986) discussed above. (See also *Kay's Tutor v. Ayrshire & Arran Health Board* (1987).) It will be remembered that the child was diagnosed with retrolental fibroplasia, alleged to have been caused by being given too much oxygen after birth. However, while excess oxygen was a possible cause of this condition there were at least five other possible causes. The child's parents were unable to establish on the balance of probabilities that it was the extra oxygen that had caused the condition in this particular case.

There are significant difficulties in other cases too, such as where the child has suffered brain damage and consequent disability, for example in cerebral palsy cases, and it is alleged that this was caused by mismanagement of labour resulting in lack of oxygen reaching the child. Prematurity is often associated with cerebral palsy and it may be difficult to establish whether it was this rather than the decisions made during delivery that caused the condition in the child. Other factors too, such as family history or lack of fetal growth during pregnancy, may be relevant and can further cloud the issue of the exact cause of the condition. (For a more detailed consideration of this issue see Harpwood 1996: 181–186.) Since the burden of proof is on the claimant, if it cannot be established that it is more likely than not that it was negligence in delivery that caused cerebral palsy, the claimant will fail.

There are some legal presumptions that may help claimants, however. One is that where negligence materially contributed to injury being caused, even if it was not the sole precipitating factor, the defendant may be found liable (*McGhee v. National Coal Board* (1973)). Therefore, where there are a number of factors which taken together caused the condition, if the contribution made by the health carer is regarded as sufficiently significant, liability can be imposed. However, this may still be difficult for a patient to establish.

There is a further complication where compensation is being sought for loss of a chance of a good outcome. For example, some people would recover well if an operation was performed timeously, whereas others would not. Even if negligence resulted in delay in surgery, the patient cannot necessarily recover damages. This will depend on how likely recovery would have been. If, for example, there is generally only a 25% chance of recovery as opposed to 75% non-recovery even if the operation had been performed when it should have been, then usually the patient cannot succeed. This is because s/he cannot establish that, on the balance of probabilities, s/he would have been more likely to recover than not. If, on the other hand, there is normally a 51% chance of recovery as opposed to a 49% chance of non-recovery, s/he would be likely to succeed as it would now be deemed to be more likely than not that s/he would have benefited from the operation. Of course there may be particular factors that would make an individual patient's chances of recovery better or worse; however, these special factors would have to be established to displace this presumption. This principle is set out in *Hotson v. East Berkshire Area Health Authority* (1987).

Establishing harm

This issue is seldom problematic, in that the result of medical negligence is generally physical injury which is easily recognised as being a form of harm. If physical injury has been caused, damages are recoverable for this and for resulting losses, such as loss of income, cost of care and so on. However, there may be some situations where the result of medical negligence is less easily characterised as a harm. Where, for example, women have become pregnant following failed sterilisation, they have sought compensation, not only for the pain and suffering of pregnancy and childbirth and costs during pregnancy, but also for the financially much more significant costs of bringing up the child. These cases are referred to as 'wrongful birth' cases. This is an evolving area of law, but suffice it to say here that recent cases have held that damages can only be awarded for upkeep of the child if the child is born with disabilities or additional problems are caused by the fact that the mother is disabled. (See *McFarlane v. Tayside Health Board* (2000); *Parkinson v. Seacroft University Hospitals NHS Trust* (2001); *Rees v. Darlington Memorial Hospital NHS Trust* (2003).) The reasoning in these cases is complex and confused, but is based in large part on the courts' general reluctance to view the birth of a healthy child as amounting to a harm or the view that awarding significant damages for the upkeep of a healthy child would be disproportionate to the degree of negligence involved.

Equally, the courts in the UK have declined to accept the legitimacy of so called 'wrongful life' actions. The usual kind of situation where this action might be contemplated would be where there had been a failure to communicate properly the results of tests conducted in pregnancy. Although the parents in this case might succeed in a wrongful birth action, a wrongful life action is brought by the child.

Thus, the child would have to show that the failure caused the harm complained of; in this case, life with disabilities. This kind of action has not been entertained by British courts for a number of reasons, such as the fear that it would encourage doctors to seek to persuade women to mitigate loss by terminating pregnancy and concern that this might devalue the lives of those with disabilities (*McKay v. Essex Area Health Authority* (1982)). Another chief issue of concern in the courts has been the alleged difficulty in calculating damages. Thus, the courts say, they would have to be able to compare the harm of being born with disabilities to not being born at all. As in wrongful birth actions, the courts will additionally hold that, save in the most exceptional circumstances, it must be regarded as a benefit rather than a harm to be born. However, it has been said that "[T]he legal and philosophical arguments in favour of rejecting the wrongful life action are powerful but can be challenged" (Mason *et al.* 2002: paras. 6.38–6.54) and reasons for doing so are discussed elsewhere. Wrongful life claims are commonly thought to be excluded now in England and Wales by the Congenital Disabilities (Civil Liability) Act 1976 s1(2)(b). Some commentators have expressed doubt as to whether the statute does completely exclude wrongful life actions (Mason *et al.* 2002: para. 6.44). There is, for example, an interesting possibility that a wrongful life action might be brought under the statute, where the action complained of is in the selection of an embryo under the new section.1A (see note 6). This matter has not been judicially considered.

Much of the foregoing has assumed that the person bringing the action for negligence is the woman seeking compensation for injuries she has suffered during pregnancy and labour. However, equally significant may be claims for negligence that harmed the fetus in utero, resulting in it being delivered dead or surviving with injuries.

Negligence causing death of a fetus before birth

In the case of the child delivered dead, as a matter of civil law the child has never been a legal person and so any claim would have to be made by the woman or both parents on their own behalf, rather than in the name of the child. Their claim would be analogous to the kinds of claims discussed above, in that the parents would have to prove that they were owed a duty of care that was breached and in this case that the breach of care caused the death of the fetus. The harm they have suffered would be the distress caused by the loss of their child. However, they cannot be awarded bereavement damages. This is a specific small sum of money that can be awarded as part of damages for the death of a relative. However, as the child has never been a legal person, bereavement damages cannot form part of any award (*Bagley v. North Hertfordshire Health Authority* (1986)). It is only where a child is delivered alive and subsequently dies of antenatal injuries that parents can claim bereavement damages (*Hamilton v. Fife Health Board* (1993)).

Negligence causing a child to be born injured

In any case where a child is the claimant it is probable that his/her parents will be bringing the claim on his/her behalf. However, it will still need to be established on the balance of probability that harm was caused to the child, either negligently or deliberately by an act or omission of the defendant. Furthermore, if the claim is based on negligence, the defendant must have owed the child a duty of care. However, where the act or omission occurred before the birth of the child, there is a potential conceptual difficulty in reconciling the idea of a duty of care being owed to an entity that has no legal personality (a fetus). If it is not legally recognised, how can it be owed a duty of care?

The need to consider this issue arose as a matter of urgency after the births of children with severe disabilities to women given thalidomide during pregnancy as a means of avoiding severe morning sickness. Although claims against the manufacturer were eventually dealt with by out of court settlements, so that the issue of liability for antenatal injury was not ruled upon, the need to establish whether such claims could be brought in future cases was clear. The law was reviewed in England and Wales and in Scotland (Law Commission (1974); Scottish Law Commission (1973)). As a result of the English review, a new statute, the Congenital Disabilities (Civil Liability) Act 1976, was passed. In fact, subsequent case law found that such actions were possible under the common law in England and Wales, *Burton v. Islington Health Authority, de Martell v. Merton and Sutton Health Authority* (1992). However the statute supersedes the common law position.

This statute provides that a person has a right of action if born with deformity, disease or abnormality, including any predisposition to physical or mental defect, due to the intentional act, negligence or breach of statutory duty of anyone before his or her birth. Being 'born' is defined as being born alive, 'the moment of a child's birth being when it first has a life separate from its mother' but the child must live for at least 48 hours in order for an action to be competent.[5]

The harm suffered by the child must be due to an occurrence which:

i. affected the mother or father in their ability to have a normal, healthy child, or
ii. affected the mother during her pregnancy, or
iii. affected the mother or her child in the course of its birth, so that the child is born with disabilities that would not otherwise be present.[6]

The child cannot bring an action unless the parent was owed a duty of care by the person alleged to be at fault. This is because the child's action is derivative from

---

[5] ss. 4 (2) (a) and 4 (4) CD(CL)A 1976.
[6] A new provision, section 1A, was subsequently added to the CD(CL)A 1976 by s. 44 of the Human Fertilisation and Embryology Act 1990. This concerns disabilities caused as a result of the selection, storage or use of embryos or gametes in fertility treatment, including artificial insemination.

the obligations owed to the parents (although no physical injury need actually be suffered by the parent).[7]

There are a number of statutory defences open to a defendant, as well as those normally available. Firstly, if the alleged wrongful act occurred before the child's conception the defendant is not liable to the child if either or both of the parents knew of this particular risk of their child being born disabled.[8] Liability under the Act is therefore excluded where either parent knew of the particular risk of disability and chose to proceed with a pregnancy.

Secondly, if the defendant was treating or advising the parent in a professional capacity then s/he is not liable to the child for any act or omission provided that s/he took reasonable care in accordance with what was then received professional opinion. However, a defendant is not to be taken as answerable to the child only because he departed from received opinion.[9] This statutory re-statement of the *Bolam* test was probably unnecessary but seems to have been included, in line with the overall intention of the statute, for the avoidance of doubt.

Liability to the child can be excluded by contract with the affected parent, but only to the same extent that liability to the parent could be excluded (e.g. any contractual terms would be subject to the provisions of the Unfair Terms in Consumer Contracts Regulations 1994).[10] Contributory negligence of the affected parent enables damages against the defendant to be reduced to the extent that the court thinks just and equitable.[11]

However, one class of persons is specifically excluded from the scheme of liability under the statute, the child's mother.[12] The woman was generally to be exempted from liability to her child, according to the Law Commission, because of the fear of disruption to the relationship between mother and child and also the potential for lawsuits on behalf of children to be used as ammunition in matrimonial disputes between the child's parents. There is one exception under section 2 where negligence leading to the injuries to the child were caused by the mother driving a motor vehicle, if she knew, or ought reasonably to have known, that she was pregnant. The reason for this exception is based upon the practical consideration that all motor vehicle drivers are legally required to have third party insurance.

Liability under the Congential Disabilities (Civil Liability) Act 1976 and wrongful life actions

The statute must also be considered in conjunction with actions for 'wrongful life' since, according to the scheme of the Act, a child can claim compensation for being born with disabilities due to acts or omissions before its conception as well as before

---

[7] s. 1(3) CD(CL)A 1976.   [8] s. 1(4) CD(CL)A 1976.   [9] s. 1(5) CD(CL)A 1976.
[10] s. 1(6) CD(CL)A 1976.   [11] s. 1(7) CD(CL)A 1976.   [12] s.1(1) CD(CL)A 1976.

its birth. Although wrongful life actions have not been accepted in UK courts, it might at first sight be suggested that the terms of the 1976 Act in fact permit exactly these kinds of claims to succeed. However, the difference between wrongful life actions and those permitted by the legislation is that under the statute, liability arises for wrongful acts or omissions that cause the child to be born with disabilities '*which would not otherwise have been present*'.[13] Therefore, unlike failures in genetic counselling or failure to warn parents that exposure to rubella might have affected the child, the claim under the 1976 Act is that the defendant's breach of duty actually *caused* the disability. The contention is therefore that, but for the wrongful action of the defendant, this child could have been born or conceived without the disability in question and the policy reasons for dismissing wrongful life actions do not, therefore, apply.

The common law position in Scotland

The 1976 Act does not apply in Scotland because the Scottish Law Commission concluded that the position was covered in common law. No statute was therefore necessary to permit a child to recover damages if born injured due to acts or omissions before its birth or conception (Scottish Law Commission 1973). This view was subsequently endorsed in the case of *Hamilton v. Fife Health Board* (1993). Subsequent cases have confirmed that this is the position, although its precise legal basis remains unclear. One approach has been to manipulate the rules of negligence by basing liability for antenatal injury upon establishing the cause of the child's disabilities and whether it was reasonably foreseeable that the wrongful acts of the defender would have these consequences (*McWilliams v. Lord Advocate* (1992)). Another approach has been to adopt a legal presumption deriving ultimately from Roman law, abbreviated as the *nasciturus* principle. This principle broadly provides that a child should be deemed to have been born whenever its interests require it. If a child has survived antenatal injuries so that it is born alive, the principle allows the courts to take into account injuries caused to it before birth (*Hamilton v. Fife Health Board* (1993)).

Whichever approach is adopted, this seems to protect the legal position of the child in Scotland, although a number of matters remain unresolved. These include whether the child must survive for any particular period after birth and, importantly, whether the woman herself can be sued by her child for any injuries caused by her. This may be particularly significant where, as discussed earlier (see p. 000), a woman's decisions about antenatal care and about the delivery of her baby put the child at risk. The Scottish Law Commission believed it would be unlikely that claims would be made against mothers but did not rule this out. Policy reasons,

---

[13] s. 1(2)(b) CD(CL)A 1976 (our emphasis)

such as those offered by the English Law Commission, might make such actions unlikely to succeed, although the matter cannot be said to be settled beyond doubt (Mason *et al.* 2002: paras. 6.35–6). In particular, if the *nasciturus* principle continues to inform Scottish law, it would undoubtedly militate against restrictions on actions when harm has been established.

Reform of actions for medical negligence

Concerns about the present approach to medical negligence claims have been increasing, both from the individuals and organisations who are parties to such actions and also from the government, which must raise funds to pay for the conduct and outcome of litigation against the NHS. These concerns were highlighted in a report by the National Audit Office in 2001. It reported that as at 31 March 2000, provisions to meet outstanding clinical negligence claims were £2.6 billion for England, £38 million for Scotland, £111 million (including creditors) in Wales and £100 million in Northern Ireland. These costs were rising rapidly and substantially, causing a significant drain on the overall health budget. There were also serious concerns about the delays in providing financial help for litigants, caused by the lengthy legal process, and the stress of litigation on all parties; the problem of funding litigation for those patients not qualifying for legal aid; the legal costs outweighing the sums granted in compensation and many other practical difficulties.

In response to this report the Government announced its intention to undertake major reform of clinical negligence claims. The Chief Medical Officer for England was asked to examine the issue and report. He issued a White Paper to address this in 2003 (Chief Medical Officer 2003). There had been much speculation about possible reforms, in particular that there would be the introduction of some form of 'no-fault' liability, whereby compensation could be paid for injury caused by health care without the need to establish negligence on behalf of the healthcare providers. There are several variations on 'no-fault' schemes that operate in countries such as New Zealand, Sweden and Finland. They have their own advantages and disadvantages which are outside the scope of this chapter. For discussion on some of the merits and difficulties of no-fault schemes see, for example, Oliphant (1996); Fallberg and Borgenhammer (1997). In the event, the creation of an overall no-fault scheme for all medical injuries has not been recommended. What was proposed was a new NHS Redress Scheme, which would have four main elements: *an investigation of the incident* that is alleged to have caused harm and of the harm that has resulted; *provision of an explanation* to the patient and of the action proposed to prevent repetition; *development and delivery of a package of care* providing remedial treatment, therapy and arrangements for continuing care where needed; and *payments* for pain and suffering, out of pocket expenses and care or treatment that the NHS could not provide.

In seeking to learn from adverse incidents and addressing the practical issues facing most patients, these suggestions will no doubt be welcome. More controversial, however, are the proposals on payments. The new scheme would cover limited types of situation. It would allow patients to be awarded payment for serious shortcomings in NHS care if the harm could have been avoided and if the adverse outcome was not the result of the natural progression of the illness. Payment would be made for reimbursement of the cost of the care leading to harm or for amounts up to £30 000. Of particular significance here, though, is the specific recommendation in respect of birth-injured babies. Families of neurologically impaired babies would be eligible for the new NHS Redress Scheme if: the birth was under NHS care; the impairment was birth-related; severe neurological impairment (including cerebral palsy) was evident at birth or within eight years. Genetic or congenital abnormality would be excluded. If these conditions were met, a package of compensation would be provided in cash or kind according to the severity of the impairment, judged according to the ability to perform the tasks of daily living, and would comprise: a managed care package; a monthly payment for the costs of care; one-off lump sum payments for home adaptations and equipment at intervals throughout the child's life; and an initial payment in compensation for pain, suffering and loss of amenity. The sums payable for all of these measures would be capped.

While it is intended that this scheme will be run as an administrative matter, hence avoiding the costs and delays of court proceedings, it is still unclear how many of the important issues will be dealt with. One crucial matter is what should be the qualifying criteria for access to the scheme, the '*Bolam*' test currently used in assessing clinical negligence or a broader definition of sub-standard care? The extent to which fault need be established under these proposals, therefore, remains to be seen. It should be noted that there would be an expectation that, except in the case of children with cerebral palsy, patients would first make an application to the NHS Redress Scheme. Patients accepting awards under the scheme would have to waive their right to sue for the same claim, but use of the scheme would not be compulsory. Negligence cases therefore seem unlikely to disappear in the near future.

There are many other recommendations that cannot be discussed here and the White Paper is being consulted upon at the time of writing. It seems likely that it will be the subject of considerable debate and whether it will be translated into legislation, and in what form, remains to be seen. The White Paper is directed only at England and Wales, but an an expert advisory group in Scotland has also been looking at some aspects of compensation. Its final report came down against introducing a no-fault scheme but suggested numerous areas where changes were needed (Ross Report 2003). It is clear that serious concerns about the present state of affairs are still being raised, see, for example, the report issued by the Commons Public Accounts Committee in June 2002,[14] and some reform seems inevitable.

However, of significance in the context of obstetric practice, which has been one of the areas of medicine in which litigation is most frequent, and where damages awards are often high, there has been an unconfirmed suggestion that birth injuries might specifically be dealt with by a no-fault scheme.[15]

Conclusion

It can be seen that the management of pregnancy and labour offers significant scope for disagreement and even litigation. It can also be said that the medical advances in these areas have contributed to the generation of at least some of these potential hazards for the practitioner. However, for these reasons it is important that doctors are well informed about the limits and the extent of their actual or possible legal liability. One interesting point to note from what has been discussed is that the law should not be seen as the enemy of medical practice. Indeed, doctors have shown themselves increasingly willing to use the law to uphold and validate their clinical judgements, even in the face of their patients' antipathy. Equally, the standards set by the law in terms of information disclosure and operational negligence are demanding but not overwhelmingly so.

It is an inevitable consequence of the practice of medicine, and its increasing sophistication, that things will go wrong. It is equally likely that some patients will reject even the best medical recommendations. This, however, provides no justification for breaching the human rights of the women concerned. It is a hard fact that – irrespective of the emotional costs – the competent person has a right to make irresponsible or unintelligible decisions. The appropriate aspiration of all parties in the medical encounter must be competent practice and mutual respect. Happily, this is precisely the experience of most doctors and most patients.

REFERENCES

Annas, G. (1988) She's going to die: the case of Angela C. *Hastings Cent. Rep.* **18**(1), 23–5.
Brazier, M. and Miola, J. (2000) Bye-Bye *Bolam*: a medical litigation revolution? *Med. Law Review* **8**, 85–114.

[14] Public Accounts Committee, 13 June 2002.   [15] *The Times* 24 June 2002.

British Medical Association. (1998) *Human Genetics: Choice and Responsibility*. Oxford: Oxford Paperbacks, Oxford University Press.

(2001) *Consent, Rights and Choices in Health Care for Children and Young People*. London: BMJ Books.

Chief Medical Officer. (2003) *Making Amends*. London: Department of Health.

Department of Health. (2001a) *Reference Guide to Consent for Examination or Treatment*. London: Department of Health.

(2001b) *Seeking Consent: Working with Children*. London: Department of Health.

Elliston, S. (1996) If you know what's good for you: refusal of consent to medical treatment by children. In S. A. M. McLean, ed., *Contemporary Issues in Law, Medicine and Ethics*. Aldershot: Dartmouth, pp. 29–55.

Fallberg, L. H. and Borgenhammer, E. (1997) The Swedish no fault patient insurance scheme. *Eur. J. Health Law* **4**, 279–86.

Gallagher, J. (1987) Prenatal invasions and interventions: what's wrong with fetal rights. *Harv. Women's Law J.* **10**(9), 359–61.

General Medical Council. (1999) *Seeking Patients' Consent: the Ethical Considerations*. London: General Medical Council.

Harpwood, V. (1996) *Legal Issues in Obstetrics*. Aldershot, Dartmouth.

Kolder, V. E. B., Gallagher, J., Parsons, M. T. (1987) Court-ordered obstetrical interventions. *N. Engl. J. Med.* **316**, 1192.

Law Commission. (1974), *Report on Injuries to Unborn Children*, Report No. 60. London: HMSO.

(1995) *Mental Incapacity*, Report No. 231. London: HMSO.

McLean, S. A. M. (1989) *A Patient's Right to Know: Information Disclosure, the Doctor and the Law*. Aldershot: Dartmouth.

(1999) *Old Law New Medicine*. London: Pandora.

Maclean, A. (2002) Beyond *Bolam* and *Bolitho*. *Med. Law Int.* **5**, 205–30.

McCullough, L. B. and Chervenak, F. A. (1994) *Ethics in Obstetrics and Gynaecology*. Oxford: Oxford University Press.

Mair, J. (1996) Maternal/foetal conflict: defined or defused? In S. A. M. McLean, ed., *Contemporary Issues in Law, Medicine and Ethics*. Aldershot: Dartmouth pp. 79–97.

Marteau, T. M. (1995) Towards informed decisions about prenatal testing: a review, *Prenat. Diagn.* **15**, 1215–26.

Mason, J. K., McCall Smith, R. A. and Laurie, G. T. (2002) *Law and Medical Ethics*, 6th edn. London: Butterworths.

Mattingly, S. (1992) The maternal-fetal dyad: exploring the two patient obstetric model. *Hastings Cent. Rep.* **22**, 13–18.

National Audit Office. (2001) *Handling Clinical Negligence Claims in England*. Report of the Comptroller and Auditor General, HC 403 Session 2000–2001.

Oliphant, K. (1996) Defining 'medical misadventure': lessons from New Zealand. *Med. Law Review* **4** (1), 1–31.

Polkinghorne Report. (1989) *Report on the Review of the Guidance on the Research Use of Foetuses and Foetal Material*. Cmd 762, London: HMSO.

Reid, S. (1999) Res ipsa loquitur: A chameleon in medical negligence cases *J. Law Med.* **7**, 75–86.

Robertson, J. and Shulman, J. (1987) Pregnancy and prenatal harm to offspring: the case of mothers with PKU. *Hastings Cent. Rep.* **17** (4), 23–33.

Ross Report. (2003) *Report of the Expert Advisory Group on Financial and Other Support.* Edinburgh: Scottish Executive.

Scottish Executive. (1999) *Making the Right Moves: Rights and Protection for Adults with Incapacity.* Edinburgh: HMSO.

(2002) *Code of Practice for Persons Authorised to Carry Out Medical Treatment or Research Under Part 5 of the Act*, SE/2002/73. Edinburgh: HMSO.

Scottish Law Commission. (1973) *Liability for Antenatal Injury*, Report No.30. Edinburgh: HMSO.

(1995) *Report on Incapable Adults*, Report No. 151. Edinburgh: HMSO.

Seymour, J. (2000) *Childbirth and the Law.* Oxford: Oxford University Press.

Solomon, R. I. (1991) Future fear: prenatal duties imposed by private parties. *Am. J. Law Med.* **17**, 411–34.

Teff, H. (1998) The standard of care in medical negligence – moving on from *Bolam*? *Oxf. J. Leg. Stud.* **18**, 473–84.

Warnock Report. (1984) *Committee of Inquiry into Human Fertilisation and Embryology.* Cmnd 9314, London: HMSO.

CASES

B v. An NHS Hospital Trust [2002] Lloyd's Reports Medical 265

Bagley v. North Hertfordshire Health Authority [1986] New Law Journal Reports 1014

Blyth v. Bloomsbury Health Authority [1993] 4 Medical Law Reports 151

Bolam v. Friern Hospital Management Committee [1957] 2 All England Law Reports 118, (1957) 1 Butterworths Medico-Legal Reports 1, (1957) I Weekly Law Reports 582

Bolitho v. City and Hackney Health Authority [1997] 4 All England Law Reports 771, (1997) 39 Butterworths Medico-Legal Reports 1, [1998] Appeal Case 232, HL

Burton v. Islington Health Authority, de Martell v. Merton and Sutton Health Authority [1992] 3 All England Law Reports 833, (1992) 9 Butterworths Medico-Legal Reports 69

Cassidy v. Ministry of Health [1951] 2 King's Bench Division 343

Chatterton v. Gerson [1981] Queen's Bench Division 432, [1981] 1 All England Law Reports 257

Corley v. North West Herefordshire HA [1997] 8 Medical Law Reports 45

Crawford v. Board of Governors, Charing Cross Hospital, (1953) The Times, 8th December

DeFreitas v. O'Brien [1995] 6 Medical Law Reports 108

Devaney v. Greater Glasgow Health Board (1987) Greens Weekly Digest 6–96

Devi v. West Midland Regional Health Authority [1981] CA Transcript 491

Donoghue or M'Alister v. Stevenson [1932] Appeal Cases 562

Gillick v. West Norfolk and Wisbech Area Health Authority [1985] 3 All England Law Reports 402, HL

Gordon v. Wilson (1992) Scots Law Times 849*Halushka v. University of Saskatchewan* (1965) 53 Dominion Law Reports (Canada) (2d) 436

Hamilton v. Fife Health Board (1993) 13 Butterworths Medico-Legal Reports 156

Hussain v. Houston (1995) Scots Law Times 1060

Hotson v. East Berkshire Area Health Authority [1987] Appeal Cases 750, [1987] 2 All England Law Reports 909 (HL)

Hunter v. Hanley (1955) Scottish Cases 200, (1955) Scots Law Times 213

In re AC (1990)573 A 2d 1235 (District of Columbia Appeals Court)

In re Madyyun (1986)114 Daily Washington Law Reporter 2233 (Washington DC Supreme Court)

Jefferson v. Griffin Spalding County Hospital 274 SE 2d 457 (Georgia 1981)

Kay's Tutor v. Ayrshire & Arran Health Board [1987] Queen's Bench Division 730, [1988] 1 All England Law Reports 871,

Lybert v. Warrington Health Authority [1996] 7 Medical Law Reports 71

McFall v. Shimp 10 Pa D & C 3d 90 (Pennsylvania1978)

McFarlane v. Tayside Health Board [1999] 4 All England Law Reports 961, [2000] 2 Appeal Cases 59, HL

McGhee v. National Coal Board (1973) Scottish Cases 37, (1973) Scots Law Times 14, HL

McKay v. Essex Area Health Authority [1982] Queen's Bench Division 1166, [1982] 2 All England Law Reports 771, CA

McWilliams v. Lord Advocate (1992) Scots Law Times 1045

Mahon v. Osborne [1939] 2 King's Bench Division 14, [1939] 1 All England Law Reports 535, CA

Malette v. Shulman (1990) 67 Dominion Law Reports (Canada) 321

Marshall v. Curry [1933] 3 Dominion Law Reports (Canada) 260

Maynard v. West Midlands Regional Health Authority [1985] 1 All England Law Reports 635

Moyes v. Lothian Health Board (1990) Scots Law Times 444

Murray v. McMurchy [1949] 2 Dominion Law Reports (Canada) 442

Newell and Newell v. Goldenberg [1995] 6 Medical Law Reports 371

Norfolk and Norwich Healthcare (NHS) Trust v. W (1996) 34 Butterworths Medico-Legal Reports 16

Parkinson v. Seacroft University Hospitals NHS Trust [2001] 3 All England Law Reports 97, (2001) 61 Butterworths Medico-Legal Reports 100, CA

Paton v. British Pregnancy Advisory Service [1979] 1 Queen's Bench Division 276

Pearce v. United Bristol Healthcare NHS Trust (1998) 48 Butterworths Medico-Legal Reports 118, CA

Re A (mental patient: sterilisation) (2000) 53 Butterworths Medico-Legal Reports 66

Re C (adult: refusal of treatment) [1994] 1 All England Law Reports 819

Re D (a minor) v. Berkshire County Council [1987] 1 All England Law Reports 20

Re F (mental patient: sterilisation) [1990] 2 Appeal Cases 1

Re F (in utero) [1988] 2 All England Law Reports 193

Re MB [1997] 8 Medical Law Reports 217

Re P (a minor) [1986] 1 Family Law Reports 272

Re R (1992) 7 Butterworths Medico-Legal Reports 147

Re S (1992) 9 Butterworths Medico-Legal Reports 69

Re T (adult) (refusal of medical treatment) [1992] 4 All England Law Reports 649

Re W (a minor) (medical treatment) [1992] 4 All England Law Reports 627

Rees v. Darlington Memorial Hospital NHS Trust [2003] United Kingdom House of Lords 52, CA

St George's Healthcare NHS Trust v. S [1998] 3 All England Law Reports 6

Schloendorff v. Society of New York Hospital 105 NE 92 (New York, 1914)

Sidaway v. Board of Governors, Bethlem and Royal Maudsley Hospital [1985] 1 Appeal Cases 871, [1985] 1 All England Law Reports 643

Smith v. Tunbridge Wells Health Authority [1994] 5 Medical Law Reports 334

Taft v. Taft 446 NE 395 (Massachusetts 1983)

Tameside and Glossop Acute Services Trust v. CH (1996) 31 Butterworths Medico-Legal Reports 93

Whitehouse v. Jordan [1981] 1 All England Law Reports 267

Wilsher v. Essex Area Health Authority [1986] 3 All England Law Reports 801, CA

X v. Austria (1980) 18 DR 154

14

Treating the preterm infant – the legal context

Sarah Elliston

University of Glasgow

Introduction

The delivery of a preterm infant can produce some of the most difficult practical challenges in obstetric and paediatric practice, amply illustrated by other chapters in this book. However, these practical challenges must at the same time proceed with consideration for the perhaps even greater challenge of deciding whether what can be done, should be done. Ordinarily, as explained in the previous chapter, decisions about acceptable medical care are expected to be taken in partnership between patients and their healthcare team, with patients setting limits on the care that they would find acceptable and that which they do not feel would be appropriate for them. Where decisions must be made on behalf of others, in this case premature babies, deciding what interventions should be attempted and when treatment should be discontinued needs the utmost care and transparency, since we cannot appeal to respecting the autonomous wishes of the individual as the touchstone for commencing or ceasing treatment.

When making such decisions, there is an inevitable tension between the desire to do everything possible to save the life of a vulnerable new person and the equally strong desire to avoid causing pain and distress or allowing suffering to continue without prospect of improvement. The way in which these sometimes opposing convictions are resolved is through attempting to weigh up the relative burdens and benefits of treatment to the child and reaching a conclusion on what course of action will cause the child the greatest benefit or the least harm. Doing so will often involve an assessment of the utility, or put another way the futility, of treatment and the likely prognosis for the child, often termed a quality of life judgement. All of these terms, and the meanings that they bear, have been the subject of much debate and disagreement and there is an unavoidable degree of imprecision in their application, since one person's view on the expected benefit or harm from treatment may differ markedly from another's. Nevertheless, that is not

Preterm Labour Managing Risk in Clinical Practice, eds. Jane Norman and Ian Greer. Published by Cambridge University Press. © Cambridge University Press 2005.

to say that these concepts have no value. The way in which they have been approached by the courts and by professional organisations gives broad guidance on how these kinds of decisions should be approached even if it cannot give a precise formula by which to arrive at a universally accepted answer in each case.

The fact that there is scope for a genuine difference of opinion based upon the differing weight given to predicted benefits and harms of treatment, and indeed in deciding what is a benefit or a harm in the circumstances, also makes it important to consider who has the authority to make this assessment. Unlike competent adults, children automatically have proxy decision-makers in the form of their parents so it is plausible to suggest that parents should have the first and the last word on treatment for their babies. Parents, it may be assumed, are in the best position to judge what is right for their child and their family will be most intimately concerned with the effects of any decision made. However, matters are rarely so simple, as one commentator notes:

> Some have argued that parents should have the right to make medical decisions on behalf of their children since they must live with the consequences of the decision. But, it has also been pointed out that having to live with the consequences is also an excellent basis for arguing that parents should not have the right to decide; i.e. there is a conflict of interest. (Bartholomew 1981: 272)

While it would be far from accurate to suggest that a conflict of interest is an inevitable or even a common concern, it does recognise that there may be circumstances where a degree of detachment might be necessary, whether provided by those professionally caring for the child or, as a last resort, provided by a court, which will be the ultimate decision-maker where there is disagreement on what the best interests of the child require.

Finally, there is the consideration of whether it is right to consider only the needs and interests of the preterm infant when faced with the vexed and ever present question of scarce resources. In an ideal world it might be hoped that all people would have access to all treatment that might benefit them, provided these benefits outweighed any probable harm to them. The reality is that health carers must make decisions about how their time, skills and the available resources are shared between the people in their care. Some might suggest that the time and intensive care spent on nursing one very premature infant who is unlikely to survive more than a few weeks would be better spent elsewhere. This chapter cannot hope to address all of the complex and difficult questions raised by seeking a just distribution of resources, but a brief mention will be made of how such issues have been approached by the courts.

General legal principles for treatment

Once the child is born alive or resuscitated,[1] it is legally recognised as a separate patient who undoubtedly has rights and is owed duties, like any other patient. As with any other patient, it is normally necessary to have consent before treatment is given but clearly here consent must be sought from another source than the patient. The child's parents are the obvious people to have authority to give consent on behalf of their child and this natural expectation is supported by the common law and in the form of statutes that give people with parental responsibility legal rights to make such decisions. (See, for example, *Gillick v. West Norfolk and Wisbech Area Health Authority* (1985).)[2]

However, it is important to remember that not all people who we think of as being parents will have parental responsibility, and hence the legal authority, to give consent to treat the child. There are detailed provisions concerning who has parental responsibility and if there is any doubt advice should be sought. However, broadly speaking both parents have parental responsibilities and rights if they were married at the time of the child's conception, or birth, or at some time after the child's birth and these are not lost if they divorce. If the parents have never married, only the mother automatically has parental responsibilities and rights, although the father may acquire them in a number of ways (British Medical Association 2001, Chapters 2 and 3).[3] There have been concerns that the lack of parental rights of unmarried fathers may be in breach of the broad interpretation of rights in respect of family life under the European Convention on Human Rights[4] and the Government has announced an intention to introduce some changes to this situation.[5]

Consent need only be obtained from one parent in order to proceed with treatment. This is because consent has been described, perhaps rather unhappily, as a "flak jacket" which protects the health carer from legal action for proceeding to treat. Only one 'flak jacket' is needed so it is not necessary to have the consent of both parents (*Re W (a minor) (medical treatment)* (1992), per Lord Donaldson). Nevertheless, if there is serious disagreement between parents, which cannot be

---

[1] The position where a child is not delivered alive will be dealt with later.

[2] The relevant statutory provisions are the Children Act 1989 s3 (1); the Children (Northern Ireland) Order 1995 Art 6 (1) and the Children (Scotland) Act s1 (1).

[3] This book provides useful professional guidance on legal and ethical aspects of treating children in a wide variety of situations.

[4] Convention for the Protection of Human Rights and Fundamental Freedoms (4. ix. 1950; TS 71; Cmd 8969). The enactment of the Human Rights Act 1998 allows the rights contained in the Convention to be used in British courts. For more detailed discussion of the operation and effect of this legislation see British Medical Association (2000).

[5] Others may also acquire parental responsibilities, such as local authorities. For further guidance see British Medical Association (2001, Chapters 2 and 3).

resolved, they may seek to involve the courts and it would be prudent to seek legal advice.

While parents have the right to make treatment decisions for their child it would be wrong to think of this as representing an absolute power over the child. The recognition of parental rights over their children is instead designed to allow parents to carry out their parental responsibilities toward them and, as such, it must be exercised in accordance with the general principle of acting in the child's best interests.

In order to be able to make a proper decision on behalf of their child, parents must feel able to give or withhold their consent freely and should be given sufficient information to enable them to consider the issues properly. The kind of information that parents should be given includes the benefits and risks of the proposed treatment; what the treatment will involve for the child; the implications of the child not having the treatment; what alternatives may be available; and the practical effects on the child and the family of having, or not having, the treatment. (See Department of Health (2001b): 14 and, for general issues on consent, Department of Health (2001a)). Recent research also emphasises that parents have a need for truthful and accurate information on a poor prognosis and that attempts to avoid distressing parents by withholding painful information may have the opposite effect. The way that such information is presented obviously requires care and sensitivity, but failure to give parents sufficient information on the likely prospects for the child, and particularly the effects of the child's treatment or condition, can be perceived as cruel and disempowering rather than kind (McHaffie 2001; McHaffie *et al.* 2001). Furthermore, it has recently been held in the case of *Glass v. UK* (2004) that parents normally have a right to be involved in decision-making about their child, especially in the case of withholding and withdrawing medical treatment. They have the authority to act on their children's behalf to defend their interests, including safeguarding the child's and their own Article 8 rights to respect for private and family life, under the European Convention on Human Rights and Fundamental Freedoms (ECHR). Where doctors propose to adopt a course of action that is against the wishes of parents, they should seek a court order to authorise them to do so, unless the situation is a true emergency. (The *Glass* case will be discussed in more detail later in this Chapter.) Clearly, in almost all cases this will require information to be provided to parents about the condition of the child and the available options.

The legal principles of consent have been discussed in the previous chapter. However, it will be obvious that in the situation of delivery of a premature child, decisions may need to be made quickly once the child is born and in these circumstances there may be little time to discuss treatment with parents or to give them the opportunity to reflect upon the interventions that may be thought necessary. It may also be unclear what the condition of the child is until it can be stabilised, and hence any judgements about the best treatment for the child may be made on incomplete evidence. Where it is anticipated that the child may be born prematurely, it would be advisable to have discussions with parents to seek their views about treating the child, much as the drawing up of a birth plan is encouraged. It is of course not possible to foresee everything that might happen, but seeking parents' views before an emergency situation is in progress does at least allow options to be canvassed in a calmer atmosphere. It also gives the healthcare team advance notice if there are any procedures that are likely to be objected to or any circumstances in which the parents would not wish treatment to proceed. If the healthcare team would feel unable to comply with these wishes (whilst confrontation should be avoided since these possibilities may never in fact arise), the reasons for objections can be explored and procedures set up for seeking legal advice if it does become necessary. As noted earlier, the *Glass v. UK* (2004) case considered that a hospital must normally seek court authorisation to proceed with a course of treatment against the wishes of an incompetent child's parents.

Where advance consideration is not possible, and it is believed treatment is urgently required, health carers may be able to rely upon the doctrine of necessity in treating the child even without valid consent from parents. This doctrine allows treatment immediately necessary to save life or to prevent deterioration in the condition of an incompetent patient (*Re F (mental patient: sterilisation)* (1990)). It would allow treatment to proceed in a crisis situation, where there is no time for adequate explanation and giving of consent by parents or where, exceptionally, parents are in no condition to give a valid consent. An example of the latter given by the Department of Health might be where parents of a seriously ill child are not able to properly consider the information they are given because of extreme distress (Department of Health 2001b:17). Nevertheless, this doctrine should be appealed to sparingly, since parents should ordinarily be as fully informed as possible and authorise treatment to be given. As soon as the situation enables it, parents should be asked for their permission to continue with treatment.

Where parents and the healthcare team are in agreement over the best course of action for the child, there is rarely, if ever, any need to involve the legal system. Even so, they are not at liberty to reach any decision they like and must still act in accordance with the law and with good clinical practice. There are limitations on what may be consented to and what may be done to a child set by the criminal law.

Criminal law limitations

The first and perhaps obvious restriction on consent is that premature infants are protected under the criminal laws that prohibit murder and manslaughter (or culpable homicide in Scotland). The entitlement of people to have their lives protected is reinforced by Article 2 of the European Convention on Human Rights. This is so regardless of the child's age of gestation or of its condition and prognosis. The most famous criminal prosecution in connection with the death of an infant is that of Dr Leonard Arthur in the early 1980s (*R v. Arthur* (1981)). This case concerned the parents' wish that their newborn baby, a boy born with Down's syndrome, should not survive. Dr Arthur therefore instructed that the child be given "nursing care only" and prescribed an appetite suppressant.[6] The child was removed to a separate ward where he was given water but not fed and he died three days later. Dr Arthur was subsequently arrested and charged with murder. The charge was later reduced to attempted murder when the post-mortem examination showed that the baby had a number of congenital defects which had not been known but which could have caused the child's death.

In summing up to the jury, the judge Mr Justice Farquharson said:

However serious a case may be; however much the disadvantage of a mongol, or indeed, any other handicapped child, no doctor has the right to kill it.

There is no special law in this country that places doctors in a separate category and gives them extra protection over the rest of us. It is undoubtedly the case that doctors are, of course, the only profession who have to deal with these terrible problems. But notwithstanding that they are given no special power ... to commit an act which causes death, which is another way of saying killing. Neither in law is there any special power, facility or licence to kill children who are handicapped or seriously disadvantaged in an irreversible way. (*R v. Arthur* (1981) at p. 5).

Subsequent cases have also been unequivocal that doctors have no right to accelerate the death of patients, even terminally ill ones (*R v. Cox* (1992). (See also *Airedale NHS Trust v. Bland* (1993) and *Re J (a minor) (wardship: medical treatment* (1990).) There is therefore no legal basis, even if it were wished to do so, to deliberately take steps to end a premature infant's life. Despite the apparent invisibility of other professionals' involvement in the eyes of the judge, it would have been possible to charge the nursing staff who carried out Dr Arthur's instructions as parties to the crime, although this never happened. Possibly the same would also have been true for the parents, whose request set this tragic chain of events in progress.

Nevertheless, despite Dr Arthur's actions, the jury was able to acquit him on the basis of a distinction that was drawn between taking active steps to end the life of the child and failing to take steps to save it. In other words, it was based on the contention that setting up the circumstances in which the child died was an omission rather than an act, that he merely "allowed nature to take its course".

---

[6] This is also described as a sedative analgesic, dihydrocodeine (DF 118).

This is a somewhat curious contention since, as we shall see later, in law it is perfectly possible to found a prosecution on the basis of an omission where the person is under a legal duty to act. Parents are undoubtedly under such a legal duty and so are healthcare professionals for patients in their care (*R v. Gibbins and Proctor* (1918); *R v. Adomako* (1994)). However, in such cases it is crucial to decide what the nature and extent of the person's duty of care is. Farquharson J put it to the jury in this way, saying that the *Arthur* case:

> ... really revolves round the question of what is the duty of the doctor when prescribing treatment for a severely handicapped child suffering from a handicap of an irrevocable nature where parents do not wish the child to survive.

There may be some doubts about this formulation, since it might more properly be asked what the duty of a doctor is toward any patient in his or her care, bearing in mind that the wishes of the parent, while a factor, do not determine this issue. Nevertheless, Dr Arthur was able to provide evidence from a number of distinguished expert witnesses in his field that the practice of treating babies as he did, in accordance with parental wishes, was not regarded as being outwith the bounds of accepted professional practice. As such, it was difficult to prove that what he did was in breach of his duty of professional care, much less that it fell so far below accepted standards that he should be found criminally liable for it. While it cannot be said with certainty why the jury acquitted him, it seems likely that the statements of the judge were influential, such as this passage:

> I imagine you will think long and hard before concluding that doctors, of the eminence we have heard ... have evolved standards that amount to committing a crime. (*R v. Arthur* (1981) at p. 22).

There are several very uncomfortable ideas here. One is that it could ever have been accepted medical practice to leave babies with Down's syndrome to die simply because their parents did not want them to survive. The second, that if this was accepted medical practice, it would be upheld by the law. This suggests that it is professional practice that sets the standard of what is lawful rather than the courts. The third is that failing to provide nourishment to a child that it seems would have been perfectly capable of taking it, and where it would in the ordinary case be provided, could be regarded as allowing nature to take its course. The issue of withdrawing or withholding food and fluids will be addressed separately later (see p. 000). If it was considered acceptable practice then, as commentators have said, "it is unlikely that Dr Arthur's regime would be acceptable today and the case has lost any credibility as precedent". (Mason *et al.* 2002: para. 16.26).

Nevertheless, although the case may not now be precedent for what is considered acceptable professional practice in the treatment of infants, the distinction between actively killing and allowing to die is one that remains in the law today.

This can be seen, for example, in the fact that while it would be unlawful to give a lethal injection to a person in a permanent vegetative state intending to kill that person, it would be lawful to remove ventilation where this is believed to provide no benefit to the patient, even when it is certain that the patient will die as a result. In the latter case, the death would be said to be caused by the patient's underlying condition, not by cessation of ventilation, and the idea would be that one is not killing the patient but failing to prolong the patient's life (*Airedale NHS Trust v. Bland* (1993)). This case will be considered more fully when discussing the concept of futility, below). There are those who doubt the moral justification for drawing such a distinction, since the end result, the death of the patient, is the same in each case. It also raises particular problems in relation to withholding nutrition and hydration, which will be addressed separately later in this chapter. Despite this, the distinction now appears well established and unlikely to disappear in the near future. The notion of treating in accordance with what is regarded as good clinical practice also remains strong and continues to be highly influential with the courts, although there have been some signs, in clinical negligence cases at least, that the courts may be more willing to scrutinise the justification for professional practice rather than accepting it at face value. (See, for example, *Bolitho v. City and Hackney Health Authority* (1998); *Pearce v. United Bristol Healthcare NHS Trust* (1998).) The extent to which this apparent willingness to assess the basis of professional judgement will extend to areas outside clinical negligence is, however, uncertain.

Another distinction that the courts have drawn is between medical treatment that is intended to kill and that where, although death is foreseen, it is not intended. This concept is commonly referred to as the doctrine of double effect and also raises a number of difficulties in squaring it with traditional legal principles. Where the doctor's primary intention is to ease the patient's pain, the fact that treatment given for this may also have the effect of shortening the patient's life does not amount to murder. (See Devlin J's summation to the jury in *R v. Adams* (1957). See also *R v. Cox* (1992).) This doctrine was referred to in *Airedale NHS Trust v. Bland* (1993) by Lord Goff who said:

[It is] the established rule that a doctor may, when caring for a patient who is, for example, dying of cancer, lawfully administer painkilling drugs despite the fact that he knows that an incidental effect of that application will be to abbreviate the patient's life ... Such a decision may properly be made as part of the care of the living patient, in his best interests and, on this basis, the treatment will be lawful. (*Airedale NHS Trust v. Bland* (1993) BMLR 64 at 114. See also *Re J* (1991) per Lord Donaldson MR at p46C-D).

Again, this kind of approach is curious since generally we are taken in law to intend consequences that we foresee and may be held liable for them, even if the consequences are themselves unwanted or unintended. In the usual case, knowing that the consequence of our deliberate action would lead to the death of another, even if this death was unwanted or unintended, would suffice for a murder charge or at the least one of manslaughter or culpable homicide (*R v Woollin* (1999). See also the discussion in *Re A (children) (conjoined twins: surgical separation)* (2001)). Here, however, ordinary legal principles are ignored or at least departed from in the context of medical treatment. For this reason it appears that it is lawful to give palliative care to a premature baby, even if this treatment may shorten the child's life. Even so, the care that is given must be in accordance with acceptable medical practice and the intention must be to relieve pain and allow the child to die with dignity, not simply or even primarily to bring about the child's death.

As mentioned earlier, it is possible for health carers to face a criminal prosecution for gross negligence that causes serious harm to the patient although such prosecutions are extremely rare. As discussed, it depends upon there being found to be such a serious breach of care and such serious harm caused that the criminal law is regarded as a suitable means of dealing with the matter. The basis for a conviction was described in this way:

> . . . the jury might properly find gross negligence on proof of indifference to an obvious risk of injury to health or of actual foresight of the risk coupled with a determination nevertheless to run it or with an intention to avoid it but involving such a high degree of negligence in the attempted avoidance as the jury considered justified conviction or of inattention or failure to advert to a serious risk going beyond mere inadvertence in respect of an obvious and important matter which the defendant's duty demanded he should address. (*R v. Adomako* (1994) at p. 83).

This is a high standard to meet as befits the serious nature of a criminal conviction. It is therefore inapplicable to a carefully made decision about the care of an infant made on the basis of best available evidence.

Finally there is a statutory offence of child neglect in England and Wales under section 1 of the Children and Young Person's Act 1933 and child cruelty in Scotland, under s12 of the Children and Young Persons (Scotland) Act 1937. These are aimed at providing criminal sanctions against parents who neglect their children, for example, by failing to seek appropriate medical assistance. There has been some suggestion that the statutes might also be applicable to healthcare professionals who fail to provide appropriate treatment for children in their care although no such cases have been brought. (See Davies (1996): 292–3, although this is doubted by Kennedy and Grubb (2000): 2165.)

Best interests, benefits and burdens and quality of life

Within the limits set by the criminal law, however, there is still scope for disagreement over how the premature child should be treated. These disagreements can usually be resolved without the need for legal action but when cases have reached the courts the basic principles that ought to be applied have been the subjects of much debate.

It has already been said that parents are the ones who are primarily entrusted with the responsibility for making decisions on behalf of their children and that they must exercise this responsibility in the best interests of the child. Here we come to some of the principal difficulties in this area: how to decide what the best interests of the child require and the circumstances in which decisions made by parents can be challenged. Although, as the Royal College of Paediatrics and Child Health puts it, "Parents are almost always their children's first, best and fiercest advocates" (Royal College of Paediatrics and Child Health 2000: 9), there may be circumstances where the healthcare team responsible for the care of the child find themselves unable to agree with parents' decisions.

The first major case to reach the English courts was known as the Baby Alexandra case (*Re B (a minor) (wardship: medical treatment)* (1981)). Like the child in *R v. Arthur* (1981), the baby girl here had Down's syndrome. However, it was known that she had an intestinal blockage that could be corrected with surgery. This surgery would normally be undertaken but the parents refused to agree to it, believing that God had found "a way out" for their daughter. Hospital staff wishing to provide treatment sought the opinion of a court on whether they could proceed without parental consent.

The case was complicated by the fact that there was a difference of opinion even amongst the doctors as to whether the operation should be performed. The local authority was involved and the child was made a ward of court. The case was eventually decided in the Court of Appeal where Lord Justice Templeman set out the principles to be followed:

It is a decision which of course must be made in the light of the evidence and views expressed by the parents and the doctors, but at the end of the day it devolves on this court in this particular instance to decide *whether the life of this child is demonstrably going to be so awful that in effect the child must be condemned to die, or whether the life of this child is still so imponderable that it would be wrong for her to be condemned to die.* There may be cases, I know not, of severe proved damage where the future is so certain and where the life of the child is so bound to be full of pain and suffering that the court might be driven to a different conclusion, but in the present case the choice which lies before the court is this: whether to allow an operation to take place which may result in the child living for 20 or 30 years as a mongoloid or whether (and I think this brutally must be the result) to terminate the life of a mongoloid child because she also has an intestinal complaint. Faced with that choice I have no doubt that it is the duty of this court to decide that the child must live. [Emphasis added]. (*Re B (a minor) (wardship: medical treatment)* (1981) at p. 1424).

Given that the prognosis for this child was still so uncertain, the decision was therefore made to permit a willing doctor to proceed with the operation.

Subsequent cases also followed this approach, attempting to determine what the prognosis for the child would be with and without the treatment in question, taking into account the pain, discomfort and distress to the child that would be likely to result in each case (*Re C (a minor) (wardship: medical treatment)* (1989); *Re J (a minor) (wardship: medical treatment)* (1990)). As such the courts are involved in performing a balancing test of the relative benefits and burdens to the child of a particular course of action. This approach is sometimes described as making a judgement on the quality of life of the infant and as such risks placing a lower value upon the lives of those who may be in most need of protection, the young, the sick and those who cannot speak up for themselves. (See, for example, Gunn and Smith 1985).

Indeed, in a case following shortly after Baby Alexandra, the argument was made that it was inappropriate to make such judgements and that respect for the principle of the sanctity of life should mean an evaluation of the expected quality of the life of the child should never be undertaken (*Re J (a minor) (wardship: medical treatment)* (1990)). The child in this case was described by one of the judges as having suffered "every conceivable misfortune" (per Lord Donaldson MR at p. 932g). He had been born at 27 weeks and weighing 2lb. Having been ventilated for a month he was now able to breathe unassisted but had suffered a series of convulsions and episodes of apnoea and brain scans showed severe hydrocephalus. He was likely to be blind and deaf and to have spastic quadriplegia but, despite the brain damage, it seemed he was able to experience pain. It was thought improbable he would survive until teenage years. The hospital treating him had sought permission not to ventilate him if he stopped breathing again. At the court of first instance, this permission was granted, although it was agreed that other treatment such as the administration of antibiotics should be given. The Official Solicitor, appointed to represent the child's interests, appealed against this decision.

The first contention was that the court should uphold the principle of the sanctity of life and should never grant permission for the withholding of life-saving or life-prolonging medical treatment. The consequence of such an approach could be to require that all possible steps must be taken to attempt to save the life of an infant regardless of the likely outcome of treatment or prognosis for the child. The Court of Appeal rejected this approach. Lord Donaldson put it this way:

> There is without doubt a very strong presumption in favour of a course of action which will prolong life, but … it is not irrebuttable. As the court recognised in *Re B*, account has to be taken of the pain and suffering and quality of life which the child will experience if life is prolonged. Account has also to be taken of the pain and suffering involved in the proposed treatment itself. (Per Lord Donaldson MR at p. 938e and f).

The Official Solicitor's alternative contention was that, following the Baby Alexandra case, it would have to be demonstrated that this baby's life would be so demonstrably awful that he should be condemned to die. He suggested that this boy's existence could not be regarded as being so burdensome that it would be better not to treat him. Again the Court of Appeal upheld the view of the court of first instance which had applied a balancing test of the relative burdens and benefits of treatment. Of particular note was the distress that mechanical ventilation itself might cause the child, which seems to be the reason why, by contrast, the administration of antibiotics in this case was recommended to continue. Weighing these factors up the court concluded that the burdens of treatment, poor prognosis and the likely further deterioration that would accompany future respiratory failure outweighed any benefit to the child in prolonging his life by ventilating him. Therefore, they authorised the hospital not to ventilate him again if the situation arose.

Other cases too have sought to weigh the benefits and burdens of treatment for severely disabled infants. (See, for example, *Re C (a minor) (wardship: medical treatment)* (1989); *Re C (a minor)(medical treatment)* (1997).) So, in the case of a terminally ill child, it has been explained that the duty of health carers is not to provide all treatment that may be available, but to provide care and comfort in the dying process. This may of course raise additional questions, such as when a child with a short life-expectancy should be described as being terminally ill. However, the critical issue is not simply the imminence of dying; this is but one factor to be taken into account when deciding whether the possible invasiveness and distress of treatment is justified by the benefit it will provide to the child in the short and the longer term. The outcome for the child with or without the treatment is therefore a central issue that falls within in the concept of a "quality of life" judgement.

What the cases have sought to make clear is that it is not the value of the child's life to others that is at issue but the quality of life that the infant may be expected to have. Even formulated in this way, however, problems remain. How is one to judge the quality of life of another person? As the Royal College of Paediatrics and Child Health say, "many people with severe handicap describe a life of high quality and say they are happy to be living it". They continue:

Disabled children and adults may not view residual disability as negatively as some able bodied people do, provided adequate support is available. It is important that society does not devalue disabled people or those living with severe impairments. (Royal College of Paediatrics and Child Health 1997: para. 2.71).

The passage clearly recognises the dangers of people making decisions about the quality of life of disabled infants. This problem can be illustrated by the legal writer Glanville Williams who famously wrote:

If a wicked fairy told me that she was about to transform me into a Down's baby (or a Down's adult) and asked me whether in these circumstances I should prefer to die immediately, I should certainly answer yes. (Williams 1981: 1020).

This approach shows how important it is to distinguish what a person would want for him or herself from what is right for this particular child. This question cannot be answered from the perspective of what the decision-maker, with his or her own experiences, values and preferences would want. It also fails to take into account the fact that the child has not felt the loss of abilities or had an existence without the disabilities with which it is born.

One way of attempting to make a better evaluation of the right thing to do for an incompetent patient is to try to make a substituted judgement, in other words, to try to make a decision as you think the person in question would make it. This approach has been unpopular with the British courts in most contexts yet, surprisingly, it has found some favour with them in the context of making decisions about the treatment of babies and young children (*Re J (a minor) (wardship: medical treatment)* (1990)). This is doubly surprising, since it is in this context that the idea of a substituted judgement is most logically difficult to sustain.

The basis of a substituted judgement is that the decision-maker tries to don the mantle of the person who is presently unable to make a decision about medical treatment. It is perhaps most applicable in the case of normally competent adults who become unable to make decisions, for example, through being in a permanent vegetative state.[7] The decision-maker attempts to decide, based on evidence about the individual's known wishes, values and preferences, what decision s/he would make were s/he able to do so. As such it is generally speculative, since one cannot know that the decision made does represent what would have been decided. There is some evidence that prediction can be very flawed even where the person making the decision knows the person well, let alone where the decision-maker is a stranger such as a health carer or a judge. (See, for example, Cohen-Mansfield *et al.* 1991.)

In the context of a premature infant, the difficulty in making a substituted judgement would appear to be even more manifest. Here we have no evidence of past preferences or values to go on and the child has never known any existence other than the one it now has, nor has any concept of a future. For a decision-maker to imagine herself a premature infant, with whatever disabilities the child has, and to attempt to state what that child would decide if it were able to form a rational judgement on proposed treatment is no easy task.

Nevertheless, it was said by Lord Donaldson in *Re J* (1990) that:

where a ward of court suffered from physical disabilities so grave that his life would *from his point of view* be so intolerable if he were to continue living that he would choose to die if he were

---

[7] This approach is taken in the USA in relation to withdrawal of treatment from those in a permanent vegetative state, as in *Cruzan v. Director, Missouri Department of Health* (1990).

in a position to make a sound judgement, the court could direct that treatment without which death would ensue from natural causes need not be given to the ward to prolong his life, even though he was neither on the point of death nor dying. (Re J (a minor) (wardship: medical treatment) (1990) at p. 938) [emphasis added]

Despite the practical and, indeed, logical difficulties of the substituted judgement test in this type of situation it does have some merits over the traditional formulation of the best interests test in that it focuses attention on the perspective of the child, rather than that of others. It asks decision-makers to consider not what they would want in such a situation nor what the parents want but what, to the best of our abilities, we think that the child itself would want. There are clear limitations of this approach but it does help to emphasise who should be the focus of our enquiry. It also appears to be more in line with the approach favoured when considering human rights principles, focusing as they do on the individual as a bearer of rights. The development of the law since the passing of the Human Rights Act 1998 will be considered later (see p. 000). However, for the moment there remain further problems with making judgements on behalf of premature infants.

These may arise from the fact that there is rarely certainty in the prognosis for the child. Some infants of low birth weight seem to thrive better than others who may be in a better condition at delivery; some complications may not be apparent or develop until later while others may be completely unexpected. In addition, there may also be lack of consensus about the relative efficacy of treatments, especially since it can be difficult to gain agreement from parents to involve their babies in clinical trials. Given these practical problems, some practitioners may be more willing to attempt measures to treat very premature infants than others and there is likely to be variation in practice. These kinds of variations may cause distress to parents if they believe that their baby might have been treated more or less, depending on the circumstances. There are some national evidence based guidelines on best practice (such as the Royal College of Paediatrics and Child Health, Guidelines 1998). These are useful as a guide to what is normally expected and courts are likely to refer to them in the event that a treatment decision is challenged. Nevertheless, it must be remembered that guidelines are just that, and there may be good reasons for departing from them in individual cases, although this will need careful justification.

The courts have so far, however, refused to dictate to individual doctors how they should treat their patients, seeing this as being a matter for professional judgement. The Court of Appeal has said that it would not make an order to force a health carer to "adopt a course of treatment which in the bona fide clinical judgement of the practitioner concerned is contraindicated as not being in the best interests of the patient". (Re J (1992), per Lord Donaldson at p. 622h). There is, therefore, scope for a difference of professional opinion over what treatment is in the child's best interests and should be provided, as long as the professional does not fall below minimum acceptable standards.[8] This issue came to the fore in a case involving an older child, Jaimee Bowen (*R v. Cambridge District Health Authority* (1995)). The case achieved publicity chiefly because of an allegation of inappropriate rationing of health care. However, the hospital concerned claimed that it was not simply the question of the high cost of experimental treatment for the child's leukaemia that had led them to refuse to fund it, but that it was mainly due to the opinion of its doctors that the treatment was so unlikely to work that it would not be appropriate to attempt it. It was also based on their assessment of the likely side effects of treatment upon the child, although the child herself had not been consulted. The issue of resource allocation will be returned to later. However, for the moment, it is important to note that although the hospital was required to review its decision, at no stage was there any suggestion that the doctors should be compelled to provide treatment against their clinical judgement. After a donation of funds from a member of the public, the child was treated privately and survived for several months before succumbing to the cancer.

The Jaimee Bowen case does raise some difficult issues about whether parents should have the right to seek other opinions and transfer their child to other hospitals or other doctors who would be willing to treat their child differently. This difficulty is compounded because in none of the cases have the courts ordered that a particular treatment must be given or that it must be withheld. They have simply authorised a course of action to proceed. So there remains a possibility that if a doctor is authorised not to treat, but another doctor would be willing to do so, a parent could seek to have the child transferred to the care of the willing doctor. To date no case has been reported where a parent has tried to do this and has been challenged. It is worth noting here that it has recently been held that courts may be willing to order doctors or a hospital to transfer the care of the patient (*R v. GMC and others, ex parte Burke*, (2004). This case is discussed in more detail later. See also *Re S (hospital patient: court's jurisdiction* (1996)). It would perhaps be clearer if courts made orders stating that this or that treatment must or must not be given. However, to do so would be to fetter the discretion of clinicians to treat a child as they think appropriate if circumstances change and also, as explained above, it could be seen as ordering doctors to treat in a way incompatible with their clinical judgement. This the courts have so far not been prepared to do. If it came to a situation where the courts believed the welfare of the child required it, it would be possible for courts to issue a specific order that a child should not be treated in such a way, but this would be an unprecedented step.

---

[8] This is generally judged by professional practice (*Bolam v. Friern Hospital Management Committee* (1957)) although, as indicated earlier, there may be some signs that the courts may be more willing to make an independent assessment of the minimum level of care expected.

Futile treatment

This brings us to the separate but closely related issue of the concept of futile treatment. If treatment is described as futile, this may also be used as a justification for not starting or continuing treatment. However, there are various ways in which a treatment may be regarded as futile and the courts have taken a particular approach to this. One way in which a treatment may be thought of as futile is where it could not achieve its intended purpose in a narrow physiological sense. An example would be where an infection is resistant to an antibiotic. Administration of the antibiotic would be ineffective and so attempting this treatment would be futile. A second sense would be where, although the treatment may be physiologically effective, it would achieve no overall benefit to the patient. An example here might be where a patient can be resuscitated but his/her condition is so poor that s/he is likely to suffer repeated respiratory failure and there is no hope of improving his/her condition. In such a case, while the treatment itself can achieve its intended aim in a narrow sense, when the treatment is considered in terms of the overall benefit it will provide, it may be thought of as futile. It is generally this second, broader meaning of futility that the courts have employed when saying that futile treatment need not be provided.

The difference between the evaluation of futility and the considerations of the benefits and burdens to the child already discussed is that treatment may be regarded as futile even if it does not seem to be burdensome to the patient. For example, in the case of *Re J (a minor) (wardship: medical treatment)* (1990) discussed earlier, withdrawal of ventilation was authorised since it was held that the burden of this treatment in terms of the distress it might cause the child outweighed any benefit that the child might obtain. By contrast, the administration of antibiotics to control infection was not believed to be burdensome and hence it was recommended to continue. However, it might have been possible to argue that, although not burdensome to the child, the provision of antibiotics would be futile since it would not amount to any overall benefit for him.

Even though the term "futility" was not used in it, a case that illustrates this kind of approach is that of *Re C (a minor) (wardship: medical treatment)* (1989). It concerned a baby with severe hydrocephalus who was believed to be dying. The paediatrician caring for her gave evidence that in his opinion the objective of treatment should be to ease suffering rather than attempt to prolong life. At first instance the judge made an order stating that the hospital should be at liberty to treat the baby to die; to give treatment to relieve her from pain, suffering and distress but that it should not be necessary to prescribe and administer antibiotics for serious infection nor to set up means of artificial feeding. Although the Court of Appeal changed the wording of the order so that the words to treat her "to die" were replaced with "to allow her life to come to an end peacefully and with dignity", the rest of this part of the order stood.

Indeed, there have even been some judicial statements that suggest that giving futile treatment might be regarded as being an assault, since the justification for giving treatment to people who cannot consent to it themselves is that it is for their benefit. (*Airedale NHS Trust v. Bland* (1993)). If there is no benefit to be gained from treatment, the justification for giving it is absent. A possible concern with this is that it seems to shift the burden of justification from those who wish to withhold or withdraw treatment to those who wish to provide it, which would strike many as being contrary to the normal expectation that the first duty of health carers is to seek to treat. However, the important point is whether there is likely to be a benefit to the individual, since, as has been discussed, the duty to treat is not an absolute one but is to treat in a manner that is beneficial to the patient. Even so, the difficulties that arise will be obvious. We are once more faced with the problem of the certainty of diagnosis and prognosis and with the judgement of the extent to which providing treatment will result in a benefit or harm to the child.

Making this judgement in the case of so called futile treatment is likely to be particularly controversial given that if the treatment may not itself be considered harmful, the main issue may in fact be whether the child's continued survival is believed to be a benefit or a harm to it. There are those who suggest that unless the child is in the process of dying, continued survival is always on balance a benefit to the child so that if treatment is not burdensome it should always be given. (See, for example, Davis (1994).) Others disagree and suggest that quality of life considerations can permit life-saving or life-prolonging treatment to be withheld, even if the treatment would not itself be unduly burdensome (such as Harris (1994)). With the acceptance of the withholding of ventilation and other forms of treatment from patients in a permanent vegetative state, who by definition cannot be aware of any burden of treatment, and who might survive for many years if such treatment was continued, the courts appear to have accepted the latter approach. This has also been endorsed in professional guidance issued by the Royal College of Paediatrics and Child Health that will be discussed later (see p. 000). Nevertheless, such judgements need the utmost caution, since, as has been shown, there are serious dangers and difficulties in judging the actual and future quality of life of a premature infant.

Parental disagreement with professional opinion

Despite the fact that the assessment of the benefits and burdens of treatment involves more than an assessment of the clinical benefits of treatment, in the cases that have been reported it is clear that medical opinion weighs heavily with the courts. In fact there is only one reported case in which the courts have upheld parents' wishes against strong medical opinion (*Re T (a minor) (wardship: medical treatment)* (1997). This case involved an infant rather than a baby. He had been born with bilary atresia and had undergone surgery that had not proved effective. However, the consensus of medical opinion was that the boy would be a suitable candidate for a liver transplant. His parents would not agree to this and the courts became involved. At first instance the hospital was authorised to proceed with a transplant as soon as a donor became available. The Court of Appeal overturned this judgment, holding that insufficient weight had been given to parental objections, which included their concern over the risks of the surgery and its effects in terms of pain and distress for their son as opposed to the likely long-term prognosis. The court also emphasised the need for the parents to be committed to providing the post-operative care the child would need. One of the judges in this case counselled caution when courts considered whether to override parental decisions about their children. He stated that:

> ... the greater the scope for genuine debate between one view and another, the stronger will be the inclination of the court to be influenced by a reflection that in the last analysis the best interests of every child include the expectation that difficult decisions affecting the length and quality of its life will be taken for it by the parent to whom its care has been entrusted by nature. (*Re T (a minor) (wardship: medical treatment)* (1997) per Waite LJ at pp. 253–4).

Given the parents' views, the Court held that it would not be in the interests of the child to undergo surgery.

This case may be regarded as exceptional, turning on an unusual set of facts. The parents lived abroad and would have had to return to England or live apart for the duration of the child's treatment. Another factor was that both parents were themselves healthcare professionals, so the suspicion is that this may have given their views more status than would ordinarily be accorded to parents. It will be remembered that the courts have not previously placed such significance on the need for parents to be committed to the aftercare of their child. However, this unusual case apart, generally medical opinion will be decisive, regardless of parental wishes. To some, the usual preference given to medical opinion represents no more than an acknowledgement that parents will be less knowledgeable about the conditions that the child is born with than practitioners. This may be especially so in the case of neonates, where most parents will have little experience of what the prognosis for the child will really mean. So it has been said that in the vast majority of cases parents

> have no yardstick by which to judge the child's quality of life ... It is only the neonatologist who can base his or her prognosis on experience, and only the neonatologists know their limitations. (Mason 1999: 282).

To others, it provides yet another example of the courts being too ready to agree with professional opinion. It is undoubtedly true that most parents are likely to have little or no experience of caring for a premature baby or a severely disabled child, unlike those who do so as professionals. However, it can be forcefully argued that there is nothing particular in the training or experience of healthcare professionals that makes them better judges of the balance of benefits and burdens for a child of being given certain treatments or of the desirability of living life in a particular condition or for a certain length of time. It must also be said that the experience of caring for a child on a short-term professional basis may be a world away from caring for a child as a member of a family. Nevertheless, the courts have not drawn a sharp distinction between professionals as experts on what is possible and experts on what is desirable and there seems little sign of this changing at present. It should be noted that even though *Glass v. UK* (2004) held that the hospital should have sought a court order before commencing a course of treatment objected to by a parent, it did not say that the parent's wishes should have been complied with. This was a matter that the UK court should have been given the opportunity to rule on. The ECHR also refused to criticise the actual decision reached by the hospital, as it was 'not its function to question the doctors' clinical judgment as regards the seriousness of the [child's condition or the appropriateness of the treatment they proposed' (*Glass v. UK* (2004): para. 87). However, deciding what properly comes within the scope of clinical judgement may not, as we have seen, always prove an easy matter.

Professional guidance

Professional organisations have understandably sought to follow the legal approach, which leads to a certain circularity, given the courts' reliance on professional opinion. Nevertheless, such organisations have sought to give practical guidance on seeking and obtaining consent from parents, how to attempt to resolve disagreement and how the issues raised by ceasing further treatment should be addressed. (See, for example, British Medical Association (1999), (2001); Department of Health (2001b); General Medical Council (2002).) Particularly interesting is the guidance issued by the Royal College of Paediatrics and Child Health. This describes five situations in which it believes it may be appropriate not to provide life-prolonging treatment (Royal College of Paediatrics and Child Health 1997: 7). The first two (that of the brain-dead child and the child in a permanent vegetative state) are unlikely to be at issue in neonatal care. More relevant are the remaining three, described as follows:

The "no chance" situation. The child has such severe disease that life-sustaining treatment simply delays death without significant alleviation of suffering.

The 'no purpose' situation. Although the patient may be able to survive with treatment, the degree of physical or mental impairment will be so great that it is unreasonable to expect them [sic] to bear it. The child in this situation will never be capable of taking part in decisions regarding treatment or its withdrawal.

The "unbearable" situation. The child and/or family feel that in the face of progressive and irreversible illness further treatment is more than can be borne. They wish to have a particular treatment withdrawn or to refuse further treatment irrespective of the medical opinion on its potential benefit.

The "no chance" and "no purpose" situations may be seen as broadly equating with the notion of futility and best interests accepted by the courts. The "unbearable" situation is rather more controversial. While it might be regarded as wholly appropriate to allow a child who is properly able to do so to make a judgement for him or herself on what is unbearable, as we have seen the courts have generally not permitted parental opinion to prevail when faced with medical opinion on the benefit of treatment for children unable to express themselves.

The guidance advocates a consensus approach, both within the healthcare team and also between them and the parents. It does, however, clearly place priority on the relative experience of professional practice of the individual team members and places the final responsibility with the consultant in charge of the child's care (Royal College of Paediatrics and Child Health 1997: 23). The need for independent second opinions and, in the last resort, the opinion of a court to resolve disagreement is also considered. These guidelines were quoted with approval in *Re C (a minor) (medical treatment)* (1997) where artificial ventilation and non-resuscitation of a 16 month infant with spinal muscular atrophy, type 1, was authorised. Here, despite the views of the parents, the court agreed with the evidence given by paediatric neurologists that the child was in a "no chance" situation and that ventilation in the event of future respiratory arrest would not be in the child's best interests (*Re C (a minor) (medical treatment)* (1997)).

Finally, it might be suggested that if a decision has been made that further treatment is not in the best interests of the child and that the child should be enabled to die with dignity, that a dignified death should be possible to achieve by providing some positive means of accelerating death, rather than by withdrawal or withholding of treatment. We have seen already that this is prohibited by the criminal law but it may be argued that there may be nothing inherently more dignified about dying as a result of untreated opportunistic infection than due to a lethal dose of sedative. Some commentators have attempted to draft legislation that would provide for neonaticide in specific circumstances (Kuhse and Singer 1985: 195). Against this approach, there is general recognition that, whatever the logical difficulties of distinguishing between allowing a child to die when it could be treated and giving a lethal injection, health carers and others do see a distinction. There has been little professional or political enthusiasm for introducing such measures and at present they remain largely a matter of academic consideration.

Nutrition and hydration

Up until now, the discussion has focused upon the provision of medical treatment. However, it may be particularly important in the situation of the premature infant to consider whether nutrition or hydration properly falls within the sphere of medical treatment, in which case it may be considered according to the same rules and principles as other medical treatment, or whether it is more appropriately described as basic care, in which case it may be argued that, along with providing adequate warmth and hygiene for the infant, it should never be withdrawn.

We have already seen that failing to feed an infant with Down's Syndrome has led to a prosecution for attempted murder, although this case resulted in an acquittal (*R v. Arthur* (1981)). The issue of nutrition has, however, been considered in a number of subsequent cases, although these have been civil cases generally concerning adults in a permanent vegetative state (PVS). Nevertheless, the approach that has been taken has relied on some principles that seem applicable to the premature infant. The general thrust of these cases has been to distinguish between the method of administration and to say that artificial nutrition and hydration should be regarded as medical treatment. Accordingly, where its administration is regarded as being futile (or unduly burdensome, where the patient is capable of experiencing this), it may be ceased.

Lord Goff in the case of Anthony Bland stated that he regarded tube-feeding as:

providing a form of life support analogous to that provided by a ventilator which artificially breathes air in and out of the lungs of a patient incapable of breathing normally, thereby enabling oxygen to reach the bloodstream. (*Airedale NHS Trust v. Bland* (1993) at p. 117).

This approach is not uncontroversial. A House of Lords Select Committee on Medical Ethics was set up after the Anthony Bland case and asked to consider a number of issues, including provision of nourishment to patients. Evidence given by a number of witnesses, in healthcare professions and outside them, diverged sharply on whether the provision of nutrition and hydration was something that properly came within the sphere of medical treatment or basic care (House of Lords Select Committee on Medical Ethics 1993–94). The Select Committee itself confessed it could not reach a conclusion on the matter and rather fudged the issue. It suggested that if other forms of care that were unquestionably medical treatment, such as the administration of antibiotics, were withdrawn, then the issue of withdrawal of food or fluids would be unlikely to arise, unless their administration was evidently burdensome to the patient (House of Lords Select

Committee on Medical Ethics 1993–94: para. 257). It may be that the most appropriate way of considering this issue is that suggested by Kennedy and Grubb:

The solution to the problem does not lie in the process of labelling the intervention as 'treatment' or 'care' or indeed anything else. Instead, the solution lies in reminding ourselves that the doctor's obligation is to act in the 'best interests' of the patient which [in some cases] means that the patient be allowed to die. (Kennedy and Grubb 2000: 2144).

Nevertheless, despite its possible lack of logic, it would seem that failing to feed a child who is capable of being fed by mouth, through the normal swallowing mechanism, would not be considered acceptable whereas failing to commence or ceasing so called artificial nutrition and hydration may be. The former would not be considered to be medical treatment while the latter would. The approach of the courts, therefore, requires an assessment of the overall benefit to the patient and suggests that any life-prolonging medical treatment, which may include artificial nutrition and hydration, that is of no benefit to the infant may be withdrawn. The British Medical Association suggests that additional safeguards are required for decisions of this kind such as a second opinion from a senior clinician unconnected with the treatment of the patient; details of cases where artificial nutrition and hydration has been withdrawn being made available for clinical audit; and that where the patient is in PVS or a state closely resembling PVS legal advice should be sought (British Medical Association 1999: 57–9). According to these guidelines, it would therefore seem crucial to consider any distressing effects that withdrawal of nutrition or hydration will have for the child, since this will form part of the assessment of the burdens and benefit to the infant. This area is given added significance with the consideration of human rights principles, such as the absolute prohibition on torture, inhuman and degrading treatment, under Article 3 of the ECHR. However, similar professional guidelines have recently been challenged in the case of *R v. GMC and others ex parte Burke* (2004). This case involved an adult suffering from a progressively degenerative disease that would eventually require him to receive artificial nutrition and hydration. He objected to the General Medical Council (GMC) guidelines, which he feared would allow artificial nutrition and hydration to be removed without his consent. The court was critical of some of the passages in the GMC guidelines, particularly those concerning the withdrawal of artificial nutrition and hydration from patients who were not dying.

Where the patient is sentient, the court stated that the proper approach to be applied was as follows:

If ANH is providing some benefit it should be provided unless the patient's life, if thus prolonged, would from the patient's point of view be intolerable. (*R v. GMC and others, ex parte Burke* (2004): para. 179)

To the extent that the court stressed that 'intolerability' judged from the patient's perspective was central, this reflects the approach taken in the cases concerning severely disabled children, discussed at length earlier. However, the suggestion made in this case is that providing artificial nutrition and hydration to a person who is not in a coma or otherwise insensate is not likely to be deemed to be intolerable, whereas dying of lack of nutrition or hydration may well be, and consequently would be a breach of Article 3 of the ECHR. The court did not explicitly address the situation of neonates but this appears implicitly to apply to them as much as it does to adults, although the mental distress felt might not be comparable to that which Mr Burke claimed he would suffer, knowing that artificial nutrition and hydration was being removed against his wishes. In the case of incompetent patients, the test remains whether treatment is in the patient's best interests but this is to be judged by reference to the question of the intolerability of the treatment from the patient's perspective.

However, in addition the court also held that:

Treatment is capable of being "degrading" within the meaning of Article 3, whether or not there is awareness on the part of the victim. However unconscious or unaware of ill-treatment a particular patient may be, treatment which has the effect on those who witness it of degrading the individual may come within Article 3. It is enough if judged by the standard of right-thinking bystanders it would be viewed as humiliating or debasing the victim, showing a lack of respect for, or diminishing, his or her human dignity.

Even where the patient is unaware of the treatment or withdrawal of treatment, then, his or her human rights may be breached unless the course of action is judged to be in the patient's best interests, according to the approach set out by the court.

The court also stressed that it is a legal requirement, not simply a matter of best practice, to obtain a court order in a number of situations. The most relevant here are:

Where there is any dispute amongst clinicians as to condition and prognosis, the patient's best interests or the likely outcome of withdrawing or withholding artificial nutrition and hydration.

Where the patient (even if a child or incompetent) has resisted the proposed withdrawal of artificial nutrition or hydration.

Where there is any opposition from those with a reasonable claim to be heard as to a patient's best interest.

Significantly, where a clinician does not feel able to comply with requests for continued artificial nutrition and hydration the court held that doctors must be prepared to arrange for care to be taken over by doctors who are willing to provide it and the courts may be willing to issue orders to compel them to transfer patient care. It was held that the GMC guidelines were incompatible with ECHR rights on a number of points. The decision is controversial for several reasons, not all explored here, and the case is being appealed by the GMC.

Human rights principles

The implementation of the Human Rights Act 1998 has already begun to introduce new ways of discussing treatment issues. The focus of this legislation is to allow people in the UK to rely upon the articles of the European Convention on Human Rights in our own countries rather than having to have cases referred to the European Court of Human Rights in Strasbourg. There had been doubts whether withdrawal of life-prolonging treatment would be considered in breach of Convention Rights, in particular Article 2 (Everyone's right to life shall be protected by law) and Article 3 (No one shall be subjected to torture or to inhuman or degrading treatment or punishment.). The first UK case to discuss this issue concerned a child who had been delivered at 31 weeks' gestation when the mother developed pre-eclampsia (*A National Health Service Trust v. D and Ors* (2000)). The baby subsequently required intubation and ventilation but developed ventilator-induced lung injury. Tests also showed that the baby had structural abnormalities in his brain, a range of serious disabilities including heart and kidney dysfunction, and a very short life-expectancy. His condition continued to deteriorate and when the child was a year and a half old, the paediatricians treating him felt it would not be in the child's best interests to subject him to resuscitation using artificial ventilation in the event of respiratory failure. The boy's parents opposed this, believing such a decision to be premature. The judge considered the evidence of the nature of the boy's condition and prognosis as well as the likely effects of treatment and authorised medical staff not to resuscitate. Despite the fact that the case was heard before the coming into force of the Human Rights Act 1998, the judge considered human rights principles and stated that there was a strong obligation in favour of taking all steps capable of preserving life, save in the most exceptional circumstances. Nevertheless, he concluded that failing to commence life-prolonging treatment (in this case resuscitation and artificial ventilation) would not be in breach of Article 2 if giving that treatment would not be in the patient's best interests.

Subsequent case law has expanded on this approach, holding that the obligation to protect life under Article 2 does not entail an absolute obligation to treat the patient if the treatment would be futile (*NHS Trust A v. M, NHS Trust B v. H* (2001)).

This effect of the implementation of the Human Rights Act 1998 has thus been explained by the British Medical Association as follows:

To the extent that best interests remain central to the decision-making process, this reflects an extension, rather than a change, of existing good practice. Since the introduction of the Human Rights Act, however, the way in which best interests are assessed and the factors taken into account in reaching those decisions are likely to be open to far greater scrutiny. Doctors must be able to show that the patient's right to life was specifically considered and, where treatment is not provided, to demonstrate legitimate grounds for not taking steps to enforce that right. (British Medical Association 2000).

In the cases so far discussed, Article 3 has also been used to assert a right to die with dignity (*A National Health Service Trust v D and Ors* (2000); *NHS Trust A v. M, NHS Trust B v. H* (2001)). Another case also illustrates this principle and the obligation to ensure that proper medical care is provided, although the circumstances are far removed from those of the premature infant (*D v. UK* (1997)). The case concerned a man who had lived most of his life in St Kitts. He came to the UK and being convicted of drug offences was imprisoned, where he developed HIV. On his release he was going to be deported to St Kitts but challenged this on the basis that he would not be able to receive adequate medical care there. The European Court on Human Rights held that deporting him would be in breach of Article 3 as this would expose him to a real risk of dying under most distressing circumstances which would amount to inhuman treatment.

It had been held that Article 3 requires the victim to be aware of the torture or inhuman and degrading treatment. An insensate patient is unaware that treatment is being provided and would be equally unaware of its withdrawal (*NHS Trust A v. M, NHS Trust B v. H* (2001)). However, this approach has been called into question by *R v. GMC and others, ex parte Burke* (2004) as discussed earlier. What can be said with certainty is that the ability of a premature infant to experience pain or suffering must always be taken into account when considering the treatment to be given, the consequences of withholding or withdrawing treatment and the appropriate care to be given to enable a terminally ill child to die with dignity.

As a corollary to this, it may also be possible for the inappropriate giving of medical treatment to be in breach of Article 3. In judging whether giving treatment breaches Article 3, the European Court of Human Rights has said:

> ... as a general rule, a measure which is a therapeutic necessity cannot be regarded as inhuman or degrading. The court must nevertheless satisfy itself that the medical necessity has been convincingly shown to exist. (*Herczegfalvy v. Austria* (1992) at para. 82).

Article 8 (Everyone has the right to respect for his private and family life) has already been briefly mentioned but it is worth reiterating that it requires family integrity to be protected. The European Court on Human Rights has held that parents have the right to be involved in significant decisions about their children and there can probably be no more significant decision than whether to allow a child to die without further treatment (*W v. UK* (1987)). The case of *Glass v. UK* (2004) has already been mentioned. It concerned disagreement between hospital staff and the family of a severely mentally and physically disabled boy. Hospital staff considered that the child was dying and should not be resuscitated in the event of respiratory collapse and proposed giving him diamorphine. This was vigorously opposed by the boy's mother but no court order was sought by the hospital to act against parental objections. Despite the regime adopted by the hospital the boy survived and notwithstanding the mother's complaints about medical staff's behaviour, no disciplinary action was taken by the GMC or any prosecution instituted. The mother claimed that her son's and her own right to respect for private and family life had been breached by these events and the case eventually reached the European Court of Human Rights. Here it was held that a failure by a hospital to seek permission of a court where it proposed a course of treatment opposed by the mother was indeed a breach of the parent's and the child's Article 8 rights under the ECHR, although this did not mean that the mother's views on treatment should have been determinative. Unlike Article 3, which is an absolute right, and Article 2, which has specified exemptions (for example, self-defence), Article 8 is a qualified right, which means that it may, in some circumstances, be legitimate to interfere with a person's right to respect for private and family life. There is a range of factors that may be taken into account such as national security but the most significant here is likely to be the protection of health and protection of the rights and freedoms of others. So, for example, as already discussed, parents do not have absolute rights to make decisions for their children. Children have their own human rights that must be protected. However, any interference must be limited to that which is necessary in a democratic society and that which is lawful to achieve the protection sought.

Other Convention rights may also in individual cases become important, such as the right to a fair trial (Article 6), freedom of thought, conscience and religion (Article 9), freedom of expression (Article 10) and the prohibition of discrimination (Article 14). In the context of medical treatment, so far the approach of the courts does not indicate a significant change since incompetent patient's best interests remains central. However, it will be necessary to demonstrate that the child's human rights, and those of the family, have been fully considered and that any decision made can be shown to be in accordance with these principles. The British Medical Association puts it this way:

> In addition to the range of questions considered in the past, there are two further questions to ask in each case:
>
> Are someone's human rights affected by the decision? And, if so,   Is it legitimate to interfere with them? (British Medical Association 2000).

Resuscitation at birth

As discussed in the previous chapter, for a child to be regarded as being a person in law it must have been born alive (*Paton v. British Pregnancy Advisory Service*

Trustees (1979); *In re F* (*In utero*) (1988); *Kelly v. Kelly* (1997)). Consequently, where a premature child is delivered but is not breathing nor has a beating heart it could be suggested that there is no duty to the child to attempt to resuscitate it, since the child is not recognised as a legal person. However, this argument depends upon how the law defines the child being "born alive". For the purposes of registration, a stillbirth is defined as:

> Where a child issues forth from its mother after the 24th week of pregnancy and which did not at any time after being completely expelled from its mother breathe or show any signs of life.[9]

All stillbirths must be registered.[10] If the fetus is delivered before the 24th week of pregnancy and shows no signs of life, there are no registration requirements (unless the fetus had been electively aborted). If the child does show any signs of life but subsequently dies, its birth and death must be registered.

The difficulty of course may be in establishing whether or not the baby breathed or showed any signs of life, since these terms are not further defined in legislation. There are examples of cases giving a variety of criteria for determining whether the fetus should be taken as being born alive, such as the need for independent circulation (*R v. Enoch* (1833)), that it had breathed (*R v. Handley* (1874)) or at least was able to breathe through its own lungs (*R v. Brain* (1834)). These cases are, however, extremely elderly. A more recent case considering them and the legislation on registration of births and deaths concluded that for a child to be regarded as "a person in being" it must be fully extruded from the woman's body and be

> breathing and living by reason of its breathing through its own lungs alone, without deriving any of its living or power of living by or through any connection with its mother. (*Rance v. Mid-Downs Health Authority* (1991) per Brooke J at p. 817).

This description was upheld in a prosecution for assault upon a pregnant woman that caused injuries to the fetus from which it subsequently died (*Attorney-General's Reference (No.3 of 1994)* (1997)). The definition is clearly problematic when the child under consideration is a premature infant who may be separated from the mother and who is yet to draw breath or is incapable of breathing without ventilatory support and the courts have not considered this precise situation in recent times. However, if a child is not regarded as being born alive, it seems there can be no duty owed to the baby itself to resuscitate it and failing to resuscitate could not be charged as murder, manslaughter or culpable homicide. In England and Wales there is a separate offence of child destruction under the Infant Life Preservation Act

---

[9] S41 Births and Deaths Registration Act 1953 Act, s12 of the Births and Deaths Registration Act 1926 and s56(1) of the Births, Deaths and Marriages (Scotland) Act, as amended by the Still-Birth (Definition) Act 1992.

[10] Registration of Births, Deaths and Marriages (Scotland) Act 1965; Births and Deaths Registration Act 1926 and Births and Deaths Registration Act 1953.

1929, where a person intending to destroy the life of a child capable of being born alive, by any wilful act causes a child to die before it has an existence independent of its mother. However, this may not be applicable either to the situation of the premature infant that has been delivered but is not yet breathing.

If the child is not regarded as being born alive, it seems likely that any legal duty to resuscitate would have to be founded upon the practitioners' duty of care toward the parents. While the nature and extent of such a duty may be difficult to define, there are good reasons for suggesting as a practical matter that the general rule should be that resuscitation should be attempted. When children are born prematurely their prognosis is likely to be uncertain and unless a trial of treatment is undertaken, commencing with resuscitation, there is no sensible way of determining whether this child will survive nor in what condition. While endorsing such an approach commentators have said:

The difficulty of such a rule is that, while resuscitation may be successful, the end result may be a severely handicapped survivor . . . (Mason *et al.* 2002: para. 16.86)

There may be cases that are clearer, where it is plain that the gestational development of the child has been interrupted too early for it to be able to be supported until it can sustain its own life. More likely, however, is that an assessment of whether resuscitation is appropriate will need to be made in accordance with the general principles already discussed, including the views of the parents and professional judgement. There is some limited legal support for this approach in the form of two unreported Scottish Fatal Accident Inquiries, where in both cases the decision of health carers not to attempt to resuscitate was declared to be a reasonable clinical decision, and by implication one that the clinician was entitled to make in the exercise of professional judgement. (See the discussion in Mason *et al.* (2002): paras. 16.86–16.87.) If this approach is followed, account will now also need to be taken of human rights principles although only a live person can presently have interests or rights.

Resource allocation

The final issue to be considered here is that of just resource allocation. While the discussion so far has centred upon the rights and interests of the premature infant, it cannot be forgotten that health carers will be concerned with the rights and interests of many patients and families and also have a role to play in the just allocation of healthcare resources. While this latter obligation may be one that is uncomfortable and even unwanted, it is inescapable if a principal concern is allocating care on the basis of medical need. The problem there may be in dealing with severely compromised infants has been starkly put:

We are all extremely reluctant to admit that there is a limit to how much we should pay to save a life. We want to believe that a human life is worth more than any amount of money, and we readily agree to sweeping statements to that effect ... With finite resources, we cannot make infinite provision for every life. More money for severely handicapped infants will mean less money for others in need. (Kuhse and Singer 1985: 165–6).

It must of course be said that money spent on any single category of patient will lead to less being available for others: this is true in all areas of health care and indeed in all areas of public funding. Relatively few cases have reached the courts on this issue and when they have the courts have shown themselves reluctant to intervene. In *R v. Central Birmingham Health Authority, ex parte Walker* (1987) the parents of a baby who required heart surgery were told by the medical staff that they lacked a sufficient number of nurses to treat the child. The couple sought leave to bring judicial review against the health authority, but the Court of Appeal refused to permit this. In the words of Sir John Donaldson MR, 'It is not for this court, or indeed any court, to substitute its own judgment for the judgment of those who are responsible for the allocation of resources'. The court would only intervene if the decision of the health authority was one that no reasonable public body could have reached.

Similarly, in the case of Jaimee Bowen already referred to it was said:

I have no doubt that in a perfect world any treatment which a patient, or a patient's family, sought would be provided if doctors were willing to give it, no matter how much it cost, particularly when a life was potentially at stake. It would, however, in my view, be shutting one's eyes to the real world if the court were to proceed on the basis that we do live in such a world ... Difficult and agonising judgments have to be made as to how a limited budget is best allocated to the maximum advantage of the maximum number of patients. That is not a judgment which the court can make.

Implicit is the recognition that resources are finite and that sometimes harsh choices will need to be made. We are faced with the problem of determining which cases are more or less appropriate for treatment and, in part, this will depend upon just the kinds of assessment of quality of life and outcome for the child as before. Here, however, what is being measured in addition is this in comparison with the quality of life and outcome for others and this is what renders the issue particularly problematic. Much has been written on how this issue should properly be approached and it is impossible to canvass all these arguments here. (For professional guidance see, for example, General Medical Council, *Priorities and Choices* (2000).) However, it is clear that this is an area where human rights may also come to be important, although no cases have yet discussed this issue in the context of the provision of medical treatment. The British Medical Association, for example, suggest that failing to provide treatment that would lead to a real, perhaps inevitable, and immediate risk of death where that treatment was likely to avert that risk could be held to be in breach of Article 2. However, they acknowledge that only reasonable and appropriate steps to avoid death are necessary. Any decision to withhold or withdraw treatment on the basis of scarce resources must, however,

be transparent, logical and able to withstand scrutiny. The decision must also be non-discriminatory; a blanket age restriction on treatment such as cardiopulmonary resuscitation, for example, is likely to contravene Article 14 . . . (British Medical Association 2000).

If this is correct, then policies stating that resuscitation of infants born below a certain age should never be attempted may be open to challenge. While a general guideline may be appropriate, it seems likely that health carers must be able to show that they have considered each infant's individual circumstances and human rights, although this will of course be based upon their experience of dealing with other infants. This being said, there will inevitably be cases where scarcity of resources is a factor that may legitimately be taken into account.

In conclusion, deciding how best to treat the preterm infant requires professionals to exercise judgement with the highest degree of skill, sensitivity and compassion. Such decisions cannot be made according to a formula, since the circumstances of each case are infinitely variable and each child and family must be given individual consideration. Nevertheless, a wide range of professional and legal guidance is available on the appropriate factors to be taken into account. The human rights and welfare of the infant will continue to be central in these complex and challenging situations.

REFERENCES

Bartholomew, W. (1978) The child-patient: do parents have the "right to decide"? In S. F. Spicker, J. M. Healy Jr and T. Engelhardt Jr, eds., *The Law-Medicine Relation: a philosophical exploration. Proceedings of the eighth trans-disciplinary symposium on philosophy and medicine held at Farington, Conneticut, 9–11 1978.* Dordrecht: Reidel pp. 272–8.

British Medical Association. (1999) *Withholding and Withdrawing Life-Prolonging Medical Treatment: Guidance for Decision Making.* London: BMJ publishing.

  (2000) *The Impact of the Human Rights Act 1998 on Medical Decision Making.* London: BMJ publishing.

  (2001) *Consent, Rights and Choices in Health Care for Children and Young People.* London: BMJ publishing.

Cohen-Mansfield, J., Rabinovich, B. A., Lipson, S. *et al.* (1991) The decision to execute a durable power of attorney for health care and preferences regarding the utilization of life-sustaining treatments in nursing home residents. *Arch. Int. Med.* **151**, 289–94.

Davies, M. (1996) *Textbook on Medical Law*, 2nd edn. London: Blackstone Press.

Davis, A. (1994) All babies should be kept alive as far as possible. In R. Gillon, ed., *Principles of Health Care Ethics*. London: John Wiley & Sons, pp. 629–

Department of Health. (2001a). *Reference Guide to Consent for Examination or Treatment*. London: Department of Health.

(2001b). *Seeking Consent: Working with Children*. London: Department of Health.

General Medical Council. (2000). *Priorities and Choices*. London: General Medical Council.

(2002). *Withholding and Withdrawing Life Prolonging Medical Treatment*. London: General Medical Council.

Gunn, M. J. and Smith, J. C. (1985). Arthur's case and the right to life of a Down's Syndrome child. *Crim. L. R.* 705–15.

Harris, J. (1994) Not all babies should be kept alive as far as possible. In R. Gillon, ed., *Principles of Health Care Ethics*. London: John Wiley & Sons pp. 643–55.

House of Lords Select Committee on Medical Ethics (1993–94). *Select Committee on Medical Ethics: Report Together with Oral and Written Evidence, Volume II – Oral Evidence*. London: HMSO.

Kennedy, I. and Grubb, A. (2000) *Medical Law*, 3rd edn. London: Butterworths.

Kuhse, H. and Singer, P. (1985). *Should the Baby Live? The Problem of Handicapped Infants*. Aldershot: Oxford University Press.

McHaffie, H. E. (2001) Withdrawing treatment from infants: key elements in the support of families. *Journal of Neonatal Nursing* **7**(3), 85–9.

McHaffie, H. E. in association with Fowlie, P. W., Hume, R., Laing, I. M., Lloyd, D. J. and Lyon, A. J. (2001) *Crucial Decisions at the Beginning of Life: Parents' Experiences of Treatment Withdrawal from Infants*. Oxford: Radcliffe Medical Press.

Mason, J. K. (1999) *Medico-Legal Aspects of Parenthood and Reproduction*, 2nd edn. Ashgate: Dartmouth.

Mason, J. K., McCall Smith, R. A. and Laurie, G. T. (2002) *Law and Medical Ethics*, 6th edn. London: Butterworths.

Royal College of Paediatrics and Child Health. (1997) *Withholding or Withdrawing Life Saving Treatment in Children: a Framework for Practice*. London: British Paediatric Association (Expected to be replaced by new guidance in the near future).

1998 *Guidelines for Good Practice: Management of Neonatal Respiratory Distress Syndrome*. London: British Paediatric Association (Expected to be replaced by new guidance in the near future).

Royal College of Paediatrics and Child Health, Hodgkin, R. (2000). *Advocating for Children*. London: Royal College of Paediatrics and Child Health.

Williams, G. (1981) Down's Syndrome and the duty to preserve life. *New Law J.* **131**, 1020.

CASES

A National Health Service Trust v. D and Ors (2000) 55 Butterworths Medico-Legal Reports 19

Airedale NHS Trust v. Bland (1993) 12 Butterworths Medico-Legal Reports 64, HL

Attorney-General's Reference (No.3 of 1994) [1997] 3 All England Law Reports 936

Bolam v. Friern Hospital Management Committee [1957] 2 All England Law Report, (1957) 1 Butterworths Medico-Legal Reports 1, [1957] 1 Weekly Law Reports 582

Bolitho v. City and Hackney Health Authority [1997] 4 All England Law Reports 771, (1997) 39 Butterworths Medico-Legal Reports 1, [1998] Appeal Cases 232, HL

Cruzan v. Director, Missouri Department of Health (1990) 497 United States Supreme Court 261

D v. UK [1997] 24 European Human Rights Reports 423, ECHR

Gillick v. West Norfolk and Wisbech Area Health Authority [1985] 3 All England Law Reports 402, HL

Glass v. UK (2004) 39 European Human Rights Reports 15

Herczegfalvy v. Austria (1992) 15 European Human Rights Reports 437

Kelly v. Kelly [1997] 2 Family Law Reports 828, (1997) Scots Law Times 896 CS (IH).

NHS Trust A v. M, NHS Trust B v H [2001] 2 Weekly Law Reports 942, [2001] 1 All England Law Reports 801, (2001) 58 Butterworths Medico-Legal Reports

Paton v. British Pregnancy Advisory Service Trustees [1979] Queens Bench 276

Pearce v. United Bristol Healthcare NHS Trust (1998) 48 Butterworths Medico-Legal Reports 118, CA

R v. Adams (1957, unreported), discussed by Palmer, H. in [1957] Criminal Law Review 365.

R v. Adomako [1994] 3 All England Law Reports 79

R v. Arthur (1981) Butterworths Medico-Legal Reports 1

R v. Brain (1834) 6 Carrington and Payne 349

R v. Cambridge District Health Authority (1995) 23 Butterworths Medico-Legal Reports 1, CA

R v. Central Birmingham Health Authority, ex parte Walker (1987) 3 Butterworths Medico-Legal Reports 32

R v. Cox (1992) 12 Butterworths Medico-Legal Reports 38

R v. Enoch (1833) 5 Casrington & Payne 329

R v. Gibbins and Proctor (1918) 13 Criminal Appeal Reports 134, CCA

R v. GMC and others ex parte Burke (2004) 79 Butterworths Medico-Legal Reports 126.

R v. Handley (1874) 13 Cox Criminal Cases 79

R v. Woollin [1999] 1 Appeal Cases 82

Rance v. Mid-Downs Health Authority [1991] 1 All England Law Reports 801

Re A (children) (conjoined twins: surgical separation) [2001] 57 Butterworths Medico-Legal Reports 1, CA

Re B (a minor) (wardship: medical treatment) [1981] 1 Weekly Law Reports 1421

Re C (a minor) (wardship: medical treatment) [1989] 2 All England Law Reports 782, CA

Re C (a minor)(medical treatment) (1997) 40 Butterworths Medico-Legal Reports 31, [1998] 1 Family Law Reports 384

In re F (In utero) [1988] Family Division (Law Reports) 122

Re F (mental patient: sterilisation) [1990] 2 Appeal Cases 1

Re J (a minor) (wardship: medical treatment) [1990] 3 All England Law Reports 930, CA

Re J [1991] Family Division (Law Reports) 33 *Re J* [1992] 4 All England Law Reports 614

Re S (hospital patient: court's jurisdiction) [1996] Family Reports 1

Re T (a minor) (wardship: medical treatment) [1997] 1 Weekly Law Reports 242

Re W (a minor) (medical treatment) [1992] 4 All England Law Reports 627

W v. UK (1987) 10 European Human Rights Reports 29

Index

abortion, previous 11–12
academic infrastructure 313–14
acidosis, neonatal 227
  hypoxia 270–1
  metabolic 277
actin 28
activating transcription factor family (ATF) 93–4
activator protein 1(AP-1) 94–5
  NF-κB cross-coupling 95
cyclic adenosine monophosphate (cAMP) 30
  signalling 93–4
cyclic adenosine monophosphate response element-
    binding protein (CREB) 85–6, 93–4
cyclic adenosine monophosphate response elements
    (CRE) 85–6
adolescence
  outcomes 127
  respiratory symptoms 122–3
adrenal insufficiency, steroid therapy 203
adrenaline
  dosing regimes 270
  hypotension 277
  mode of administration 270
  neonatal resuscitation 270
β-adrenergic agents 223–4
  anaesthesia in preterm labour 250–1
  see also β sympathomimetics
β2-adrenergic receptor agonists 160
adrenergic receptors 30
adult respiratory distress syndrome (ARDS) 243–4
adults, outcomes 127
advance authorisations 324–5
age
  at death 112–13
  see also gestational age
airway, resuscitation 265–6

albumin, serum levels 283
alcohol abuse 16
  social deprivation 156
alcohol consumption 15, 16
alpha fetoprotein (AFP), maternal serum 145–6
ambulatory monitoring, maternal 319
amnio drainage 217
amniocentesis, materno-fetal infection diagnosis
    172–3
amnioinfusion 183
amnion 48–9, 49–50
  prostaglandin source 84
amniopatch 183
amniotic fluid
  culture 172–3
    positive 8–9, 173
  proinflammatory cytokines in infections 144
  volume 177–8
anaemia of prematurity 280
  risk factors 280
anaesthesia
  Caesarean section 245
  corticosteroid use 249
  fetal heart rate 237
  fetal monitoring 237
  general 235
    avoidance 256
    cardiovascular changes 242
    pre-eclampsia 245
  ideal 254–7
  inevitable delivery 248–9, 253
  local 238–9
  miscarriage risk 237
  planned preterm delivery 239–48
  premature delivery risk 237
  preterm labour 249–52

anaesthesia (cont.)
  provision 252–7
  regional 239
    Caesarean section 245
    choice 256
    hypotension 251
    restrictive lung disease 246–7
  risks 235
  surgery during pregnancy 239
  tocolysis 249–52
anaesthetic management 236
  liaison with team 240
anaesthetists 235, 239
  expertise 242
  planned preterm delivery 240
  preterm delivery risk factors 248
analgesic management 236
  ideal 254–7
  incidental effects 371–2
  patient-controlled analgesia 238–9
  provision 252–7
  spinal analgesia 242
  timing 253
  see also epidural analgesia
anandamide (ANAN) 156
anhydramnios 194
annexins 79
antenatal care 17–18, 154–5
antepartum haemorrhage 159
antibiotics
  hazards of use 181
  as medical treatment 384
  neonatal infections 286
  pPROM 180–1, 204
  preterm labour prevention 56, 204
  prophylactic 164
    pPROM 180–1
anticoagulation, maternal 246
antiphospholipid syndrome 17
antiprogesterones 45–6
  labour onset 53–4
anxiety, maternal 237, 239
anxiolytics 237
apoptosis
  cervical ripening 48
  membrane rupture 51
arachidonic acid 55–6, 77–8, 83
arachidonoyl ethanolamine (AEA) 156
Arthur case 369–70
aspirin, anaesthetic implications 251

assault 330
  treatment as 380
assisted reproduction 4–5, 12–13
  multiple births 114
asthma, maternal 246
atosiban 160, 197–8
  anaesthetic implications 252
  multiple pregnancies 217
  pre-eclampsia 223–4
attention deficit hyperactivity disorder (ADHD) 124–5
autism, retinopathy of prematurity 125–6
autoregulation 289

β sympathomimetics 182, 195–7
  anaesthesia in preterm labour 250–1
  contraindications 196–7
  diabetes mellitus 196–7
  medical emergencies 237
  multiple pregnancies 217
  pulmonary oedema 217
Baby Alexandra case 373–4
bacteraemia, fetal 173
bacterial endotoxin 55–6, 79–80, 83
  fetal exposure 182
bacterial vaginosis 6–7
bacteriuria 55–6
  asymptomatic 9–10, 158
bag and mask device 266
bed occupancy 309–10
bed rest, multiple pregnancies 212–13
behavioural outcomes, school age
    children 123–6,
benzodiazepines 237
bereavement damages 353
best interests of child 373–5, 377
  rejection in Scotland 342–3
betamethasone 182–3
  lung maturation enhancement 183
  maternal therapy 202–3
birth
  management 338–9
  NHS Redress Scheme for injuries 358
  wrongful 352
birthweight 109
  economics of low 318
  outcome 110
  see also extremely low birthweight babies; very
    low birthweight babies

Bland case 369, 370–2
  feeding 384
bleeding, acute episodes in neonates 280
blindness 117, 118–19, 121
body weight
  maternal 16
  neonates 272, 277
    monitoring 277
Bolam test 331, 347–8
Bolitho case 348
Bowen, Jaimee (case) 378, 392
brain, fetal
  acquired disorders 287–90
  development 288
    postnatal steroids 274–5
  injury 116, 122
    perinatal 175–6
    vulnerability 292
    white matter 175–6, 183
  sensitisation to hypoxia-ischaemia 184
  white matter
    injury 175–6, 183
    vulnerability to injury 292
brain, maternal
  brain death 246
  damage and intrauterine death in multiple
    pregnancy 216–17
breathing, neonates
  air versus oxygen 267
  resuscitation 266–8
  see also ventilated babies, surfactant therapy;
    ventilation, mechanical
breaths, rescue 266
breech delivery 323–4
  mode in preterm 205
bronchopulmonary dysplasia *see* lung disease,
  chronic
bupivacaine 255

Caesarean section 5–6
  anaesthesia 245
    provision 253
  combined surgical procedures 241
  communication necessity 255–6
  counselling 323–4
  elective 205
    IUGR 228
    pre-eclampsia 225
  hypoxic fetal stress avoidance 184–5
  internal cardiac compression 245–6

intracranial trauma risk 254
IUGR 228
maternal hypertension 242–3
multiple births 218
  diamniotic preterm first twin breech 220
  diamniotic very low birth weight 219
  higher order 220–1
  limits of viability 221
placental abruption 216
refusal 338
viability limits 178–9
caffeine intake 16–17
calcitonin gene-related peptide (CGRP) 30
calcium, uterine contractions 28–9
calcium channel(s) 29
  receptor-operated 32–3
calcium channel blockers 160, 198–9
  anaesthetic implications 252
  multiple pregnancies 217
calcium-calmodulin 28
cannabis 156
capnography 239
carbon dioxide pneumoperitoneum 239
cardiac arrest in pregnancy 245–6
cardiac compression, internal 245–6
cardiac disease, maternal 241–2
cardiac transplantation 247–8
cardiopulmonary resuscitation, maternal 245–6
cardiotocography 227
  contraction strength 191
  erroneous interpretation 237
  immature fetal cardiovascular physiology
    204–5
cardiovascular system, neonates 275–7
cardioversion, direct current 245–6
care
  breach of 372
  obligation for dying with dignity 388
  see also duty of care
carotid artery, internal 288
catecholamines, endogenous 237
causation 348, 351–2
C/EBP family 81
C/EBP site on COX-2 gene 85–6
cephalosporins 181
cerebral arteries, pattern 288
cerebral palsy 118, 175–6
  causation 351
  quadruplet risk 220–1
  risk in monochorionic twins 291

cerebral palsy (cont.)
  spastic 184
  triplet risk 220–1
cerebrovascular accidents, pre-eclampsia
    223
cervical cerclage 163–4, 183–4
  emergency 201
    multiple births 221
  multiple pregnancies 211–12, 213
cervical index 137
cervical length 163–4
  digital examination 136
  fetal fibronectin combination 147
  high-risk women 140
  measurement 138
    cost effectiveness 320
  mid-trimester 138
  multiple pregnancies 141, 211–12
  predictive ability 139–42,
  predictive value 146
  threatened preterm labour 141
  ultrasound imaging 163–4, 171–2, 193
cervical os, internal
  opening 171–2
  ultrasound-identified dilatation 193
cervical ripening 37–48
  collagen structure 89–92
  control 43–8
cervical stitch retention 183–4
cervical therapy 163–4
cervix
  appearance change 137–8
  dilatation 171–2
  funnel length/width 137
  funnelling 137, 171–2, 211–12
  incompetence 10
  myometrial contractions 89–92
  pregnancy 35, 39–42
  relaxin in maturation 143–4
  secretions 134–5
  smooth muscle 39
  structure 38–9
  suprapubic pressure 137–8
  transfundal pressure 137–8
  ultrasound imaging 136–42
    dilatation 171–2
    transvaginal 159–60
chest compressions 268
child destruction offence 390–1
childbearing, delayed 4

children
  competence 343–5
  legal recognition 366, 389–90
  terminally ill 375
Chlamydia trachomatis 7–8, 55–6
chondroitin sulphate 38–9, 41
chorioamnionitis 8–9, 174–5, 175–7
  amniotic fluid volume 177–8
  expectant management 179
  multiple pregnancies 216, 221
  periventricular leukomalacia 291–2
  preterm delivery risk 248–9
  subclinical 173
  temperature increase 248–9
  treatment 181
chorion 48–50
chorionicity 210
circulation, neonates 268
clindamycin, mode of action 181
clinical judgement 378
clinical trials, parental agreement 377
clomiphene 12–13
Clostridium difficile 181
clotting screen, intrauterine death
    216–17
clumsiness *see* dyspraxia
coagulopathy in pre-eclampsia 244–5
co-amoxiclav 180–1
  hazards of use 181
  necrotising enterocolitis 181
  preterm labour use 204
cognitive ability
  school age children 123–4
collagen
  cervical ripening 89–92
  cervical structure 38–9, 40
  fetal membranes 48–50
  fibroblast production 45
collagen graft 183
collagenases 9, 36–7, 40, 89–92
  relaxin stimulation 143–4
colony-stimulating factors 286
common law
  competence 340
  Scotland 356–7
compensation, loss of good outcome
    351–2
competence 339–45
  absence 340–2
  children 343–5

common law 340
  treatment refusal 343–4
  young people 343–5
complications, development 377
Congenital Disabilities (Civil Liability) Act (1976)
    353, 354
  liability under 355–6
congenital malformations, lethal 115
connective tissue disorders 158
connexin-26 27–8
connexin-43 27–8
  gene 94
  upregulation in labour 96
consent 329–32
  legal validity 330
  parental 366–8
consultants 312–14,
continuous positive airway pressure (CPAP) 267–8,
    274
contraction-associated proteins 76
contractions, preterm 144
cord entanglement 220
  multiple births 220–1
cordocentesis 173
  IUGR 227
corticosteroids
  anaesthesia in preterm labour 249
  antenatal use 111–12, 182–3, 271
  contraindications 203
  fetal lung maturity 223–4
  gestational age 203
  IUGR 227
  magnesium sulphate combination 224–5
  maternal therapy 202–3
  multiple pregnancies 214–16
  postnatal 274–5
  repeated doses 202–3
  surfactant therapy 203
corticotrophin-releasing hormone
  labour onset 54
  predictive value 143
  prostaglandin synthesis stimulation 85
corticotrophin-releasing hormone receptors 54
corticotrophin-releasing hormone-binding protein
    (CRH-BP) 54
cortisol, labour onset 52–3
cost effectiveness of management strategies 318–20
costs in negligence claims 357–9
counselling 295–6, 320–5
  Caesarean section 323–4

labour 323–4
  preliminary discussion 323
  pre-pregnancy 159–60
  resuscitation 324–5
  transfer 324
courts
  authorisation of course of action 378
  doctors' professional judgement 377–8
CRE modulator protein (CREM) 93–4
C-reactive protein 173
  neonates 284–5
  pregnancy risk 194
creatinine, maternal levels 247
criminal law limitations 368–72
critical care services 312
cryoprecipitate 183
cryotherapy, retinopathy of prematurity 287
cyclo-oxygenase (COX) 33–4, 77–8, 83–6
cyclo-oxygenase 1 (COX-1) 200
cyclo-oxygenase 2(COX-2)
  gene C/EBP site 85–6
  gene expression in uterine tissue 85
  gene induction 85–6
  myometrial expression 84–5
  promoter 85, 85–6
  role in labour 83–6
  selective prostaglandin inhibitors 200
  transcription mediation 86
cyclo-oxygenase 2 (COX-2) inhibitors
    161, 200
cyclosporin 247–8
cytokines
  cascade 55–6
  inflammatory 9
    cervical changes 76–7
    fetal exposure 182
    predictive value 144–5
  myometrial contraction 34
  neonatal assay 285
  pro-inflammatory 36–7, 46–7, 176–7
    periventricular leukomalacia 175–6

damages
  Scottish law 356–7
  wrongful life actions 353
death
  acceleration 383–4
  age at 112–13
  allowing 370–1
  dignified 383–4, 388

decision-making
  parents 367
    involvement 367–8
  proxy 365
  quality of life 375–6
  treatment 364–5
decorin 41
deformities, right of action 354–5
delivery
  iatrogenic 1, 2, 4, 5–6
  immediate versus delayed 177–9, 194
  management 204–5
  mode 184–5
    anaesthesia provision 252
    intracranial trauma risk 254
    IUGR 228
    pre-eclampsia 225
    preterm breech 205
    vertex presentation 205
  pre-eclampsia 225
  see also preterm delivery
dermatan 38–9
dermatan sulphate 41
dermatan sulphate proteoglycan II 41
developmental quotient (DQ) 118
dexamethasone
  anaesthesia in preterm labour 249
  antenatal use 182–3
  IL-8 inhibition 91
  maternal therapy 202–3
  NF-κB effects 91
diabetes mellitus 158
  anaesthesia in preterm labour 249
  β sympathomimetics 196–7
  prophylactic medical care 159–60
  steroid contraindications 203
diacylglycerol 34–5
digital examination
  membrane rupture diagnosis 171–2
  preterm labour 191
disability 109, 117
  outcome 116
  overall severe 117–18
  prematurity 174–5
  quality of life 375–6
  rate 109–15
  substituted judgement 376–7
  see also neurological disability
discharge arrangements for neonates
  293

disclosure, doctors to patients 331–2
disease, right of action 354–5
disseminated intravascular coagulation (DIC)
  intrauterine death 216–17
  pre-eclampsia 244–5
diving reflex 289
dobutamine 276
doctors
  clinical judgement 378
  developments in practice 349–50
  disclosure to patients 331–2
  duty of care to parents 391
  junior practitioner 350–1
  newly qualified 350–1
  obstetricians 322–3
  professional judgement 377–8
  professional opinion differences
    377–8
doctrine of necessity 341
  Scotland 342–3
  treatment of child 368
doctrine of *res ipsa loquitur* 350
doctrine of strict liability 346
dopamine 276
double-stranded oligodeoxynucleotides (ODN)
  97
drugs
  administration
    neonates 269–71
    pregnancy 238–9
  pharmacology in pregnancy 238
drugs, recreational 154–6
ductus arteriosus
  patent 275–6
    adverse effects 275–6
  premature closure 199–200
duty of care 345–6
  breach 346, 349
  developments in practice 349–50
  nature and extent 370
  negligence 346
  to parents 391
dyspraxia 123

eclampsia 222
economic evaluations 315–16
  stages 315–16
  types 315
economics of service provision 315–20
  interest 317–18

eicosanoids 36–7
elastase 36–7, 40
elastin 39–42
elective delivery *see* iatrogenic delivery
embryo
    decisions made by mother 334
    legal standing 334
emergency treatment 343
emotional support, maternal 254
encephalopathy
    Caesarean section risk 184–5
    neonatal with IUGR 227
endoscopic repair of membranes 183
endothelin receptors 34–5
endothelins
    myometrial contraction 34–5
    myometrial stimulation 53
endotoxins 9
    intra-amniotic 176–7
enteral nutrition 277–8
    minimal 279–80
environmental pollution 17
ephedrine 242
epidural analgesia
    fetal temperature increase 248–9
    post-operative 239
    preterm labour 254, 255
    vasodilatation 242
epidural haematoma 246
epinephrine, *see* adrenaline
erythromycin
    mode of action 181
    preterm labour use 204
    prophylactic 180–1
erythropoiesis 280
erythropoietin, recombinant 281
Escherichia coli 283–4
ethics, status of fetus/embryo 334
European Convention on Human Rights 338, 387
    entitlement to life 368–9
    parental responsibility 366
    parental rights 388–9
expert evidence 347–8
extended perinatal mortality rate (EPMR) 114
extremely low birthweight babies
    behavioural outcomes 125
    cognitive ability at school age 123–4
    deaths 112–13
    motor function 123
extremely preterm infants

feeding problems 122
    peri-viable 294–5

Family Law Reform Act (1969) 344
family life, respect for 388–9
feed tolerance 279–80
feeding
    difficulties 121–2
    failure to 384–5
    intolerance 279
    neonates 277–83
    problems 122
fentanyl 255
fetal distress
    intrapartum 227
    labour with pre-eclampsia 223
fetal membranes 48–9
    changes in labour 76–7
    relaxin in maturation 143–4
    tensile strength 48–9
    see also membrane rupture; premature rupture of
        membranes; preterm premature rupture of
        the membranes (pPROM)
fetal monitoring
    anaesthesia 237, 253
    intrapartum 204–5
    parents' wishes 323–4
fetus
    compromise in maternal pulmonary
        hypertension 240
    decisions made by mother 334
    deteriorating condition 5
    growth restriction 154–5
    inflammatory response 171
    legal standing 334–5, 339
    management recommendations 321
    maternal behaviour modulation 336–7
    medical intervention 337
    negligence causing death 353
    safeguarding 336–7
    treatment as person with rights 335–6
    ultrasound imaging 214–16
    viability 1
    wellbeing in multiple pregnancies 214–16
fibroblasts, cervical 39
fibronectin, fetal 320
    bedside testing 134–5
    cervical length combination 147
    cervico-vaginal secretions 134–5, 192–3
    clinical utility 134–5

fibronectin, fetal (cont.)
  membrane content 48–9
  multiple pregnancies 212
  predictive value 134, 146
  preterm uterine activity 147
fluids
  management guidelines 278
  neonates 277
  withdrawing/withholding 370–1
  see also hydration
folic acid supplementation 293
follow-up compliance 115
food *see* nutrition
forced expiratory volume in 1 second (FEV1)
    122–3
forced vital capacity (FVC) 122–3
fungaemia 283–4
funnelling of cervix 137, 171–2

galanin 30
gamete intrafallopian transfer (GIFT) 158–60
gap junctions 27, 37
Gardnerella vaginalis 6, 55–6
gastrin-releasing peptide 30
gastrointestinal colic 194
gastro-oesophageal reflux 122
genital tract infection 154–5
  multiple pregnancies 216
germinal matrix
  bleeding 287–90
  haemorrhage 289–90
gestational age 1, 110
  calculation 324
  determination 3–4
  legal definitions 2
  lower limit 2–3
  multiple birth delivery 211, 219
  preterm delivery risk 133
  preterm labour 191
  steroid benefits 203
Geudel airway 265–6
Gillick competence 343–4
glucocorticoids 86, 97
  antenatal 183
glyceryl trinitrate 36, 160
glycosaminoglycans 38–42
  fibroblast production 45
G-proteins 30
granulocyte colony-stimulating factor (G-CSF)
  predictive value 145

growth
  catch-up 126–7
  restriction 110, 114
  school age children 126–7

haematological scoring systems, neonatal 284–5
haemodialysis, chronic 247
haemoglobin 280–1
haemostatic function 199–200
harm
  establishment 352–3
  liability 346
  serious 372
healthcare team
  consensus approach 383
  disagreement with parents 373
  see also doctors; nurses; staff, hospital
health-related quality of life 126
hearing impairment 119
heart disease, congenital maternal 241
heart rate, fetal
  anaesthetic drugs 237
  auscultation 214–16, 323–4
  continuous electronic monitoring 227
heat loss 261–5
  neonates 272
HELLP syndrome (haemolysis, elevated liver
    enzymes and low platelets) 222, 224
  delivery 245
  pre-eclampsia 244–5
heparan sulphate 38–9
heparin 38–9
home uterine activity monitoring (HUAM)
    135–6
home-based care 320
hospitals
  admissions 317
  bed occupancy 309–10
  service economics 317
  see also staff, hospital
host defences, immature 284
human chorionic gonadotrophin (hCG) 161
human rights 338
  decision-making 377
  parental responsibility 366
  principles 387
  see also European Convention on Human Rights
Human Rights Act (1998) 387–8
humidification, environmental for neonate 272
hyaluronic acid 38–9, 41

hydralazine 243
hydration 202, 384–5
    benefits 385
    burdens 385
    as medical treatment 384
    withholding 370–1
hydrocephaly, post-haemorrhagic 290
hydrocortisone 277
17α-hydroxyprogesterone caproate 32
15-hydroxyprostaglandin dehydrogenase (PGDH)
        34, 77–8
    expression 88
    function 88–9
    isoforms 88–9
    promoter 88–9
hyperactivity 125
hyperbilirubinaemia 283
hypercaloric feeding 279–80
hyperoxia 267
hypertension
    anaesthesia in preterm labour 249
    planned preterm delivery 242–5
    pre-eclampsia 222–3
    pregnancy 158
hyponatraemia 277
hypotension
    neonates 276–7
    regional anaesthesia 251
hypothermia prevention 261–5
hypovolaemia correction 276
hypoxia 37
    fetal 177
    fetal stress 184–5
    intrapartum 228
    IUGR 227, 228
    neonatal acidosis 270–1
    placental bed 222–3
    resistance 288–9
hypoxia-ischaemia, brain sensitisation 184

iatrogenic delivery 1, 2, 4, 5–6
    preterm 225, 228
ibuprofen 276
idiopathic preterm delivery 6
    black population 155
IκB kinase complex (IKK) 81–2, 97
IκBβ protein 95, 97
ileal perforation, indomethacin-induced 199–200
immaturity 109–10
    blindness 118–19

immunosuppressive treatment 247–8
incubators
    temperature control 272
indomethacin 160
    anaesthetic implications 251
    medical emergencies 237
    patent ductus arteriosus closure 276
    polyhydramnios 217
    renal function 199–200
    tocolysis 182, 199–200
Infant Life Preservation Act (1929), child
        destruction offence 390–1
infections 6–10, 54–6
    amniotic fluid proinflammatory cytokines 144
    cause of death 174–5
    clinical signs 173
    extra-uterine 9–10
    fetal
        assessment 173
        biophysical score 173–4
        hypoxia-ischaemia combination 184
    genital tract 154–5
    intra-amniotic 171
    intrauterine 8–9, 287–90
    lower genital tract 6–8
    lower respiratory tract 122
    materno-fetal 171
        diagnosis 172–4
    neonatal 283–6
        prevention 286
        prophylactic antibiotics 180–1
        susceptibility 284
    nosocomial with parenteral nutrition 277–8
    organism cultures 285–6
    systemic 158
inflammation/inflammatory response, fetal 171
    assessment 173
    detection 173–4
inflammatory cells 76–7
inflammatory mediators 46–7
    myometrial contraction 36–7
information for parents 367
inhibitory proteins (IκBs) 81–2
inositol 1,4,5-triphosphate 32–3, 34–5
inpatient management of preterm labour 194
insulin release 196–7
intellectual impairment 118
intensive care
    adult facilities 312
    see also Neonatal Intensive Care Unit

interleukin 1(IL-1)
  membrane rupture 50–1
  prostaglandin production 53
interleukin 1β (IL-1β) 36–7, 46–7
  bronchopulmonary dysplasia 176–7
  up-regulation in labour 96
interleukin 6 (IL-6) 36–7, 46–7
  amniotic fluid levels 144
  bronchopulmonary dysplasia 176–7
  neonatal assay 285
  periventricular leukomalacia 175–6
  prostaglandin production 53
interleukin 8 (IL-8) 36–7, 46–7, 77, 89–92
  bronchopulmonary dysplasia 176–7
  neonatal assay 285
  production 90
    during labour 91–2
  promoter binding sites 90–1
interleukin 8 (IL-8) gene 90
  expression 90
interleukin 10 (IL-10) 97
interventions for benefit of adult 342–3
intraparenchymal haemorrhage 289–90
intrauterine death, multiple pregnancies
    216–17
intrauterine growth restriction (IUGR)
    159, 225–8
  aetiology 225–6
  corticosteroids 227
  definition 225–6
  delivery 228
    elective 228
  diagnosis 226
  extremes of viability 228
  incidence 226
  management 226–8
  monitoring 227
  placental insufficiency 223
  pre-eclampsia 223
  tocolysis 226–7
  transfer to neonatal intensive care 227–8
intrauterine infection 8–9, 287–90
intraventricular haemorrhage 174–5, 289–90
  antenatal glucocorticoids 183
  patent ductus arteriosus 275–6
  steroid prophylaxis 182–3, 202–3
intubation, neonates 267–8
in vitro fertilisation (IVF) 158–60
IQ levels 118, 127
iron supplementation 281, 293

jaundice
  causes 282
  neonates 282
  risk factors 282
  side effects of treatment 283
  treatment threshold 283
judgements, substituted 376–7
jugular vein, internal, cannulation 243–4

kernicterus 283
killing
  active 370–1
  intentional 371–2
Kleihauer test 191
kyphoscoliosis 246–7

labetolol 243
labour
  induction 225
    maternal hypertension 242–3
  management 204–5, 329, 338–9
  onset
    transcription factors 93
    triggers 52–3
  precipitation risk 236–9
  term 52–4
  see also preterm labour
labour-associated proteins 76–7
laparoscopic surgery 239
laser therapy for retinopathy of prematurity 287
left handedness 123
legal issues see treatment, legal issues
leukocytes 36–7, 46–7
  cervical ripening 53
  protease-producing 45
liability, no-fault 357–8, 359
life, obligation to protect 387
life-prolonging treatment 382–3
lifestyle modification 154–8
lipopolysaccharide 55–6, 79–80, 83
Listeria monocytogenes 9
litigation costs 308
L-NAME 47–8
London Regional Specialised Commissioning
    Group (LRSCG) 308–11
lung(s)
  fetal maturity 214–16
    corticosteroids 223–4
    cost effectiveness 319–20
  inflation pressure 266–7

injury 176–7
maturation enhancement 183
see also pulmonary *entries*
lung disease, chronic 120–1, 122–3
adolescents/young adults 127
CPAP use 267–8
fetal exposure to inflammation 176–7
materno-fetal infection 171
mechanical ventilation 273–4
school age children 122–3
steroid therapy 274–5
lung disease, restrictive in pregnancy 246–7
lung function tests
adolescents/young adults 127
school age children 122–3
luteolysis induction 83

macrophages 55–6
magnesium sulphate 160
adverse effects 200–1
anaesthetic implications 251
corticosteroid combination 224–5
medical emergencies 237
pre-eclampsia 224–5, 244
tocolysis 182, 200–1
malabsorption, short bowel syndrome 121–2
malpresentation
IUGR 228
multiple births 220–1
managed clinical networks 309–10, 314
guidelines 310
management strategies, cost effectiveness 318–20
manslaughter prohibition 368–9
marital status 14
maternal age 13–14
maternal disease management 158–60
maternal/fetal conflict 338
maternal-placental perfusion 216
maternity services 310–11
guidelines 310–11
matrix metalloproteinase (MMP) 40, 46–7
membrane rupture 50–1
preterm prelabour 51
matrix metalloproteinase 8 (MMP-8) 89–92
upregulation in labour 96
matrix metalloproteinase 9 (MMP-9) 145
medical emergencies 236–7
preterm labour prevention 237
medical practice
practitioner responsibilities 349–50

technique varying 350
membrane rupture 48–52
biochemical events 50–1
diagnosis 171–2
endoscopic repair 183
morphological changes 49–50
zone of altered morphology 49–51
see also premature rupture of membranes;
preterm premature rupture of the
membranes (pPROM)
Mental Incapacity Bill 341–2
mesenteric artery, superior, flow velocity 279
mifepristone 32
miscarriage
risk with anaesthesia 237
see also stillbirth
morbidity
bias 110
maternal 310
neonatal 179
pulmonary insufficiency 177–8
short-term 119–22
mortality
bias 110
outcome studies 115
prematurity 174–5
rate 112–13
steroid prophylaxis 182–3
studies 116
time of death 112–13
motor coordination, fine 123
motor disability, periventricular leukomalacia 292
multi-organ dysfunction 222–3
multiple births 4, 13
Caesarean section 218
diamniotic preterm first twin breech 220
diamniotic very low birthweight 219
higher-order 220–1
limits of viability 221
risks 221
care in different neonatal units 307
cord entanglement 220–1
delivery
gestational age 211, 219
limits of viability 221
mode 218–21
diamniotic
preterm first twin breech 220
very low birth weight 218–19
limits of viability 221

multiple births (cont.)
  locking 220–1
  malpresentation 220–1
  medical staffing 221
  monoamniotic 220
  outcome assessment 114
  resuscitation equipment 261–3
  triplets 220–1
  vaginal delivery 218
    risks 222
  see also twin pregnancy
multiple pregnancies 12, 13, 37, 210–21
  aetiology 210–11
  bed rest 212–13
  cervical cerclage 211–12, 213
  cervical length 141
  chorioamnionitis 216, 221
  complications 214
  corticosteroids 214–16
  fetal fibronectin 212
  genital tract infection 216
  home uterine activity monitoring 212
  incidence 210–11
  intrauterine death 216–17
  investigations 215
    threatened preterm labour 214–16
  observations 215
  perinatal morbidity/mortality 210–11
  placental abruption 216
  polyhydramnios 217
  prenatal care 212
  preventive strategies for preterm labour 212–14
  risk prediction 211–12
  tocolysis 213, 217
  transfer to neonatal unit 217–18
  treatment of threatened preterm labour
    216–18
  ultrasound assessment 211–12
  uterus over-distension 211
  see also twin pregnancy
murder
  attempted 384–5
  prohibition 368–9
mycoplasmas, genital 8
myometrial contractions 26
  cervical tissue 89–92
  fundally dominant 76
  metabolic modulation 37
  oxytocin stimulation 32–3
  strength 191

myometrium
  cholinergic stimulation 30
  electrical activity 28
  function control 30, 31
  hormonal modulation 30–7
  labour onset 76
  neuronal modulation 30
  oxytocin sensitivity 197–8
  smooth muscle 27–8
    contractility 161–2
  stretch 94–5
myosin 28
myosin light chain kinase (MLCK) 28, 29
myosin light chain phosphatase (MLCP) 161–2
myosin light chains, dephosphorylation 29

naloxone 270
naproxen 251
nasal intermittent positive pressure ventilation
    (NIPPV) 274
nasciturus principle 356
national cohorts 111
necrotising enterocolitis 121–2, 278–80
  co-amoxiclav 181, 204
  indomethacin-induced 199–200
  patent ductus arteriosus 275–6
negligence
  causation 351–2
  causing death of fetus 353
  child born injured 354–5
  contribution to injury 351
  costs of claims 357–9
  duty of care 345, 346
  gross 372
  liability in obstetric care 345–57
  medical professional 347–8
  reform of actions 357–9
  relationship between wrongdoer/harmed 346
  Scottish law 356–7
  statutory offence 372
Neisseria gonorrhoeae 55–6
neonatal care categories 308–9
Neonatal Intensive Care Unit
  admission 271–2
  cot blocking 307
neonatal life support algorithm 263–4
neonatal management, differences over time
    111–12
neonatal services, specialist 313
neonatal unit needs 307

neonates
  abnormalities and right of action 354–5
  born injured through negligence 354–5
  cardiovascular system 275–7
  discharge arrangements 293
  electrolytes 277
  feeding 277–83
  fluids 277
  infections 180–1, 283–6
  jaundice 282
  long-term follow-up 295–7
  management
    recommendations 321
    until discharge 271–82
  neurological screening 287–90
  nutrition 277–83
  outcome
    interventions 182–4
    predelivery interventions 201–4
    prophylactic antibiotics 180–1
  peri-viable 294–5
  physiological condition 254
  predischarge arrangements 287–93
  respiration 272–5
  support withdrawal 324–5
  thermal environment 272
  transfusion 280–2
  see also resuscitation
neonaticide 383–4
neonatologists, obstetrician collaboration 322–3
Neopuff flow-controlled pressure-limited device 266
neurological disability
  IUGR 227
  materno-fetal infection 171
  NHS Redress Scheme 358
neurological screening of neonates 287–90
neuronal migration abnormalities 287–90
neuropeptide Y 30
neutrophils 89–90
  neonatal transfusion 286
NF-κB 81–2, 94–5
  activation in amnion in labour 95
  amnion cells 88–9
  AP-1 cross-coupling 95
  bacterial endotoxin 83
  binding blocking 97
  COX-2 promoter 85–6
  dexamethasone effect 91
  double-stranded oligodeoxynucleotides 97
  functions 95

inhibition 96–8
  pathway 82–3
  PGDH downregulation 88–9
  preterm delivery prevention 96–8
  therapeutic target 97
NHS Redress Scheme 358
nifedipine 160, 243
  anaesthetic implications 252
  dosage 199
  maternal side effects 198–9
  multiple pregnancies 217
  tocolysis 198
nimesulide 200
Nitrazine test 171–2
nitric oxide
  L-arginine system 47–8
  cervical ripening 47–8
  donors 35, 36, 160, 201
  myometrial contractility 35–6
nitric oxide synthase 35–6
'no chance' situation 382–3
'no purpose' situation 382–3
no-fault liability 357–8, 359
non-resuscitation 383
non-steroidal anti-inflammatory drugs (NSAIDs)
    77, 238–9
nuclear factor kappa B *see* NF-κB
nurses
  recruitment/retention 312–13
  specialist 307
nutrition 16, 384–5
  artificial 384
  benefits 385
  burdens 385
  as medical treatment 384
  neonates 277–83
  withdrawing/withholding 370–1
nutritional status 154–5

obstetricians
  neonatologist collaboration 322–3
  preliminary discussion 323
obstetrics
  economics 317–18
  liability for negligence 345–57
occupation, maternal 16, 154–5
oestradiol 45
  labour onset 52–3
  pregnancy levels 241–2
17β-oestradiol 30–2

oestriol (E3) 30–2, 142–3
oestrogen
  cervical ripening 45
  myometrial contractility 30
oestrogen receptors 142–3
oligohydramnios 175
  indomethacin-induced 199–200
  IUGR 228
  neonatal outcome 183
  prognosis for survival 178
  ultrasonography 171–2
  umbilical cord compression 177
oliguria 243–4
operative delivery 5–6
  see also Caesarean section
opiate abuse 16–17
opioids 238–9
organ transplantation 247–8
osteonectin 49–50
osteopenia of prematurity 277–8
outcome(s) 3
  oligohydramnios 183
  resource allocation 392–3
  reviews 109–15
outcome measurement 1
  adolescence 127
  adults 127
  denominator 112
  disability 116
  follow-up compliance 115
  growth restriction 114
  hospital-specific 110–11
  lethal congenital malformations 115
  mortality rate 115
  multiple births 114
  national cohorts 111
  peri-viable neonates 294
  racial characteristics 114–15
  regional-specific 110–11
  school age 122–7
  time period of study 111–12
outpatient management of preterm labour 194
oxygen
  dependency 119, 120–1
  home 120–1, 295–7
  resuscitation 267
  saturation level 293
oxytocin
  delivery expediting 178
  myometrial contraction 32–3

myometrium sensitivity 197–8
oxytocin antagonists 160, 197–8
  multiple pregnancies 217
  tocolysis 182
oxytocin receptor 33, 77, 92–3
  AP-1 binding site 94
  mRNA downregulation 93
  promoter 92–3

pacemaker cells, myometrial 28
packed red blood cell transfusion 280
pain, human rights issues 388
palliative care 371–2
parens patriae jurisdiction 340–1
parenteral nutrition 277–8
parents
  advance authorisations 324–5
  best interests of child 373–5
  clinical trials agreements 377
  consensus approach 383
  consent 344, 366–8
  decision-making 321–3, 367
    involvement 367–8
    treatment 365
  disagreement
    with healthcare team 373
    with professional opinion 380–1
  fetal monitoring 323–4
  human rights 388–9
  information
    needs 367
    presentation 295–6
  post-operative care commitments 381–2
  preliminary discussion 323
  preparation for preterm labour 202
  preterm infant discharge 293
  quality of life judgement for child 381–2
  responsibility 366
  rights over children 367
parity 12
patient-controlled analgesia 238–9
patients
  decision-making 332
  information
    requirements 330–2
    on risks 331
  medical advice acceptance 337
  refusal to cooperate 337
D-penicillamine 287
penicillin, mode of action 181

perinatal centres 311
  accommodation of mother 311–12
  transfers 324
perinatal mortality, extended rate 114
periventricular haemorrhage 287–90
  autoregulation 289
  classification 289
  clinical features 290
  complications 290
  phenobarbital 204
periventricular leukomalacia 175–6, 287–90
  betamethasone 183
  chorioamnionitis 291–2
  histopathological changes 291
  lesion distribution 291
  motor disability 292
  prevalence 291
permanent vegetative state 376, 380, 385
peroxisome proliferator activator receptor (PPAR) 82–3
  bacterial endotoxin 83
peroxisome proliferator response elements (PPREs) 82–3
pH, uterine 37
phenobarbital 204
phosphate supplementation 277–8
phospholipase A_2 9, 77–83
  activation 79–80
  C/EBP binding sites 81
  cytosolic 78–9, 80
    binding sites 80–1
    promoter 80
    rapid 80
    $sPLA_2$ gene induction 82
  expression 79
  secretory 78–9, 81
    bacterial endotoxin 83
    gene induction 82
phospholipases 55–6, 77–8
phosphorus metabolites 37
phototherapy 283
placental abruption 51, 223–4
  Caesarean section 216
  multiple pregnancies 216
  pPROM 177
placental bed, hypoxia 222–3
placental dysfunction, viral infections 8
placental insufficiency, pre-eclampsia 223
placentation, abnormal 222–3
planning, advance for complex cases 322–3

plasminogen activators 36–7
platelet activating factor (PAF)
  myometrial stimulation 53
  prostaglandins
    production 53
    synthesis stimulation 85
platelets 183
pneumoperitoneum, carbon dioxide 239
pneumothorax
  patent ductus arteriosus 276
  surfactant administration 269
pollution, environmental 17
polyhydramnios, multiple pregnancies 217
postgraduate training 313–14
post-operative care, parental commitment 381–2
postpartum haemorrhage, multiple births 221
prediction of preterm labour
  cervical ultrasound 136–42
  endocrine factors 142–5
  fetal fibronectin 134–5
  marker combination 146–7
  risk scoring 133
  uterine activity monitoring 135–6
predischarge arrangements, neonates 287–93
pre-eclampsia 222–5
  aetiology 222–3
  clinical features 243
  coagulopathy 244–5
  criteria 224
  definition 222–3
  delivery 225
  general anaesthesia 245
  gestation
    greater than 34 weeks 223
    up to 34 weeks 223–4
  hypertension 222–3
  iatrogenic preterm delivery 225
  incidence of preterm labour 223
  indications for delivery 244
  intrauterine growth retardation 223
  magnesium sulphate 224–5
  management of preterm labour 223–5
  placental insufficiency 223
  planned preterm delivery 242–5
  severe 223–4
  tocolysis 223–4
pregnancy
  behaviour of women 334
  brain death 246
  cardiac arrest 245–6

pregnancy (cont.)
cervix 35, 39–42
competence absence 340–2
complications 194
drug administration 238–9
hypertension 158
interval 12
management 329, 332–7
medical disorders 158
persistent vaginal bleeding 159
previous second trimester loss 159
problems 337
prophylactic medical care 159–60
screening 332–4
stress 156–7
see also multiple pregnancies
premature rupture of membranes 48
C-reactive protein 173
see also preterm premature rupture of the
membranes (pPROM)
prematurity 174–5
prenatal care of multiple pregnancies 212
preterm delivery
causes 5–10
counselling 323–4
definition 1–3
economics 318
iatrogenic 225, 228
idiopathic 6
black population 155
incidence 1, 4–5, 153–4
management recommendations 320–5
planned 239–48
fetal reasons 240
maternal reasons 240–8
previous 10–11
risk factors 248–9
risk with anaesthesia 237, 248–9
team planning 240
preterm labour
anaesthetic implications 249–52
clinical assessment 191, 192
counselling 323–4
detection 319
diagnosis 191–4
differential 194
investigations 192–3
incidence with pre-eclampsia 223
inevitable 248–9, 253
investigations 191–3

management
economics 319–20
pre-eclampsia 223–5
onset prevention 160–2
problems 254
preterm premature rupture of the membranes
(pPROM) 8–9, 48, 51, 171
between 25 and 31 weeks gestation 178–9
at 32–6 weeks 179
amnioinfusion 183
cervical cerclage 183–4
conservative management 178–9
delivery mode 184–5
diagnosis 171–4
endoscopic repair 183
before fetal viability 177–8
IL-6 levels 144
immediate versus delayed delivery 177–9
inpatient management 179–80
materno-fetal complications 174–7
outpatient management 179–80
perinatal survival 177–8
previous 11
prophylactic antibiotics 164
private life, respect for 388–9
professional guidance, legal opinion 382–4
professional opinion
differences 377–8
parental disagreement 380–1
progesterone
cervical ripening 45–6
functional withdrawal 96
IL-8 inhibition 91
isoforms 96
labour 95–6
myometrial contractility 30
cPLA$_2$ inhibitor upregulation 80
withdrawal theory 53–4
progesterone receptors 32
function 96
prognosis 364–5
lack of certainty 377
uncertain 373–4
prognostic significance 2
prostaglandin(s) 9
amnion as source 84
biosynthetic pathway 77–8
cervical changes 76–7
cervical ripening 44–5
delivery expediting 178

ductus arteriosus patency 199–200
   glucocorticoid inhibition 86
   labour onset 53
   myometrial contraction 33–5
prostaglandin D synthase (PGDS) 87
prostaglandin D_2 77–8
prostaglandin dehydrogenase 88–9
   chorionic 53
prostaglandin E synthase (PGES) 87
   membrane-associated 87
prostaglandin E_2 34, 77–8
   cervical ripening 44–5
   MMP activity 50–1
   production inhibition 86
   synthesis 33–4
prostaglandin F synthase (PGFS) 87
prostaglandin $F_{2\alpha}$ 34, 77–8
   cervical ripening 44–5
   MMP activity 50–1
prostaglandin I synthase (PGIS) 87
prostaglandin I_2 77–8
   cervical ripening 44–5
prostaglandin synthases 87
prostaglandin synthesis inhibitors 199–200
   haemostatic function 199–200
   side effects 200
prostaglandin synthetase inhibitors 251
proteases 9, 51
protein kinases 80
proteoglycan, cervical 41–2
pseudomembranous colitis 181
psychiatric disease 15
psychological stress 156–8
pulmonary dysfunction, adolescents/young adults 127
pulmonary hypertension
   maternal 240, 241
   persistent 199–200
pulmonary hypoplasia, oligohydramnios 175
pulmonary insufficiency 174–5
   morbidity 177–8
pulmonary oedema
   β-adrenergic agent therapy 250–1
   β sympathomimetics 217
   magnesium sulphate with corticosteroids 224–5
   maternal hydration effect 202
   pre-eclampsia 223–4, 243–4
pyelonephritis 9, 158

quality of life
   decision-making 375–6

disability 375–6
evaluation of expected 374–5
expectation 375–6
judgements 364–5, 374, 375
life-saving/prolonging treatments 380
objective 126
parental judgement 381–2
resource allocation 392–3
school age children 126

race of mother 14–15, 155
racial characteristics 114–15
referral centres 110–11
rehospitalisation 122
relaxin 46
   predictive value 143–4
relaxin receptors 143–4
renal disease 158
   maternal 247
renal function 199–200
reproductive disorders 158–60
res ipsa loquitur doctrine 350
research
   base 314
   economics of obstetrics 318
resource allocation 365, 391–3
   Jaimee Bowen case 378
   outcomes 392–3
   quality of life 392–3
respiration, neonates 272–5
respiratory disease, maternal 246–8
respiratory distress syndrome 111–12, 174–5
   anaesthesia in preterm labour 249
   lung injury 269
   prematurity-related 179
   prevention 134–5
   risk 269
   steroid prophylaxis 182–3, 202–3
respiratory support, air versus oxygen 267
respiratory symptoms, chronic at school age
   122–3
respiratory syncytial virus (RSV) 122
resuscitation 260–71
   air versus oxygen 267
   airway 265–6
   anticipation 260–1
   at birth 389–91
   breathing 266–8
   counselling 324–5
   decision not to 295, 324–5, 383

resuscitation (cont.)
  equipment 261–3
  futile treatment 379–80
  high-risk infants 260–1
  human rights issues 387
  hypothermia prevention 261–5
  initial assessment 265
  limit absence 294–5
  personnel 261–4
  preparation 261–4
  procedure 261
retinopathy of prematurity 117, 118–19, 121
  autism risk 125–6
  interventions 287
  ophthalmological surveillance 295–7
  patent ductus arteriosus 276
  risk 287
review groups 308–9
Rho A 161–2
Rho associated coil-forming protein kinase (ROCK
  I and II) 161–2
Rho kinase inhibitors 161–2
risk factors for preterm delivery 3, 10–18
  epidemiological 153, 154
  maternal 10–18
ritodrine 160, 195–6
  anaesthesia in preterm labour 250–1
  fetal effects 197
  infusion 197
  maternal effects 196–7
  pre-eclampsia 223–4
  side effects 196

sanctity of life principle 374–5
sarcoplasmic reticulum 29
school age, outcomes 122–7
scoring system, preterm delivery risk 133
Scotland
  children 344–5
  common law 356–7
  doctrine of necessity 342–3
  emergency treatment 343
  interventions for benefit of adult 342–3
  young people 344–5
screening tests 332–4
  availability 333–4
  choice 333
  preterm delivery risk 133
selection bias 112
sepsis 283–4

  maternal 178
  neonatal clinical features 284–5
service(s)
  guidelines 310
  integrated 309–10
  requirements 307–14
service infrastructure 309–10
  change implementation 314
service provision economics 315–20
  hospitals 317
sex, fetal 17
short bowel syndrome 121–2
small for gestational age fetus 225–6
smoking 15, 16
  risk factor 154–5
  social deprivation 156
smooth muscle
  cervical 39
  contractility 161–2
social support, enhanced 157–8
sociodemographic risk factors 13–15, 17
socioeconomic factors 154–5
  stress 157–8
socioeconomic status 4, 14–15
sodium bicarbonate 270–1
spinal analgesia 242
spiral artery conversion failure 222–3
spontaneous delivery 1
staff, hospital 272
  counselling 295–6
  requirements 312–13
  resuscitation 261–4
  see also doctors; nurses
standard of care 346–50
standard practice, departure from 349
staphylococci, coagulase-negative 283–4
Staphylococcus aureus 283–4
steroid hormones 95–6
  see also corticosteroids
stillbirth
  definition 390
  IUGR 227
strabismus 121
streptococcus group B 7
stress 15
  pregnancy 156–7
  psychological 156–8
  socioeconomic factors 157–8
strictures, intestinal 121–2
subclavian vein cannulation 243–4

subependymal haemorrhage 289–90
substance abuse 16–17
substance P 30
succinylcholine 251
suffering, human rights issues 388
sulindac 217
surfactant therapy 269
  antenatal steroids 271
  neonates 272–3
  racial characteristics of babies 115
  steroid use 203
  types 269
  ventilated babies 111–12
surgery
  fetal monitoring 237
  laparoscopic 239
  service organisation 308
survival
  benefit to child 380
  harm to child 380
  neonatal 153–4, 174–5
  oligohydramnios prognosis 178
  perinatal following pPROM 177–8
  rate 109–15
  resuscitation 260–1
swallowing problems 122
symphysis pubis pain 194
systemic lupus erythematosus (SLE) 17, 158
  prophylactic medical care 159–60

tachycardia 275
tachypnoea 275
temperature, environmental for neonates 272
temperature, fetal increase with epidural analgesia
  248–9
terbutaline 160
Δ^9 tetrahydrocannabinol (D^9 – THC) 156
thalidomide 354
Thames Regional Perinatal Group (TRPG)
  308–11
thrombin, placental abruption 51
thrombocytopenia 224
  neonatal sepsis 284–5
  pre-eclampsia 244–5
thromboembolism, maternal 246
  risk 247–8
thromboxane 77–8
thromboxane synthase (TXS) 87
thyrotrophin releasing hormone
  (TRH) 203–4

tissue inhibitors of metalloproteinase (TIMP) 46–7
  membrane rupture 50–1
tissue use constraints 324–5
tocolysis/tocolytic agents 31
  anaesthesia in preterm labour 249–52
  beneficial effects 195
  cervical ripening 38
  chorioamnionitis treatment 182
  contraindication 182
    placental abruption 216
  intrauterine death in multiple pregnancy
    216–17
  intravenous access 214–16
  IUGR 226–7
  magnesium sulphate 224–5
  multiple pregnancies 213, 217
  pre-eclampsia 223–4
  preterm labour
    onset prevention 160–2
    threatened 194–201
  prophylactic 160–2
T-piece breathing device 266
training, postgraduate 313–14
transcription factors, labour onset 93
transfer
  counselling 324
  delayed with pulmonary oedema 243–4
  disadvantages 307
  intrauterine 324
    to neonatal unit 217–18
  neonatal intensive care 227–8
  postnatal 324
  pre-eclampsia 223–4
  transport services 311–12
transfusion
  neonates 280–2
  response to 280–1
  risks 281
transport services 311–12
treatment, legal issues 364–5
  assault 380
  benefits 365, 375, 379, 380, 385
  burdens 375, 379, 385
  court distinction from intentional killing 371–2
  criminal law limitations 368–72
  damages 353, 356–7
  decision-making 364–5
  disagreements 372–3
  futility 364–5, 379–80, 387
  given in best interests 341

treatment, legal issues (cont.)
  harms 365, 380
  inappropriate 388
  legal principles 366–8
  life-prolonging 380, 387
  life-saving 380
  litigation costs 308
  no-fault liability 357–8, 359
  professional guidance 382–4
  refusal 343–4
  relative efficacy 377
  utility 364–5
  withdrawing/withholding 380
    resources 392–3
  see also common law; competence; courts;
    damages; negligence; Scotland
Trichomonas vaginalis 55–6
tumour necrosis factor (TNF) 53
tumour necrosis factor α (TNFα) 36–7
  MMP-1 production 51
turquoise light phototherapy 283
twin pregnancy 159
  diamniotic 210
    delivery 218–19, 220
  dichorionic 216–17
  dizygotic 210
  locked twins 220
  monoamniotic 210
    delivery 220
  monochorionic 210, 216–17
    cerebral palsy risk 291
  monozygotic 210

ultrasound imaging 3, 4, 110
  biometry 225–6
  cervical length 163–4, 171–2, 193
  cervix 136–42, 159–60
    dilatation 171–2
  cranial 291, 291–2
  fetal assessment 173–4, 214–16
  multiple pregnancies 211–12
  oligohydramnios 171–2
  preterm labour 191
  three-dimensional 138
  translabial in membrane rupture diagnosis
    171–2
  transvaginal 136
    cervical canal length 163–4
    cervix 159–60
    membrane rupture diagnosis 171–2

umbilical artery, absent end-diastolic
    flow 279
umbilical cord compression 177
'unbearable' situation 382–3
Ureaplasma urealyticum 55–6
urinary tract infection 158
uterine activity
  contractile 26–7
  home monitoring 212
  monitoring 135–6
  preterm 147
uterus
  over-distension 211
  palpation 191
  physical abnormalities 17

vaginal bleeding, persistent in pregnancy
    159
vaginal delivery
  intracranial trauma risk 254
  maternal hypertension 242–3
  multiple births 218
    risks 222
vaginal secretions, fetal fibronectin 134–5
vaginal speculum examination 191
vaginosis, bacterial 6–7
vasoactive intestinal peptide 30
ventilated babies, surfactant therapy
    111–12
ventilation, maternal 239
ventilation, mechanical 273–4
  conventional 273–4
  high-frequency oscillatory 273–4
  human rights issues 387
  pressure effects in neonate 267–8
  pressure-cycled 273–4
  withdrawal 379, 383
  withholding 380
very low birthweight babies
  cognitive ability at school age 124
  deaths 112–13
  dyspraxia 123
  home oxygen 120–1
  oxygen dependency 120–1
  racial characteristics 115
viability 3
  extremes 228
  limits and multiple birth delivery 221
viral infections 8
vitamin supplements 293

weighing
  neonates 272, 277
  see also birthweight
wheeze 122–3
white cell count 284–5
wrongful birth cases 352

wrongful life actions 352–3, 355–6

Y-27632 Rho kinase inhibitor 161–2
young people, competence 343–5

zone of altered morphology (ZAM) 49–51

Printed in the United States
By Bookmasters